One-on-One Tutoring by Humans and Computers

This page intentionally left blank

One-on-One Tutoring by Humans and Computers

Martha Evens
Illinois Institute of Technology

and

Joel Michael
Rush Medical College

Routledge
Taylor & Francis Group
LONDON AND NEW YORK

First published 2006 by Lawrence Erlbaum Associations, Inc.

Published 2021 by Routledge
2 Park Square, Milton Park, Abingdon, Oxon OX14 4RN
605 Third Avenue, New York, NY 10017

Routledge is an imprint of the Taylor & Francis Group, an informa business

Cover design by Tomai Maridou

Library of Congress Cataloging-in-Publication Data

Evens, Martha W.
One-on-one tutoring by humans and computers / Martha Evens and Joel Michael.
p. cm.
Includes bibliographical references and index.
ISBN 0-8058-4360-4 (cloth : alk. paper)
ISBN 0-8058-4361-2 (pbk. : alk. paper)
1. Cardiovascular system—Physiology—Study and teaching—Data processing. 2. Intelligent tutoring systems. 3. Tutors and tutoring. 4. Computer-assisted instruction. I. Michael, Joel. II. Title.
QP104.E945 2005
612.1'028'5—dc22 2005040097
CIP

ISBN 13: 978-0-8058-4360-6 (hbk)

This book is dedicated in memoriam to
Allen Rovick: friend, colleague, and collaborator.
His contributions to the CIRCSIM-Tutor project
will be evident to all who read this book.

This page intentionally left blank

Contents

This page intentionally left blank

Preface

This book tells how we built an intelligent tutoring system, CIRCSIM-Tutor, that has the capability of generating a natural language dialogue with a student. Its domain happens to be cardiovascular physiology and the goal is to help first-year medical students learn to solve problems via causal reasoning, but we think that the story we have to tell is applicable to the development of intelligent tutoring systems (ITS) that address the educational needs of many different student populations in a wide variety of scientific disciplines and domains.

Successful implementation of a one-on-one tutor that communicates in natural language required that we (a) investigate the behavior of expert human tutors, and (b) solve the many problems that arise in implementing such a system.

We believe that educators, educational researchers, and computer scientists will find something of interest here. What you take away with you will, of course, depend on your individual interests and background, but we have tried to present our ideas in a way that will allow all our readers to get something of value here, wherever they are coming from.

We realize that readers may not know a great deal about the cardiovascular system, and so we have provided the minimum physiology background that is needed to understand the many issues here that relate in a direct way to the particular domain of our ITS.

The organization of this book, in some sense, reflects the diverse audience that we want to address.

In Part I (Introduction), we have provided a brief history and overview of the CIRCSIM-Tutor project (Chapter 1) and the necessary background about the domain and the problem being solved by the students (Chapter 2).

In Part II (Studies of Expert Human Tutors), we discuss our methodology for studying human tutoring (Chapter 3), the language used in tutoring sessions in our domain (Chapter 4), the domain knowledge used by students and tutors (Chapter 5), the planning for tutoring that occurs (Chapter 6), how tutors carry out a tutoring session (Chapter 7), the generation of hints by tutors (Chapter 8), and then we present the analysis of one extended tutoring session (Chapter 9). We conclude this section with a general discussion of the effectiveness of human tutoring including some of our own studies (Chapter 10).

In Part III (Building CIRCSIM-Tutor), we first discuss the architecture of our system (Chapter 11) and then describe each of the major system modules: the planning modules (Chapter 12), the input understander (Chapter 13), the student modeler (Chapter 14), the domain knowledge base and problem solver (Chapter 15), the dialogue generator (Chapter 16), and finally, the screen manager (Chapter 17).

In Part IV (What Have We Learned?), we begin by describing the results of actually using CIRCSIM-Tutor in the classroom (Chapter 18). Then we discuss other current research efforts and how they have demonstrated the value of using natural language in tutoring (Chapter 19). We provide a discussion of future directions for research and development (Chapter 20). Then we end with a summary of the secrets of our success and a final take-home message (Chapter 21).

With the encouragement of our publishers, we are including a CD-ROM with the human tutoring transcripts and the source and object versions of the system from the 2002 experiments. We also include the log files from the student trials in 1999 and 2002. We have added a list of our publications and theses, many of them available from our Web site at Illinois Institute of Technology.

We are especially grateful to the Cognitive Science Program of the Office of Naval Research (ONR) for its financial support of our work under Grant Number N00014-94-1-0338 and N00014-02-1-0442 to Illinois Institute of Technology, and Grant Number N00014-00-1-0660 to Stanford University. The content of this book does not reflect the position or policy of the government and no official endorsement should be inferred.

The research described here would never have been done, and this book itself would not have been written, without the concern and the efforts of Dr. Susan Chipman, Director of the ONR Cognitive Science Program, which has funded much of the basic research on natural language understanding, on human tutoring, and on Intelligent Tutoring Systems over the last 20 years. She actually read our quarterly progress reports, pointed out problems, and suggested alternative solutions. With her encyclopedic knowledge of the literature, she told us where to find new ideas and approaches that we had missed. Her workshops for ONR grantees served as crash courses in research methodology and also put us in touch with people in the field who have been extraordinarily helpful throughout our project: Herbert Clark, T. Govindaraj, Dedre Gentner, Art Graesser, Johanna Moore, and Kurt Van Lehn.

Dr. Chipman encouraged us to publish throughout the course of our work and suggested possible venues. Five years ago she decided that we should write a book. It took us a little while to see the wisdom of this endeavor and even longer to put it into practice, but that is why you are reading this book today.

We also want to acknowledge that the CIRCSIM-Tutor project would never have happened without Dr. Allen Rovick, expert tutor and master teacher. He was determined to explore every kind of new technology to help his students learn and he was a central figure in the construction and use of computer-aided instruction programs (CIRCSIM, GASP, and ABASE) at Rush Medical College. His vision and his charm attracted students and colleagues to work with this project and helped bridge the gulf between physiology and computer science. He asked us tough questions about tutoring and inspired us all with the determination to look for answers about how tutoring works and why, and about how we can make it better.

We had hoped to present him with a copy of this book when it was published, but he died in December 2004, just as we were preparing to send the third and final draft off to the publishers. We miss him very much.

We have many others to thank for their special contributions. Alan Lesgold arranged for the University of Pittsburgh to ship us the Xerox Lisp Machines that ONR lent to us and then debugged them over the telephone when we could not get them to work.

Ron Kaplan (Kaplan & Bresnan, 1982) generously arranged for Xerox PARC to lend us his package of grammar-writing software; we strongly recommend this excellent tool to anyone who is thinking about using the lexical functional grammar paradigm. Mary Dalrymple helped us understand the paradigm and the software.

Erica Michael gave us major assistance in analyzing the data from the experiments reported in Chapters 10 and 18. Leonard Evens provided major computer support.

We also owe thanks to a number of experts in intelligent tutoring systems who reviewed various drafts of the manuscript: Elizabeth Owen Bratt, Susan Chipman, Diane Litman, Gregory Sanders, and Kurt VanLehn. They made many helpful suggestions that led to significant improvements.

CIRCSIM-Tutor clearly owes its very existence to the PhD students at Illinois Institute of Technology who built it. None of this would have happened without the labors of Nakhoon Kim, Yoon Hee Lee, Leemseop Shim, Chong Woo Woo, Yuemei Zhang, Jai Hyun Seu, Ru-Charn Chang, Glenn Mayer, M. Ali Elmi, Ramzan Ali Khuwaja, Gregory Hume, Gregory Sanders, Joanne Dardaine, Farhana Shah, Stefan Brandle, Hasan Abbas, Michael Glass, Jung Hee Kim, Yujian Zhou, Byung-In Cho, and Feng-Jen Yang. Several more students are currently carrying on further research and building Version 3: Chung Hee Lee, Evelyn Lulis, D. Bruce Mills, and Jay Yusko. Version 3 also owes a large debt to Dr. Reva Freedman, who earned her PhD at Northwestern University in 1996.

Several students have made important contributions as part of their master's theses or projects. Among them are Khelan Bhatt, Yong Wook Kim, Jun Li, Kumar Ramachandran, Shripriya Ramaswami, and Hyun Seok Roh.

Our employers, Rush Medical College and Illinois Institute of Technology, deserve our gratitude for providing us with facilities and laboratory space to carry out this work. We also need to thank the managers of the student computer laboratories at Rush Medical College who installed our program for us and put up with invasions by waves of implementers.

We owe still more thanks to Dr. Reva Freedman for permission to copy Figure 16.3 from her dissertation. We must also thank the Psychonomic Society and their journal, *Behavior Research Methods, Instruments, and Computers,* for permission to copy Figure 3.1 from Li, Seu, Evens, Michael, and Rovick, 1992, and the publisher, Taylor

& Francis, and their journal, *Interactive Learning Environments,* for permission to copy Figure 18.3 and Table 18.5 and Sample 18.4 from Michael, Rovick, Glass, Zhou, and Evens, 2003.

We thank Dr. Stefan Brandle for permission to copy Table 7.1 from his dissertation. We thank Dr. Byung-In Cho for permission to copy Figure 17.3 and Tables 12.7, 12.8, 12.9, and 17.2 from his dissertation. We thank AAAI Press and Dr. Michael Glass for permission to copy Tables 10.8 and 10.9 from Glass, Kim, Evens, Michael, and Rovick (1999). We thank Jay Yusko for permission to copy Figure 15.2 from Yusko and Evens (2004).

We also cannot forget the many Rush Medical College students who volunteered to participate in the CIRCSIM-Tutor program in different ways. The stipends we provided were a small price to pay for their enthusiastic cooperation with whatever we asked them to do. Their feedback, always helpful whether it was positive or negative, certainly motivated us to continue our efforts.

Finally, our publisher, Lawrence Erlbaum Associates, has been extraordinarily helpful in many ways. We particularly want to thank Judith Amsel, Anne Duffy, Bill Webber, Kristin Duch, Lori Stone, Rebecca Larsen, and Marianna Vertullo.

—Martha Evens and Joel Michael, Chicago
January 2005

This page intentionally left blank

PART I: Introduction

This book is divided into four parts. Part I, which you are reading now, provides an introduction to the CIRCSIM-Tutor project and what we have accomplished. Part II describes our studies of human, one-on-one tutoring. Part III details the process of building CIRCSIM-Tutor. Finally, in Part IV we describe the use of the system in the classroom and what we have learned from our collaboration.

The goal of Part I is to give you the background necessary to understand our research on human tutoring and the implementation of CIRCSIM-Tutor, a smart tutor able to generate a natural language dialogue. In Chapter 1 we try to explain where we are coming from and provide a brief history of the project. You will also need to have some understanding of the domain in which our tutors, both human and machine, function. Chapter 2 provides the necessary background about the cardiovascular phenomena of interest and the problems to be solved, but does not attempt to make you an expert in cardiovascular physiology!

This page intentionally left blank

1

Origins of the CIRCSIM-Tutor Project

1.0 WHAT DO WE MEAN BY TUTORING?

When it was discovered that Johnny can't read (Flesch, 1955), his parents hired a tutor to help their son master this essential skill. Colleges and universities across the country employ individuals, often fellow students, to tutor students needing assistance in mastering a course. Students at Oxford University and Cambridge University learn many academic subjects from their interaction with an assigned tutor. Students aiming for admission to Ivy League universities hire tutors to help them prepare for the scholastic assessment tests. College juniors seek similar assistance to help them prepare for the medical college admissions test (MCAT) or the law school admissions text (LSAT). Tutoring has achieved even greater prominence with the enactment of the No Child Left Behind Act of 2001 (U.S. Government, 2001), which treats tutoring under the guise of "supplemental educational services" as a panacea for students in "failing" schools.

What all these examples have in common is a one-on-one dialogue between a teacher and a student for the purpose of helping the student learn something. The conviction that tutoring is the most effective teaching modality is not new, although it has also been recognized as being extremely expensive. Some recent evidence supporting the belief in the efficacy of tutoring is presented later.

This book describes the CIRCSIM-Tutor project, an attempt by Martha Evens, Joel Michael, and Allen Rovick to develop a computer tutor that can interact with students in a one-on-one manner using natural language understanding and generation. To accomplish this, we needed to develop a better understanding of what it is that human tutors do and how they do it and then to build a system that simulates some, at least, of what we see human tutors do.

1.1 ONE-ON-ONE TUTORING IS VERY POWERFUL

Although not the first to look at the effects of tutoring in a systematic way, in 1984, Benjamin Bloom published what is probably still the most cited article on tutoring, "The 2 Sigma Problem: The Search for Methods of Group Instruction as Effective as One-on-One Tutoring." Bloom synthesized the results of studies conducted by two of his graduate students and others, and found that elementary school students who learned from a skilled tutor in a one-on-one setting, on the average, performed 2 standard deviations better than students who learned the same material in a conventional classroom setting. This meant that the average student who had been tutored performed better than 98% of the students who had learned in the classroom. Bloom went on to compare the effect of one-on-one tutoring with the effect of a number of other variables and treatments and found that none of them produced an effect as large as 2 sigma. Bloom's challenge to educators and educational researchers was to develop some method of group or classroom instruction that would be as effective as one-on-one tutoring.

Studies of one-on-one tutoring have, of course, continued since the mid-1980s. Although much of this later work supports Bloom's conclusion (if not necessarily the 2 sigma effect), there are some dissenters. We examine the literature on one-on-one tutoring in much greater detail in Chapter 10, but we can say here that there is a strong consensus about the power of one-on-one tutoring.

It is important to note that much of this early work examined the effects of tutoring by classroom teachers on acquisition of new knowledge, rather than the learning of problem solving skills. Furthermore, few of these studies controlled for, or even assessed, the level of expertise of the tutors involved. Finally, studies of the tutoring process, what tutors do when they interact with a student and how they do it, have been carried out only recently. And only recently have there been attempts to look at the differences in behavior (not outcomes) of expert versus novice tutors. We discuss these issues briefly in Chapter 10.

1.2 NATURAL LANGUAGE DIALOGUE IS IMPORTANT TO TUTORING

The idea that dialogue is important to learning is certainly not a new one. Plato's (1937) *Dialogues* are still in print, and are still widely read, presumably because of the power of such interactions to convey and clarify meaning.

What is it about dialogue that makes it so important to learning? Philosophers of science (Frawley, 1988) tell us that learning the language of a discipline is an essential part of learning the concepts of that discipline, and it is clear that real understanding of something involves, at least in part, an ability to describe the basic concepts in appropriate language (Lemke, 1990; Roth & Lawless, 2002). Chi and her associates (Chi, Bassok, Lewis, Reimann, & Glaser, 1989; Chi, de Leeuw, Chiu, & LaVancher, 1994) have shown the importance of self-explanation (putting the ideas into words) in learning. Natural language tutoring dialogue gives students a chance to formulate their explanations and to have them critiqued by an expert. Barbara Fox (1993b) has observed that tutoring involves a collaborative construction of meaning, a process that arises from a natural language interaction or dialogue between two individuals. Graesser, Person, and Huber (1993) argued that the real basis for the effectiveness of tutoring versus classroom teaching is the much greater number of deep questions raised by the student (or the tutor) in one-on-one tutoring. To raise and respond to these questions requires an environment of natural language dialogue.

The pioneer builders of intelligent tutoring systems, Jaime R. Carbonell (1970), Collins and Stevens (1980, 1982), William Clancey (1982), and John Seely Brown (J. S. Brown, Burton, & deKleer, 1982), assumed that good tutoring began with natural language dialogue. When the PACT Algebra Tutor asked students to give explanations, the students scored better on the posttest than students who used PACT without this facility (Aleven, Koedinger, & Cross, 1999).

But students stopped producing explanations when they discovered that Aleven's system did not understand them and he is now trying to add a natural language understanding capability to his system (Aleven, Ogan, Poppescu, Torrey, & Koedinger, 2004; Aleven, Popescu, & Koedinger, 2001). The experiments of Di Eugenio (2001) have demonstrated the value added by natural language generation. A system that asks the student to produce natural language responses instead of choosing from a menu, is testing recall rather than recognition. Requiring students to create a natural language response increases learning and gives the system the opportunity to do a better job of diagnosis.

Language and its use is an essential part of any learning, and tutoring is intrinsically a dialogue between the tutor and the learner. We believe the success of an intelligent tutoring system will be enhanced to the extent that it is able to carry on a natural language dialogue with the user. We pursue this idea further in Chapter 19.

1.3 HOW WE GOT STARTED

Physiology is one of the biological sciences that concerns itself with the functions of the organism. Learning physiology poses many difficulties for students: (a) It requires the application of considerable chemistry and physics to the understanding of biological phenomena, (b) some understanding of the structure of the organism at different organizational levels is essential, (c) it simultaneously deals with phenomena at many different levels of organization and complexity from the individual molecule to the whole organism, and (d) there is a high level of interaction between phenomena at all levels and between levels, including both negative and positive feedback.

Meaningful learning of physiology (learning with understanding) thus requires not only the acquisition of facts and concepts, but also the ability to integrate the acquired facts into robust, usable mental models of the phenomena being studied, and to use that knowledge to solve problems (Michael, 2001; Michael & Modell, 2003). However, such integration rarely occurs in the lecture hall, and thus teachers of physiology have typically used laboratory exercises (Modell et al., 2000) and small group problem-solving sessions (Michael, 1993) as vehicles to help students reach the level of meaningful learning. Furthermore, meaningful learning is characterized by the students' ability to use the mental models that have been built to solve problems that arise in the discipline (e.g., predict the outcome of some event, calculate the numerical value of some parameter, explain the occurrence of certain events; Michael & Rovick, 1999).

By the early 1970s, the availability of digital computers in physiology research laboratories began to suggest to physiology teachers that this technology might be used in ways that would help students integrate facts into mental models and learn how to use their models to solve problems. Shortly after Rush Medical College (Rush) reopened its doors in 1970, Michael and Rovick began exploring the use of the computer in teaching physiology.

1.3.1 MacMan

MacMan (Dickinson, Goldsmith, & Sackett, 1973) is a mathematical model of the baroreceptor reflex, those components within the cardiovascular system that maintain a nearly constant blood pressure. It was originally written as a FORTRAN program and ran on a mainframe computer at McMaster University where it was developed. It had a simple interface that allowed the user to specify the parameters to be changed in running the model, and to designate what variables would be displayed (graphically or in tabular form) as the model ran. All output was delivered via a line printer.

MacMan was first run at Rush using an acoustic coupler modem and a telephone line to connect to the computer at McMaster University (Michael, 2001). We (Michael and Rovick) were sufficiently impressed with MacMan that we requested permission to translate the FORTRAN program into TUTOR, the language for the PLATO system (Hody & Avner, 1978). We were given permission to do this, and a print copy of the program was sent to us. The Office of Computer-Based Education (as it was then called) at Rush carried out the translation. We wrote a laboratory manual that described certain experiments to be carried out (parameters to be systematically varied, outputs to be examined), provided a description of how students could design and carry out their own experiments, and included a set of questions to direct the students' attention to certain phenomena that they should observe.

However, the PLATO version of MacMan was used for only a year or 2, as we found that the program was not a particularly useful learning resource for our students. There were several reasons for this failure: (1) the students were likely to "cook-book" the experiments (carry them out in a rote fashion without any thought about what they were doing, why they were doing it, and what the results might mean; see Modell et al., 2000) just as they frequently did with "wet lab" experiments; (b) our students were so inexperienced in experimental design, and knew so little about the physiology involved, that they were unable to generate experiments that would aid them in understanding the system; and (c) thus, the success of student use of MacMan was totally dependent on continuous student interaction with a knowledgeable and skilled instructor.

The limited learning outcomes from student exploration of a unguided simulation (one with no built in scaffolding or didactic interaction) was not a phenomenon peculiar to our domain or our student population. Vockell and Rivers (1984) compared the learning that occurred with student use of guided and unguided versions of the same simulation, and found more learning with the guided version. Steinberg (1984) cautioned developers of simulations that the absence of guidance can limit the learning that results from working with a simulation. De Jong and van Joolingen (1998) have reviewed more recent studies demonstrating the same phenomenon.

1.3.2 Heartsim

Our response to this failure of a "naked" simulation (with no actual pedagogy incorporated in the program) to produce much learning was to produce Heartsim (Rovick & Brenner, 1983). This was a PLATO program made up of two components. One component was MacMan, the mathematical model. The second component was a "teaching" module. This didactic component was notable for two things. We realized that we were only really interested in assisting our students to make qualitative predictions (deciding whether a parameter would increase, decrease, or remain unchanged), because much medical decision making involves such qualitative reasoning. Also, we believe that students tend to remember the qualitative model more readily than the mathematical one. We decided that the most important thing for the students to learn was how to do this style of qualitative causal reasoning.

As a result, we introduced the Prediction Table (Rovick & Michael, 1992) as an interface to collect student input, organize the students' thinking about the problem, and to provide the basis for providing feedback about student errors. (The Prediction Table is equally useful as a paper-and-pencil exercise, and we made use of prediction tables in the baroreceptor problems that we used as pretests and posttests in our research on tutoring.) The didactic component also defined a set of experiments (procedures or problems) for the students to carry out. The program requested the students to (a) select a procedure to be done, (b) make predictions about a set of requested responses to the disturbance, (c) correct any logic errors they had made, (d) correct any relationship errors they had made, and (e) then examine the results of the procedure plotted and displayed as a table (both carried out by the MacMan component). Finally, the program compared the students' predictions with the actual results (accomplished by storing the correct predictions—not by looking at the output of MacMan) and provided text feedback to correct the students' lack of information or misconceptions. Heartsim also provided students with the option of designing their own experiments and then predicting the outcomes, although relatively few students were observed to do this. The next chapter shows the Prediction Table used in CIRCSIM and CIRCSIM-Tutor, gives a more complete description of what happens when a student solves a problem using the Prediction Table interface, and provides definitions of the two types of errors mentioned here—errors in relationships and errors in the direction of change.

The PLATO system enabled us to monitor program usage, and to our surprise, and also our delight, we found that students were using Heartsim for many more hours than were scheduled as part of the course. That is, students were coming into the computer lab on their own time to work with the program. The fact that chronically overworked medical students would devote extra time to using our program suggested that it was making some perceptible contribution to their learning. We felt we had some evidence that Heartsim "works."

In retrospect, we believe it was the introduction of the Prediction Table that caused the program to be so effective in assisting the students' attempts to understand the baroreceptor reflex and learn to predict the responses of the system to disturbances. This "device" not only helped students organize their thinking and reasoning in a powerful way, but the errors and patterns of errors that could be detected enabled us to arrange for feedback that addressed significant problems that the students encountered. We have more to say about the Prediction Table in later chapters.

1.3.3 CIRCSIM

Although Heartsim was effective, there was one major drawback. Few of our colleagues in other medical schools had access to the PLATO system, and it was therefore difficult for us to share our program with others or get peer review of it. We decided to develop a BASIC program for MS-DOS machines, which we called CIRCSIM (Rovick & Michael, 1986).

In translating Heartsim into CIRCSIM, we realized that we were actually making no use of the mathematical model (MacMan) that was embedded in Heartsim. That is to say, the most effective teaching was being generated from the stored arrays of correct predictions for each procedure, not from the quantitative outputs generated by the model. Thus, in CIRCSIM, we store only the correct predictions and the limited data needed to display (as tables and simple graphs) some of the results of each of the eight procedures. There is no mathematical model in CIRCSIM, although all the results displayed by CIRCSIM come from MacMan. Thus, the entire emphasis in CIRCSIM is on qualitative causal reasoning.

We continued to use the Prediction Table, but made extensive changes to the error checking, including checking for multi-prediction error patterns. The didactic feedback provided to students in response to errors and error patterns was also improved. Finally, to help students start to develop their thinking about the baroreceptor reflex, we rewrote the first, mandatory experiment as a guided procedure. The program directs the students in a stepwise fashion through the sequence of predictions to be made. This emphasizes the need for a chain of causal reasoning in solving such problems. This procedure then ends with a step-by-step development of a simplified model for the homeostatic, negative feedback system, the baroreceptor reflex, that regulates blood pressure. This provides additional emphasis on the importance of students' developing an algorithm for solving further CIRCSIM problems.

1.3.4 The Educational Context for the Use of Heartsim and CIRCSIM

During the development of both Heartsim and CIRCSIM, it was assumed that the students have already acquired the facts and concepts about the baroreceptor reflex from their reading, attendance at lecture, and participation in the other problem-solving exercises scheduled in the course. These programs are not intended to "deliver" that knowledge to the students although knowledge is delivered (and perhaps acquired) by means of the didactic feedback provided when student errors are detected.

The programs have been used in regularly scheduled computer laboratory sessions in which instructors are present (almost always Michael and Rovick) to interact with the students. We have thus spent over 15 years doing one-on-a-few tutoring with students in groups of two or three helping them to solve problems about the baroreceptor reflex. Because such problems also appear on the examinations that we write, we have also had considerable experience with one-on-one interaction with students preparing for an examination or wishing to discuss the examination answers.

1.3.5 The CIRCSIM Experiment

In 1992, we (Rovick and Michael) reported the results of an experiment, carried out with 50 first-year medical students, which demonstrated that using CIRCSIM did indeed help students understand the behavior of the baroreceptor reflex.

Four groups of students were studied: (a) 14 students worked at CIRCSIM, one student at each computer; (b) 15 students worked at CIRCSIM, two or three to a computer; (c) 14 students participated in the routinely scheduled CIRCSIM computer laboratory, interacting with their instructors throughout; and (d) 9 students served as a control group (they used the CIRCSIM program only after the conclusion of the experiment).

A pretest was administered to all participants at the beginning of the experiment. The pretest consisted of a paper-and-pencil Prediction Table problem describing a perturbation of the blood pressure. This was scored for the number of correct predictions (maximum score 21) and for the presence of "bugs" (patterns of predictions inconsistent with the physiology of the baroreceptor reflex; maximum score 9). Two different versions of the pretest were created (A and B); each used a disturbance that was NOT used in CIRCSIM. Half of the participants took version A and half took version B. Performance on these two versions of the pretest was found to be the same.

Participants then worked with CIRCSIM for 2 hr in a manner determined by the group to which they were assigned (Groups 1, 2, and

3), while the control group (Group 4) did nothing (that is to say, they studied cardiovascular physiology as they would normally). All students then took the posttest; those participants who had answered version A on the pretest answered version B for the posttest, and those who had answered version B on the pretest answered version B on the posttest.

One way analyses of variance (ANOVAs) were carried out on the results of the pretest and posttest. A comparison of the performance of students in Groups 1, 2, and 3 (all of whom had used CIRCSIM), with the performance of students in the control group (Group 4), showed a significant increase in the number of correct predictions (p = .016). It was interesting that a comparison of the performance of the students in Group 1 (who worked with CIRCSIM alone), with the performance of students in Group 2 (who worked in pairs or threesomes on CIRCSIM), showed that working together on CIRCSIM led to a larger increase in the number of correct predictions than working alone (p = .01).

Similar results were obtained when the data on the number of "bugs" present was examined. Working with CIRCSIM (Groups 1, 2, and 3) resulted in a larger reduction in the number of "bugs" than occurred with the control group (Group 4); the p value was .012. In addition, students who worked in the computer laboratory with an instructor present (Group 3) showed a bigger reduction in the number of "bugs" than did the students who worked with CIRCSIM without interacting with an instructor (Groups 1 and 2); the p value was .01.

We (Rovick & Michael, 1992) concluded that CIRCSIM works in that students using it improved their ability to make correct predictions about the responses of the baroreceptor reflex and decreased the number of incorrect patterns of predictions ("bugs"). When we considered why students did better in pairs than working with the program individually, we came to the conclusion that it was probably the experience of talking about the problem and its solution that made the difference. We began to think about a program that would produce questions and hints as well as explanations, and would require natural language input from the student.

1.4 THE BIRTH OF THE CIRCSIM-TUTOR PROJECT

By the late 1980s, experience working with students using CIRCSIM had convinced Michael and Rovick that although CIRCSIM was an effective learning resource for their students, there were many kinds of errors and misconceptions that it was unable to remedy, in part, because it could not detect their presence. This conviction arose from the experience of tutoring students using CIRCSIM and observing that even when few, if any, errors were being made, conversation with the students nevertheless revealed significant problems with their understanding of the baroreceptor reflex. Further, observations of students using CIRCSIM (and the results of the CIRCSIM experiment) suggested that the conversations students had with one another contributed in an important way to the learning that was taking place. It seemed to us (Michael and Rovick) that the solution to our dissatisfactions with CIRCSIM would be to write a program that could hold a conversation, a dialogue, with students while they were engaged in solving a CIRCSIM problem.

At the same time, we were aware of the growing body of work in which applications of computer science and artificial intelligence to education were beginning to yield increasingly robust and interesting results (Anderson, Conrad, & Corbett, 1989; Anderson & Reiser, 1985; Clancey, 1987; Lajoie & Lesgold, 1989; Lesgold, 1988; Russell, Moran, & Jordan, 1988; B. A. Sherwood & J. N. Sherwood, 1988; Wilensky et al., 1988; Woolf, 1988).

A colleague put Michael and Rovick in touch with his former graduate advisor, Martha Evens, a researcher in computer natural language processing who had published widely (Evens, 1988; Evens, Litowitz, Markowitz, Smith, & Werner, 1980) in this area. She had also been involved in a series of experiments with medical expert systems and the generation of case reports (Collier, Evens, Hier, & Li, 1988). After only a few meetings in which we (Michael and Rovick at Rush Medical College and Evens at Illinois Institute of Technology) discussed our mutual interests, we agreed to launch a collaborative effort to develop a smart tutor version of CIRCSIM. This effort soon received funding from the Cognitive Science Program of the Office of Naval Research under the direction of Dr. Susan Chipman.

1.5 THE OBJECTIVES OF THE CIRCSIM-TUTOR PROJECT

The overall goal was clear to the three of us. We wanted to produce a computer tutor that would assist students in learning to make qualitative predictions about the baroreceptor reflex. That is, we wanted to produce a computer tutor that could approximate the kinds of effective interactions that Michael and Rovick had with their students in the physiology computer laboratory. We wanted a computer tutor that could ask and answer questions, and, when appropriate, explain physiological mechanisms. We wanted a computer tutor that could diagnose the source of the student's learning difficulty. We wanted a computer tutor that would assist the student in achieving a level of meaningful learning about cardiovascular phenomena.

To accomplish this, we needed to develop robust computer natural language capabilities, both to understand the answers and questions generated by the students and to generate questions, answers, and explanations. We needed to develop student modeling capabilities so that the computer tutor would function with some understanding of what the student knew and didn't know. We needed to develop a planner that could decide what needed to be done next to advance student understanding. And finally, we set out to develop a set of tutoring tactics that could be utilized by the computer tutor when needed. The systems that we have developed and how we got to where we are today are described in Part III of this book.

When we looked at the available literature on tutoring, we found very little explicit and detailed information about what experienced tutors do and how they do it. We decided to try to base our system on what our expert human tutors (Michael and Rovick) do. Our first step was to capture and analyze human tutoring sessions, to try to understand what Michael and Rovick do when they tutor students or interact with them in the CIRCSIM computer lab. Part II of this book describes what we did, how we did it, and what we learned about human tutoring.

1.6 OVERVIEW OF THE CIRCSIM-TUTOR PROJECT

1.6.1 Research on Human Tutoring

Of necessity we (the CIRCSIM-Tutor project team) began by studying what happened in one-on-one tutoring sessions conducted by Michael and Rovick. We needed to know many things that were not known when we started. What language did the student use in discussing the baroreceptor reflex (we had to be able to understand the students' answers or questions)? What language did the tutor use (we needed to be able to generate some approximation of what a tutor would say)? What knowledge was required to solve a CIRCSIM problem and what knowledge was used to tutor a student solving such a problem? What tactics and strategies were employed by the tutor in a one-on-one session (we needed to be able to generate an interactive dialogue that would accomplish the same thing)?

This research was carried out by recording the dialogue that was generated by the tutor and a student as the student attempts to solve a CIRCSIM problem. A keyboard-to-keyboard system was eventually designed that enabled us to capture and analyze a large number of tutoring sessions.

1.6.2 Implementing an Intelligent Tutoring System

As our understanding of what happened in a one-on-one tutoring session grew, it became possible for us to begin to implement CIRCSIM-Tutor. It was clear from the beginning that we would need system components to accomplish a number of specific tasks. We needed an input understander so that the system could understand and respond to the students' answers or questions. We also needed a text generator to produce the tutor's side of the dialogue (ask questions, answer questions). All this text needed to be managed on the screen. We needed to be able to store the knowledge that is needed to solve a CIRCSIM problem and to tutor the solution of such a problem. CIRCSIM-Tutor needed to be able to construct a model of the student and what the student knew and did not know.

The architecture of this intelligent tutoring system evolved over the years. Equally important, the hardware on which we were developing the system changed; we began the project using Xerox work stations, eventually transferred the system to a Macintosh computer, and then transferred that system to a PC. Each change in hardware necessitated some change in our programs. In the end, it is clear that advances in the hardware available to us contributed greatly to the success of CIRCSIM-Tutor; faster processors make possible the quick response time needed to generate an effective dialogue.

1.6.3 Assessing What We Have Accomplished

As working versions of CIRCSIM-Tutor became available, it was essential that they be tested. We needed to discover whether a particular version actually worked; that is, did it correctly assess student predictions, did it understand the language input to it, was the language it generated appropriate and correct, did it carry out the expected tutoring plans? Much of this testing was carried out by the tutors (Michael and Rovick). We also need to know whether students could use the system; that is, was it sufficiently user-friendly that students (not the tutors) could learn to use it with minimal, if any, learning time. Initial student testing was informal and involved only a small group of students at a time, medical students who volunteered to assist us.

When we completed working versions of CIRCSIM-Tutor, we then had to ask how well they worked in the classroom. Several questions needed to be answered. Did the system work as planned (did it understand student input and did it generate appropriate replies)? Did students using CIRCSIM-Tutor learn to solve problems about the baroreceptor reflex? Finally, what did students think about their experience using the program; did they find it helpful, easy enough to use, and so forth? We eventually conducted four experiments with large numbers of students to answer these questions (described in Chapter 18).

1.7 ORGANIZATION OF THIS BOOK

This book is divided into four parts. Part I, which you are reading now, provides an introduction to the CIRCSIM-Tutor project and what we have accomplished. Part II describes our studies of human, one-on-one tutoring. Part III details the process of building CIRCSIM-Tutor. Finally, in Part IV, we describe what happened when we used CIRCSIM-Tutor in the classroom, what we have learned from our collaboration, and where the artificial intelligence in education community is headed—at least those of us who believe that natural language is the key to good tutoring.

1.8 GOALS OF THIS BOOK

We hope that you will take away from your reading of this book three ideas:

1. One-on-one tutoring is a powerful technique for helping students learn complex subjects and problem-solving skills.
2. Natural language dialogue contributes in a powerful way to the efficacy of one-on-one tutoring.
3. Using presently available technology, a computer tutor with natural language capabilities can be built and can serve as a valuable aid to student learning.

1.9 TAKE-HOME MESSAGE

The CIRCSIM-Tutor project arose from the perceived need by two physiology teachers (Michael and Rovick) for a learning resource that was not currently available. It was, from the start, a collaborative effort between two teachers who were both content experts and tutoring experts and a computer scientist with expertise in natural language processing. CIRCSIM-Tutor, the system that we eventually produced, was designed to be a simulation of our expert tutors, not as an instantiation for a learning theory. It was intended for routine use in the classroom and it was tested in the classroom at every major turning point in its development. Thus, it has been field-tested with real students in a real educational context.

2

What's Being Tutored: The Domain and the Problem

You do not need to know much about the underlying physiology to understand the results of our research on human tutoring or the ideas underlying the building of our Intelligent Tutoring System, but a certain minimal familiarity with the physiology of the baroreceptor reflex, particularly the concepts and the language used to describe it, is helpful to understand fully the tutoring and the tutorial dialogues that are discussed here. It is also helpful to understand the problem being solved by the students. This chapter provides the minimal necessary background in physiology. If you find this chapter difficult, you can, of course, skip ahead to the next chapter, and then come back here later if you need more information about the underlying physiology to understand the tutoring dialogues.

2.0 WHAT DOES IT MEAN TO UNDERSTAND PHYSIOLOGY?

Learning physiology, like learning any other discipline, requires the acquisition of knowledge about the subject matter of the discipline

(Michael & Modell, 2003; Michael & Rovick, 1999). The "facts" of any discipline include data about the entities that are the subject of the discipline (e.g., "the normal value of blood pressure is 120/80 mm Hg") and concepts that describe or explain the behavior of these entities (e.g., "blood pressure is determined by cardiac output and total peripheral resistance"). Learning the language of the discipline and how that language is used to frame arguments and discussion is also a part of learning the discipline (Frawley, 1988).

However, the mere acquisition of facts, regardless of the length of the "laundry list," does not constitute "understanding" of physiology (Michael, 2001; Michael & Modell, 2003). The "facts" and "concepts" that have been acquired must be organized into mental representations or mental models (Gentner & Stevens, 1983; Lesh & Kelly, 1997; Markman, 1999). These models may be nothing more than a "laundry list" with no internal structure and no relationship to other knowledge possessed by the learner, or they may be highly structured and well integrated with old knowledge. To the extent that these models are correct and more or less coherent (contain the correct collection of entities related to one another in correct ways), they can be used by the learner to solve problems of many different kinds. Problem solving is, of course, a skill that must be learned and practiced to be perfected.

Understanding physiology, achieving a measure of meaningful learning (Michael, 2001), thus requires acquisition of sufficient facts, the building of appropriate mental models of the phenomena being considered, and the ability to use these models to solve problems appropriate to the discipline (see Simon, 2001). Physicians need this kind of understanding of physiology and this kind of reasoning, even if it is not always used in arriving at a diagnosis.

2.1 THE DOMAIN: THE CARDIOVASCULAR BARORECEPTOR REFLEX

2.1.1 The Role of the Cardiovascular System

The cardiovascular system is basically a pump (the heart), a very large collection of tubes (the blood vessels), and a number of control mechanisms (components of the nervous system and the endocrine system). The function of the cardiovascular system in the economy of the body is to deliver to every cell the nutrients and oxygen it requires and to remove the waste products produced as a result of its activity. To accomplish this, the muscle that the heart is made of contracts, increasing the pressure in the system, and pumping a volume of blood out into the circulation, where it flows to all parts of the body. A more complete description of the function of the cardiovascular system can be obtained from any of a number of physiology textbooks (e.g., Berne & Levy, 1998; L. Sherwood, 2001).

2.1.2 Regulation of Blood Pressure by the Cardiovascular System

One of the challenges faced by the cardiovascular system is ensuring that all parts of the body receive the blood flow that they require to support their resting metabolic activity and their special activities that contribute to the overall maintenance of the body (e.g., muscles contract, the gastrointestinal system absorbs digested food, etc.). In brief, the appropriate distribution of flow is made possible by mechanisms that insure that the pressure in the circulation that produces flow, the mean arterial pressure (MAP), is held more or less constant, and the resistance to flow in each organ or tissue is varied to produce the needed local flow. This requires close regulation of MAP, however. These two functions, producing adequate local flow and regulating systemic MAP, must occur simultaneously.

Figure 2.1 shows a causal concept map representing the components that make up the baroreceptor reflex that regulates MAP. We now realize that in the education literature, the term *concept map* usually refers to the type of representation of the hierarchical relationship among concepts that was developed and studied extensively by Novak (Novak & Gowin, 1984). In a Novak concept map, the "links" between concepts can include many different relationships (such as "is-a," "has-parts," etc.). In a causal concept map, the links always describe a causal relationship between a parameter (the "determinant"), whose change in value causes another parameter to change its value. We began using the term concept map to mean a *causal concept map* before we were aware of Novak's use of the term and have continued our use to avoid confusing our students. CIRCSIM and CIRCSIM-Tutor are based on this same qualitative, causal model.

There are some important conventions that help in reading a causal concept map like the one in Fig. 2.1. The arrow from heart

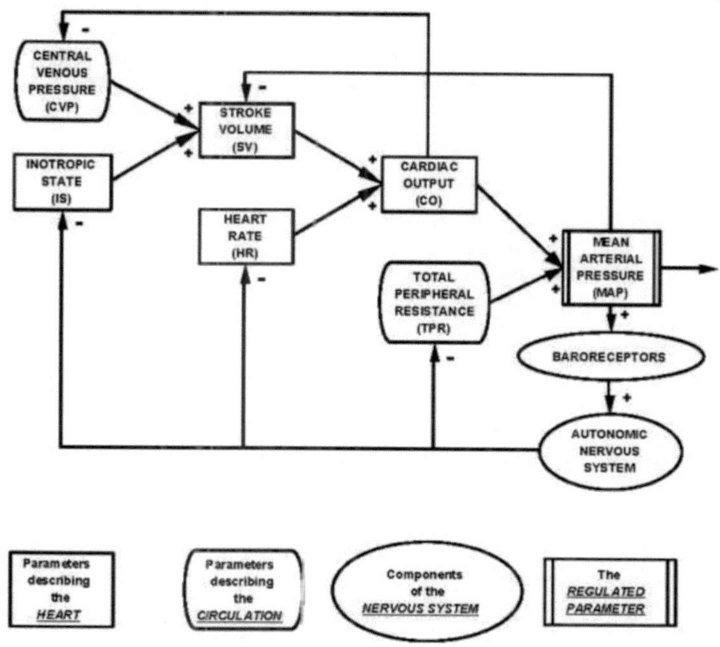

FIG. 2.1. A causal model of the baroreceptor reflex.

rate (HR) to cardiac output (CO) indicates that any change in HR causes a change in CO. The plus sign on the arrow means that those changes are always in the same direction. In other words, an increase in HR (if it is the only parameter changing) always results in an increase in CO and a decrease in HR results in a decrease in CO. Such relationships are often referred to as "direct" ones in the tutoring dialogues. The minus sign on the arrow from Cardiac Output (CO) to Central Venous Pressure (CVP) means that changes in CO cause CVP to change in the opposite direction. So if CO increases, CVP goes down, and if CO goes down, CVP goes up. These relationships are commonly referred to as "inverse" in the tutoring dialogues. Table 2.1 defines the variables and shows some of the relationships among them.

The concept map in Fig. 2.1 also contains some other information that is visually coded. The shape of the elements provides information about the anatomical nature of the element (cardiac, circulatory, or neural). In addition, the regulated variable, MAP, is visually distin-

TABLE 2.1

Cardiovascular Parameters Involved in the Baroreceptor Reflex (Whose Responses Must Be Predicted by the Students)

- Autonomic Nervous System (ANS)—The part of the nervous system that innervates the heart and the blood vessels.
- Baroreceptors (BR)—Sensory receptors (located in the carotid artery that supplies blood to the brain) that measure the hydrostatic pressure that is present; the neural signals that they generate travel to the brain carrying information about the pressure that is present.
- Cardiac Output (CO)—The volume of blood pumped out of the heart each minute; CO = SV × HR.
- Central Venous Pressure (CVP)—The pressure present in the great veins just outside the heart; determines the rate at which the ventricles (the pumping chamber) fill with blood and is thus the major determinant of SV. In some of the early tutoring transcripts, the determinant of filling is referred to as right atrial pressure or RAP, a closely related parameter that behaves in the same way as CVP.
- Heart Rate (HR)—The number of heart beats per minute; controlled by the autonomic nervous system.
- Inotropic State (IS)—Determines how much blood is pumped each beat (for any amount of ventricular filling that is present); controlled primarily by the activity in the sympathetic nerves (ANS) innervating the heart. (In some of the early transcripts, this parameter is referred to as cardiac contractility or CC.)
- Mean Arterial Pressure (MAP)—The pressure present in the aorta and major arteries; determines blood flow in the circulation and is determined by MAP = CO × TPR.
- Stroke Volume (SV)—The amount of blood pumped from the heart with each beat; determined by CVP and IS.
- Total Peripheral Resistance (TPR)—The resistance to flow posed by the entire circulation; arterial resistance (Ra), the resistance to flow posed by the arterial system, and is the largest component of TPR.

guished from the other elements. Both of these features are commonly employed in physiology textbooks to help students focus their attention on important features of the concept map.

This model is a simplified one in that it assumes that the blood returning to the heart in the veins fills the right atrium, which in turn fills the left ventricle. Thus, the right ventricle, the pulmonary circulation, and the left atrium are all assumed to be passive structures that do not affect the function being modeled (the regulation of blood pressure). This simplified model does, however, behave in a way that closely mimics the responses of the real cardiovascular system. The nature of this model and its assumptions are explained to the users of CIRCSIM and to students participating in our tutoring experiments.

2.2 THE PROBLEM: PREDICTING THE RESPONSES OF THE SYSTEM TO DISTURBANCES OF THE BLOOD PRESSURE

If some disturbance, whether caused by a change inside the body or imposed from the outside, causes blood pressure (MAP) to change, the baroreceptors will change their firing and a reflex response will be generated that will attempt to restore MAP to its original, normal value. This reflex acts very quickly, operating to bring MAP to a new steady state within a matter of 2 to 3 min, and always moves MAP toward the normal value, although it cannot fully compensate for the initial disturbance. Such baroreceptor reflex responses are elicited by a great many phenomena that occur quite normally in the body, by disease processes, and by pharmacological interventions. It is essential that medical students understand the behavior of the baroreceptor reflex, and this means that they must be able to predict how the relevant variables will change their value (increase, decrease, or remain unchanged) when a change in mean arterial pressure occurs, eliciting a baroreceptor reflex. That is to say, the students need to learn to do qualitative, causal reasoning.

The Prediction Table (Rovick & Michael, 1992) is a device that assists students to organize their thinking about causal reasoning and also serves as a device for collecting the students' predictions in CIRCSIM and CIRCSIM-Tutor (see Table 2.2). The seven parameters in the leftmost column are arranged in a sequence that supports and emphasizes the stepwise, causal reasoning process we want students to understand and employ. The three columns of predictions (DR, RR, and SS) that these systems request from the students require them to think through the response of the system as it evolves over time; each column represents a more or less definable time frame during which the system is responding in a certain way. Prediction Tables are also used in the pencil-and-paper exercises employed as pretests and posttests.

The DIRECT RESPONSE (DR) refers to the changes that occur in the system as a result of the disturbance and before any reflex re-

TABLE 2.2

The Prediction Table Used in Both CIRCSIM and CIRCSIM-Tutor (and Also Used in a Pen-and-Paper Form in Pretests and Posttests)

Parameter	*DR*	*RR*	*SS*
Inotropic State (IS)			
Central Venous Pressure (CVP)			
Stroke Volume (SV)			
Heart Rate (HR)			
Cardiac Output (CO)			
Total Peripheral Resistance (TPR)			
Mean Arterial Pressure (MAP)			

Note. DR is the Direct Response before any reflex changes occur; RR is the Reflex Response, the response to the Baroreceptor Reflex; and SS is the new Steady State that is achieved as a result of RR acting to compensate for the changes that occur in DR.

sponse occurs. Another way to think about DR is that it is what would happen in a purely passive system (one without reflexes). The individual changes that occur in DR depend entirely on the nature of the disturbance (which parameter is changed first by the disturbance). In almost every situation, the consequence of whatever is occurring during DR is that blood pressure (MAP) changes.

The REFLEX RESPONSE (RR) describes the reflex response that occurs as a consequence of the change in blood pressure. It is mediated by changes in the neural signals that innervate the heart and the circulation. RR has two basic patterns of changes in parameter values, depending on whether blood pressure is increased or decreased by the disturbance (as long as the system is intact and all parameters are free to change in a normal way).

SS then defines the new Steady State that the system reaches as the DR (and its change in blood pressure) is countered by the RR. One of the most significant features of the SS is that blood pressure is never restored to its predisturbance value although it always moves toward the normal value before the disturbance.

There are two fundamental relationships describing the cardiovascular system that students must understand (Table 2.3). The amount of blood pumped by the heart each minute, the cardiac out-

TABLE 2.3
Important Equations Describing the Cardiovascular System

Cardiac Output (CO) =	Heart Rate (HR) × Stroke Volume (SV)
Mean Arterial Pressure (MAP) =	Cardiac Output (CO) × Total Peripheral Resistance (TPR)

put (CO), is determined by (and is the arithmetic product of) the number of beats per minute (heart rate or HR) and the amount of blood pumped each beat (stroke volume or SV). Predictions must always be consistent with the equation, CO = HR × SV; one cannot predict that HR and SV will increase and also predict that CO will be unchanged or will decrease. Similarly, mean arterial pressure (MAP) is always determined by the product of cardiac output (CO) and total peripheral resistance (TPR). This means that one cannot predict that TPR will increase, CO will be unchanged, and MAP will fall. CIRCSIM checks these two relationships and, if either is violated, alerts the student to this error and asks that the predictions be brought into conformity with these relationships. Note, however, that the student's predictions can conform to both of the relationships and still be incorrect.

There is another kind of relationship that is relevant to solving a CIRCSIM problem. The Steady State (SS) can be regarded as being the "sum" of the Direct Response (DR) and the Reflex Response (RR). Logically then, one cannot predict that a particular parameter, say inotropic state (IS), will be unchanged in DR, will increase in RR, but will be decreased in SS. CIRCSIM also checks such logic errors and gives the student a chance to correct them (see Section 1.3.2).

Both CIRCSIM and the current version of CIRCSIM-Tutor present eight different problems for the student to solve. They are described in Table 2.4.

2.3 THE EDUCATIONAL CONTEXT OF THE PROBLEM

The students who participated in the CIRCSIM-Tutor project (whether in tutoring studies or trials with CIRCSIM-Tutor) were all first-year medical students at Rush Medical College in Chicago. They were enrolled in the first quarter of a two-quarter, comprehensive medical physiology course. The cardiovascular portion of this

TABLE 2.4
The Problem Set (Also Called the Procedures) for CIRCSIM and CIRCSIM-Tutor

1.	Decrease arterial resistance (Ra) to 50% of normal.
2.	Denervate the baroreceptors.
3.	Reduce Ra to 50% of normal in a denervated preparation.
4.	Increase venous resistance (Rv) to 200% of normal.
5.	Decrease cardiac contractility (CC) to 50% of normal.
6.	Hemorrhage: Remove 0.5 L (Blood volume = 4.5 L).
7.	Hemorrhage: Remove an additional 1.0 L (Blood volume = 3.5 L).
8.	Increase intrathoracic pressure (Pit) from –2 mm Hg to 0 mm Hg.

course culminates with a 2-hr computer laboratory in which students work with CIRCSIM (and, in some cases, CIRCSIM-Tutor). Our tutoring experiments were always conducted during the brief period between the end of all assigned sessions in the cardiovascular block and the scheduled CIRCSIM computer laboratory session. At this point in time, the students had participated in a 2-hr laboratory session dealing with cardiovascular phenomena, 7 hr of lecture, a 2-hr computer laboratory on hemodynamics and reflex controls, a 2-hr workshop on hemodynamics, and two 2-hr workshops in which patient-based problems are solved. Thus, the students are assumed to have acquired the "facts" about cardiovascular physiology (including those relating specifically to the baroreceptor reflex) and to have had an opportunity to begin assembling and using a robust mental model of this system to solve problems.

2.4 THE GENERALITY OF QUALITATIVE, CAUSAL REASONING

Understanding any aspect of physiology calls for knowing the causal relationships between system parameters. Understanding also calls for being able to predict the consequences of a disturbance to any one parameter on all of the other parameters (Michael & Modell, 2003; Michael & Rovick, 1999). Control systems like the baroreceptor reflex are common, with every organ system incorporating negative feedback relationships.

Qualitative, causal reasoning is not limited to physiology, however. In biology, "... students in domains such as genetics and ecology are often asked to predict outcomes resulting from the interactions of multiple variables within a dynamic system" (Hurst & Milkent, 1996, p. 542). Thus, the ability to carry out qualitative causal reasoning is essential in this discipline.

Qualitative causal reasoning in physics (see Forbus, 1988; Weld & de Kleer, 1990) is a well established discipline within the AI-cognitive science community. Further, it is being used to create sophisticated software for helping students develop a conceptual understanding of important phenomena (Forbus, 1997). In addition, the physics education community is now actively promoting the importance of students gaining a conceptual understanding of physical phenomena (see diSessa, 1993; Mazur, 1997), and assessment tools for qualitative causal understanding of force (Hestenes & Halloun, 1995; Hestenes, Wells, & Swackhamer, 1992) and electricity and magnetism (Maloney, O'Kuma, Heiggelke, & Van Heuvelen, 2001) have been developed. The availability of these assessment tools has provided the physics education community with a valuable tool for evaluating educational innovations aimed at increasing meaningful learning of physics (see, e.g., Hake, 1998).

The teaching of basic electronics also involves the same kind of qualitative approach and the same kind of causal reasoning (Kieras, 1985). Cawsey (1992, 1993) has carried out extensive studies of tutors in this domain (as part of a project to build an intelligent tutoring system) and found that they emphasize qualitative, causal reasoning. Moore and her group in Edinburgh (Core, Moore, & Zinn, 2000, 2001, 2003) have carried out further human studies of tutors in basic electronics and found similar reasoning patterns.

Qualitative causal reasoning of this kind is also central to troubleshooting equipment of many different kinds. Lesgold's (1992) SHERLOCK II project is based on the same kind of analysis of the problem to be solved. This project is a landmark because of its demonstrated success—the participants learned more in 20 hr of tutoring than in 4 years of field experience (Lesgold, Lajoie, Bunzo, & Eggan, 1992).

Since the advent of a medical science that is grounded in biology, physics, and chemistry, practitioners in medicine have used causal reasoning to arrive at diagnoses or to plan and manage therapy (Kuipers, 1987a, 1987b, 1987c; Kuipers & Kassirer, 1984). Complex, quantitative models of important medical phenomena do exist (Horn, Simonett, & Webb, 1999; Ottesen & Danielsen, 2000) and can be run on computers to yield exact results; these models can, at best, be used in a qualitative way without the computer. Thus, clinical reasoning, even when vast amounts of patient data are available, is commonly qualitative, with the physician looking for patterns of increases and decreases in key parameters.

Thus, causal reasoning is prevalent in many different disciplines. One-on-one tutoring to help students learn how to solve such problems (how to understand such domains), whether carried out in physiology or any other discipline, undoubtedly has many common features. And, a computer tutor that successfully helps first-year medical students learn about the baroreceptor reflex can be a model for other natural-language-based tutors that help students learn to solve problems using qualitative reasoning.

2.5 TAKE-HOME MESSAGE

CIRCSIM-Tutor is intended to help students acquire an understanding of the mechanisms within the cardiovascular system that regulate blood pressure (hold it more or less constant). Understanding this mechanism, referred to as the baroreceptor reflex, means that the student can predict the qualitative responses of the system to disturbances in blood pressure, whether caused by the activity of the body, exogenous disturbances, or pathology. This kind of causal reasoning is common in a number of other disciplines. Thus, the goals and the accomplishments of the CIRCSIM-Tutor project have broad applicability outside the domain of physiology.

PART II: Studies of Expert Human Tutors

A major goal of the CIRCSIM-Tutor project was obtaining an understanding of the human tutoring processes carried out by expert tutors so that we could emulate them in our system as closely as possible. This part of our book describes how we collected and studied transcripts of human tutoring sessions and what we found out in the process.

Chapter 3 discusses the collection and analysis of the transcripts. Chapter 4 describes our studies of the language used by tutors and students during the tutoring sessions. Chapter 5 addresses the domain knowledge needed for solving our problems and the (wider) knowledge of domain pedagogy used in the tutoring sessions.

Chapter 6, 7, and 8 together describe three levels of planning that take place in our sessions. Chapter 6 discusses the top-level planning of the problem-solving approach, the problems to be solved (called curriculum planning in ITS circles), and the global tutoring plans that we made. Chapter 7 deals with the tutoring strategies and tactics employed by our tutors. Chapter 8 describes the techniques that our tutors employ to deliver hints. Finally, Chapter 9 gives a detailed analysis of a small piece of dialogue that shows how these many layers of planning interact with each other.

This page intentionally left blank

3

The Collection and Analysis of Tutoring Transcripts

3.0 DIFFERENT TUTORING MODALITIES

Michael and Rovick had already developed considerable experience tutoring students solving CIRCSIM problems when this project began. Their experience and the result of the CIRCSIM experiment had convinced them that students who used the program did learn to predict the behavior of the baroreceptor reflex successfully. They were also convinced that a computer tutor with natural language capabilities would be even more useful in helping students correct their conceptual errors. To build such a tutor required that we understand how Michael and Rovick tutor students as they solve problems about the physiology of the baroreceptor reflex.

When asked for examples of tutoring to use as a basis for developing the computer tutor, Michael and Rovick recruited several student volunteers and made audiotapes of one-on-one tutoring sessions. A paper-and-pencil baroreceptor Prediction Table problem was given to the students and they were tutored as they solved the problem. A secretary in the Department of Physiology transcribed the tapes. She was experienced in transcribing letters, memos, and papers, so she corrected the language produced by the tutors and by the students whenever she could, and she omitted most of the side comments and laughter as well as most of the hesitations and restarts. Not surprisingly, she found this to be a rather big job, and it took her 3 months, working intermittently as her time permitted, to produce transcripts for six 1-hr sessions.

Seeking to capture the nonverbal cues that were obviously present, and to observe the student filling in the Prediction Table, we also tried videotaping a session. We realized as we viewed this tape that we had no experience and little understanding of how to code videotapes. Furthermore, it was clear that even if we had the resources (people and dollars) to carry out the work that would be involved (repeated viewing and reviewing very information-rich tapes), we would not be able to study many sessions, although it was clear that we needed to capture many examples of language to make useful generalizations.

At this same time, we recognized that our computer tutor would have to operate with a much narrower communications channel (the keyboard for input and the screen for output) than was available in a human face-to-face tutoring session. This limitation was a consequence of the technology readily available at the time (1989). It seemed appropriate, therefore, to collect tutoring transcripts with a comparably narrow bandwidth system. It has been amply demonstrated (Fox, 1990; Grosz, 1977, 1978; Thompson, 1980) that the same person working in the same domain will use a different sublanguage when interacting with a computer than when talking to another person. We decided that, because we were proposing that the students use a keyboard as an input device, the best possible language examples for our work would be keyboard-to-keyboard transcripts made while the student and the tutor were sitting at computers in different rooms so that none of the usual nonverbal cues would be available to either side.

In this chapter, we describe how we collected keyboard-to-keyboard transcripts and what we learned about ways to study transcripts and extract information from them over the years. Finally, we discuss some lessons learned.

3.1 COLLECTING TRANSCRIPTS OF ONE-ON-ONE TUTORING

3.1.1 The Computer Dialogue System

We started collecting transcripts long before the days of broadband communication and the Internet, when most computer communication involved telephones and modems. At that time (1989), our home institutions (and many other people) used Hayes modems, running the Smartcom III communication package, so we needed a system to run on Hayes equipment. This meant that someone had to write a program in SCOPE (the Smartcom command language). We were lucky enough to recruit Jun Li to build the Computer Dialogue System (CDS) for us (Li, Seu, Evens, Michael, & Rovick, 1992).

The initial version of CDS communicated what was typed by both users and displayed it on both screens. It also saved the dialogue on the hard disk of the tutor's PC. We deliberately made it possible for the tutor and the student to type at the same time to provide the kind of back channel responses that Barbara Fox (1988a, 1988b) described in human tutoring (with the tutor adding "mmm" and "go on" to keep the student talking). The first trial showed us what could happen when both the tutor and student typed something at the same time, not a rare occurrence. For example, when one user typed "mix" and the other typed "together," both screens displayed the string "mtogietxher" instead of "mix together." We gave up on back channel communication. Li quickly implemented a new program that forced the users to take turns typing. Both users were asked to type a particular string to signify the end of their turns. The tutor typed "xxx" and the student typed "zzz." Li also formatted the output on each computer into three labeled windows: one for the tutor input, one for the student input, and one with help information. This worked very well and we were able to capture between 60 and 90 turns an hour with this system. This is how the first eight keyboard-to-keyboard transcripts were collected in November 1989.

We were satisfied with the system in most ways but we became frustrated sometimes when the student did not answer for a long time. Li redefined the process to allow for interruptions. Either the tutor or the student could type "yyy" and the system would ask the other party to give up the turn in a pop-up window. The request could be granted or refused. Both tutors and students were observed to request interrupts, which were usually granted by the other party.

The screens were programmed so that neither party could type while the other was typing. Li also added a screen indicator to show which party is holding the turn. After we read Fox's technical reports (1988a, 1988b) about the human tutoring sessions that she observed, we realized that we should be trying to record some timing information as well. Li added facilities to CDS to report the clock time of the student input, the time elapsed between the display of the tutor input and the start of the student input and the time that the student took to type that input. This information has been very valuable in figuring out how CIRCSIM-Tutor should recognize and handle pauses. Figure 3.1 shows a screen from the version of CDS used to collect the majority of our tutoring dialogues.

By 1999, the arrival of the Internet and the revolution in telecommunications that was occurring prompted us to ask Yujian Zhou to build us a new version of CDS that embodies some of our current ideas about how to do a better job of collecting transcripts. This version does not require a telephone and a modem (it uses two networked computers) and it is written in C++, so it is much more

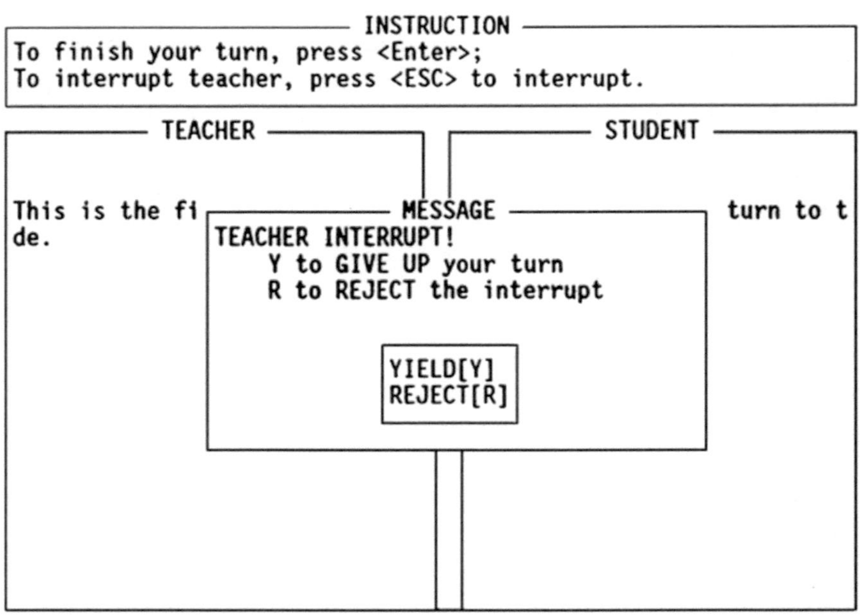

FIG. 3.1. Computer Dialogue System (CDS) screen from the version used to collect most of the human tutoring transcripts (copied by permission from Li, Seu, Evens, Michael, & Rovick, 1992b, Figure 3b, p. 537).

portable. (A copy of the most recent version of CDS is included in the CD-ROM that accompanies this book.)

Zhou also added some really valuable functionality. The new system allows the creation of another window, in addition to the text window, which can be viewed by both parties in the tutoring session. This means that we can display instructions on the screen instead of providing a paper booklet for the student. During the 25 tutoring sessions held in November 1999, we put a Prediction Table in this window to record the predictions as the student made them and any corrections made during the progress of the session. Both the tutor and the student can update this screen. Fox described human tutors working on solving problems together and coconstructing the answers (1993b). Michael and Rovick do this constantly in face-to-face tutoring. The new CDS allows some of this joint process to go on as both the tutor and the student collaborate on the task of filling in the Prediction Table. H. H. Clark's (1996) work on joint actions explains why this phase of the tutoring process is so important to both the tutor and the student. The interface that Jung Hee Kim and Michael Glass have designed and implemented for Kim's iTutor carries the coconstruction process still further—it allows the tutor and the student to coconstruct solutions to equations in algebra problems (Kim & Glass, 2004; Patel, Glass, & Kim, 2003).

Were we starting this project today, there are a number of Internet-based approaches that we could use to accomplish the goal of collecting tutoring transcripts, but CDS has served us quite well.

3.1.2 Formatting and Numbering the Transcripts

The log file for each session was not easy to read. Li wrote a C program to read the log, interleave the turns, label each sentence, and format each one so that it begins on a separate line. A sample of the output of the program can be seen in Example 3.1.

Example 3.1: A Sample From the First Keyboard-to-Keyboard Session Captured With CDS and Numbered

K1-tu-28-1: We're dealing now with the DR period.
K1-tu-28-2: That's before there are any neural, reflex changes.

K1-tu-28-3:	The TPR is neurally controlled.
K1-tu-28-4:	So what do you think would happen to it?
K1-st-29-1:	During the DR period it would remain unchanged.
K1-tu-30-1:	Correct.
K1-tu-30-2:	What other variables are neurally controlled?
K1-st-31-1:	CC, HR
K1-tu-32-1:	Again correct.

The label K1-tu-28-4 on the fourth sentence in Example 3.1 tells us that this is an excerpt from keyboard session 1, the tutor is typing, and this is turn number 28, sentence 4. This label is rather large and cumbersome, but it makes it easy to locate the context whenever we need it and to separate the student's contributions from the tutor's contributions. Sometimes when the labels take up too much space in a paper or on a slide, we cut them down to "S:" and "T:" After the numbering program is run, some hand-editing is typically needed to deal with cases when the tutor or the student sprinkled periods at the end of abbreviations and the program has been tricked into believing that it had reached the end of a sentence when it had not.

It is important to note that most of the excerpts of tutoring transcripts that are found in this book have been edited to remove typographical errors, misspellings, and idiosyncratic abbreviations, all of which would make it difficult for the reader to understand the dialogue that is occurring. We have not made changes to the grammar or the content of any transcript. The only unedited transcripts are found in Chapter 12 where we describe the input understander and how it copes with the real ill-formed input. The original unaltered transcripts can be found on the CD-ROM that came with the book.

3.2 HOW WE CONDUCTED THE KEYBOARD TUTORING EXPERIMENTS

All tutoring experiments (regardless of the type of data being extracted from the transcripts of the sessions) were conducted at Rush Medical College according to a protocol approved by the Rush Institutional Review Board. Students were recruited to participate with flyers (shown in Table 3.1) that advertised "earn while you learn." We were careful to communicate the fact that participation was strictly

TABLE 3.1

An Example of an "Earn-While-You-Learn" Flyer

EARN WHILE YOU LEARN!

We are conducting studies of student problem solving behavior in cardio-vascular physiology and the manner in which faculty can assist in the acquisition of problem solving skills.

Our next set of experiments will take place on November 13 and 14.

Control subjects will complete a 30 minute pre-test, work through a one-hour assignment, and then finish by completing a 30 minute post-test. All of this to be done at home on either Saturday (11/13) or Sunday (11/14).

Control subjects will earn $20 for their participation.

Experimental subjects will spend 2 hours at Rush (1289 Jelke) on Saturday (11/13) or Sunday (11/14), at a time that is mutually agreed upon, completing a 30 minute pre-test, a 1 hour assignment, and a 30 minute post-test.

Experimental subjects will earn $50 for their participation.

Both controls and experimental subjects can expect to learn some important cardiovascular physiology.

There is a sign-up sheet attached. If you would like to participate in this experiment, please fill it out and hand it in to Dr. Michael or Dr. Rovick. We will need your email address and phone number in order to contact you to schedule your participation.

Questions about this study can be directed to:
Joel Michael (X26426 or jmichael@rush.edu)
Allen Rovick (X26567 or arovick@rush.edu)
Department of Physiology

voluntary and that participation, or lack of participation, would have no bearing on the students' grade in the course. The number of students who failed to show up for a scheduled session, although not large, indicates that students did believe that their course grades would not be affected. However, we did suggest quite strongly that participation would help students learn something about the cardiovascular system that was important to them. This certainly contributed to the attention and effort that every student brought to their attempt to solve the problem we presented to them. Michael and Modell have both observed independently that when students perceive that what a computer program is trying to teach them is irrelevant but they agree to use it anyway to obtain a stipend, their lack of motivation results in little learning (Michael & Modell, personal communication, 12/3/94).

Sessions were usually conducted during a 2- to 3-day period after the students had completed all scheduled components of the cardiovascular block but before the regularly scheduled CIRCSIM computer laboratory (see Section 2.3 for a description of the scheduled components that make up the cardiovascular block in the course). The tutor (Michael or Rovick) usually worked in his office while the student worked in a second room some distance from the tutor. One of the experimenters (usually a graduate student in Computer Science) stayed in the room with the student to make sure that CDS functioned properly. In this way, we could make sure that the student was given help with the computer but not with the solution of the problem. In some experiments, pretests and posttests were administered to the students before and after tutoring.

Students were given a notebook containing several pages to guide them through the tutoring session. Table 3.2 details the content of this notebook and the tutoring process that was generally followed. The problem that the student was asked to solve appeared on page 3 of the student's notebook but does not appear in the transcript, although it is sometimes made clear in the initial portion of the tutoring exchange. If you are reading the transcripts from the CD-ROM you may want to look at the table of procedures that appears with them.

CDS (described in Section 3.1) proved to be a very simple system for students to learn to use, and their initial interactions with the tutor (confirming that the students had read and understood the information on each page) provided the only practice with the system that was needed.

After making sure that the student understood the problem, the tutor then initiated the interaction in a manner determined by whatever research plan was being followed (which varied somewhat over the 10 years that we collected data in this way; see Chapter 6). Tutoring most often proceeded for 1 hr (although we did conduct nine 2-hr sessions), at which time the session ended whether or not the

TABLE 3.2

Outline of the Instructions Provided to the Student for the Keyboard-to-Keyboard Sessions (Contained in a Notebook Placed Next to the Student's Computer)

Page 1	Overview of experiment
Page 2	Brief description of physiological model with which they will be working (see Section 2 1)
Page 3	Description of the problem (the disturbance that will result in a change in blood pressure)
Page 4	Definition of Direction Response (DR) phase
Page 5	Description of how to make predictions
Tutoring of DR predictions	
Page 6	Description of the Reflex Response (RR) phase
Tutoring of RR predictions	
Page 7	Description of Steady State (SS) phase
Tutoring of SS predictions	

problem had been completely solved. If time permitted, and at the request of the student, there might be some face-to-face interaction between the tutor and the student to clarify any issues that had not been dealt with during the formal keyboard interaction. This opportunity for clarification was deferred if any posttest was administered.

The constraint of having only 1 hr to tutor the solution to a problem certainly affected tutor behavior in important ways. The tutors always attempted to complete at least the first 2 phases of the problem because they felt that the most interesting tutoring took place then (the solution to the third phase—the new Steady State—can be generated in a more or less algorithmic fashion without necessarily referring to much physiology). One consequence of this time pressure is that not all of the student difficulties that became evident during tutoring could be pursued. We can observe the tutors prioritizing misconceptions as they decide which ones to attack; some are more important than others, and some may be more readily attacked with a particular student. Time constraints are always present in any tutoring situation, whether conducted by a human tutor or by an intelligent tutoring system.

3.3 ANALYSIS OF TUTORING TRANSCRIPTS

3.3.1 Reading the Transcripts and Debriefing the Tutor

In our original proposal to the Office of Naval Research, we describe a process of reading the transcripts with the tutors and debriefing them. We planned to sit down with the tutor after the session, read the session together turn by turn, and ask lots of questions. After every tutor turn, we planned to ask what that turn was meant to accomplish, what the underlying plan was, and why they phrased the turn the way they did. We planned to ask after every student turn how what the student said changed the tutor's model of what the student knew or whether it suggested the presence of some kind of student misconception or bug.

These plans did not fully succeed for several reasons. The tutoring sessions were held at the busiest time of the year for the tutors and so typically we wound up trying to debrief the tutors a month or so after the sessions were held, instead of the next day as had been planned. Also, we did not know nearly enough about interviewing techniques to do this interviewing as effectively as we desired. However, we did acquire some useful domain knowledge through the delayed debriefing sessions that we carried out. We did know something about knowledge engineering, and the tutors were accustomed to trying to convey domain knowledge to students and enjoyed trying to teach it to us. They gave us some very useful information about top-level instructional planning, but not much about language or about lower-level planning, and none at all about student modeling.

We turned to reading and rereading the transcripts. Using this approach, Yuemei Zhang (1991) produced some rules for discourse generation (see Chapter 16), and Leem Shim (1991) extracted some rules for student modeling (see Chapter 14). Chong Woo (1991) figured out rules for setting goals, and for choosing strategies and tactics to carry out those strategies (see Chapter 7). He then combined these rules with the rules derived by Zhang and Shim, to produce the first working Version 2 of CIRCSIM-Tutor (see Chapter 12). Ru-Charn Chang (1992) analyzed the structure of the tutor's sentences and wrote a sentence generation program. Yoon Hee Lee (1990) and Jai Seu (1992) analyzed the student input and wrote versions of the parsing and the spelling correction programs.

3.3.2 Marking up Tutoring Sessions With Standardized General Markup Language

For several years, we marked up paper transcripts of tutoring sessions with comments, questions, and notes. For some projects, we even used complicated coloring schemes with red, green, and blue pens, but it was not until 1994 that we started sustained, consistent use of electronic markup. Our files show that Gregory Sanders typed in the starts and the endpoints of a number of student initiatives in 1991, but he did not make a serious attempt to get us all to follow his lead. In 1994, Gregory Hume was working on identifying hints in the transcripts with Joel Michael, but he was also teaching at Valparaiso University in Indiana. He could only come to Chicago once a week, so he typed the classification of the hint on the electronic transcript next to the hint itself and e-mailed it to Joel. They began to do this regularly with excellent results. Not long afterward, Reva Freedman came back from a conference, told us about the markup being done on task-assistance dialogues, and urged us to expand the markup that Hume and Michael had started, using SGML (Standardized General Markup Language).

SGML was initially developed to mark up text for printers, but it has become a way to code text for many types of research (Barnard, Burnard, Gaspart, Price, & Sperberg-McQueen, 1995; Nakatani, Grosz, Ahn, & Hirschberg, 1995; Sperberg-McQueen & Burnard, 1994). This research methodology was then adopted by dialogue researchers working on task-assistance dialogues (Allen & Core, 1997; DAMSL, 1997; Nakatani & Traum, 1998), and motivated Freedman to start us in the same direction (Freedman, Zhou, Kim, Glass, & Evens, 1998).

Freedman persuaded Jung Hee Kim, who was just starting to work with our project at the time, to develop a plan for marking up a number of features in our sessions. Because her own focus was on planning and dialogue generation, she suggested that Kim examine tutoring strategies and tactics, so that we could expand the repertoire of methods available to CIRCSIM-Tutor. Kim embarked on a long-term study of tutoring methods in human tutoring sessions using markup as the major tool (Kim, 2000; Kim, Freedman, Glass, & Evens, 2002). She and Freedman spent many hours arguing about what features to include in the markup, how to construct a standard (Wiebe, Bruce, & O'Hara, 1999) and how to do the analysis (Dahlback & Jonsson, 1989; Galdes, Smith, & Smith, 1991).

Intensive markup is very tedious and difficult work, but it enabled us to discover facets of tutoring dialogues that we had not noticed in repeated readings. We used the excellent suite of free tools from Edinburgh (McKelvie, Brew, & Thompson, 1997) to check that the markup was correctly nested and to carry out automatic counts of members of important categories. With Freedman and Kim both urging us on, others of us started to do markup as well, especially Yujian Zhou, Feng-Jen Yang, and Evens. Kim (2000) wrote a manual to help coordinate our efforts and ensure that we were all using the same notation and carrying out our markup in a consistent manner.

We show an extended example of dialogue markup in Table 3.3. This example represents a complete markup of the passage from our numbered example in Section 3.1.2. For some purposes, we may choose to mark up just the student initiatives or just the discourse markers. Here we were trying to mark up a complete session to understand the planning at all levels and how those plans interact. This kind of nested markup allows us to identify the top-level strategy, labeled a *directed line of reasoning* or DLR by Gregory Sanders (1995), and then look at the individual tactics that the tutor uses to carry out this strategy. These individual tactics are called T-tutors-DR-info, T-tutors-mechanism, and T-tutors-value. These tactics, like most others, appear in other strategies, not just in this one. The tactics, in turn, are made up of tutor statements (T-informs) and tutor questions (T-elicits).

Markup provided us with a way to demonstrate that one major difference between experienced tutors and novices is that experienced tutors ask more questions than do novice tutors and they tell the students less (Glass, Kim, Evens, Michael, & Rovick, 1999).

TABLE 3.3

Extensive Markup of a Tutoring Episode

```
<T-tutors-variable, variable = TPR, try = first>
  <T-does-neural-DLR>
    <T-tutors-DR-info>
      <T-informs>
          K1-tu-28-1: We're dealing now with the DR period.
          K1-tu-28-2: That's before there are any neural,
                      reflex changes.
      </T-informs>
    </T-tutors-DR-info>
    <T-tutors-mechanism>
      <T-informs>
          K1-tu-28-3: The TPR is neurally controlled.
    </T-tutors-mechanism>
    <T-tutors-value>
      <T-elicits>
          K1-tu-28-4: So what do you think would happen to it?
        <S-ans, catg=correct>
          K1-st-29-1: During the DR period it would remain
                      unchanged.
        </S-ans>
      </T-informs>
        <T-ack, type = positive>
          K1-tu-30-1: Correct.
        </T-ack>
      </T-elicits>
    </T-tutors-value>
  </T-does-neural-DLR>
</T-tutors-variable>
<T-tutors-variable, variable = CC>
  <T-tutors-via-analogy, base = TPR, target = another-neural-
             variable>
<T-proposes-analogy, result = success>
      <T-elicits>
          K1-tu-30-2: What other variables are neurally
                      controlled?
        <S-ans, catg=correct>
          K1-st-31-1: CC, HR
        </S-ans>
        <T-ack, type = positive>
          K1-tu-32-1: Again correct.
        </T-ack>
      </T-elicits>
    </T-proposes-analogy>
  <T-requests-inference-from-analogy>
    . . . . . . . .
</T-tutors-variable>
```

Marking up many examples of nested strategies and tactics allows us to ultimately make generalizations about the strategies used by human tutors. This nested markup carries enough detail so that we can eventually convert these generalizations into rules for the tutoring system and generate language like this.

Another advantage of markup is that the marked-up data can easily be fed to a machine learning program, which can then make some of these generalizations for us. We describe our use of machine learning in the next section.

3.3.3 Applying Machine Learning Techniques to Studying Transcripts

It was Reva Freedman who first argued that we should be using machine learning to derive planning rules from our marked up examples (Freedman, Zhou, Glass, Kim, & Evens, 1998). Fortunately, Yujian Zhou had experience in using machine learning from her master's studies in Beijing. She taught us all how to actually make use of machine learning to discover rules for classifying student answers and for implementing some of the ideas about hinting from Hume's thesis.

Zhou used Quinlan's (1993) learning algorithm, C4.5, to discover a number of decision rules about tutoring strategies and tactics. One of the first rules to emerge (Zhou, 2000, p. 62) was the following:

If variable v1 is non-neural, then
    <t-corrects-variable, variable = v1>
        <t-tutors-via-determinants>
    </t-corrects-variable>
    <t-corrects-variable, variable = v2>
        <t-moves-forward>
    </t-corrects-variable>

This rule fits 13% of the dialogue data input. For example, in Example 3.2 we see the tutor teaching CO via its determinants and then moving forward from CO to Central Venous Pressure:

Example 3.2: Tutoring via the Determinants of a Variable

K36-tu-94-3:	Hr is the most potent determiner of CO. So what will the reflex do?
K36-st-95-1:	Reduce hr
K36-tu-96-1:	And if hr goes down, what happens to co?
K36-st-97-1:	Co decreases
K36-tu-98-1:	And if co is down what happens to rap?
K36-st-99-1:	Rap will I

This strategy is used so frequently by the tutors that Woo had discovered it and implemented in the system early on, but this output of the machine learning program gave us enough confidence in the process to persevere and expand its use.

Students frequently hedge their answers and we had not realized that the tutors paid much attention, but when Zhou fed data about response strategies to C4.5, the output was the following rule:

If student answer was correct and not hedged, then proceed.
If student answer was correct and hedged,
then give acknowledgment and proceed.
If student answer was partially correct, then give acknowledgment and proceed.
If student answer was a near miss, then introduce a nested method.
If student answer was "don't know," then give answer and proceed, etc.

Zhou (2000) used machine learning to acquire rules for the generation of hints and for the development of the student model, as well for tutoring strategies. We have found this approach very useful.

Of course, with most machine learning approaches, it is essential to formulate some viable hypotheses to test in advance. Freedman also introduced us to some of the important work on dialogue by Schegloff (e.g., Schegloff & Sacks, 1973) and the British research on conversational analysis of educational dialogue (Sinclair & Coulthard, 1975), which provided us with relevant targets.

3.4 TAKE-HOME MESSAGE

We were fortunate in being able to work with students who were highly motivated to succeed at the task we set for them, solving a problem about the baroreceptor reflex. Although some were more successful than others, all of them tried very hard. The keyboard-to-keyboard system (CDS) also proved its worth. It enabled us to collect a corpus of tutoring transcripts that became the fundamental resource for our analysis of human tutoring and for building the CIRCSIM-Tutor system.

We believe that the labeling and numbering has been worthwhile even if it is cumbersome. It has made it easier to find the context of a given turn quickly. This has been particularly helpful in our current work on analogies in tutoring, because it has taken us several tries to figure out how much context we needed to understand what triggers an analogy and how the tutor follows up on an analogy after it is delivered (Lulis, Evens, & Michael, 2004a, 2004b, 2004c).

We are beginning to see more uses for the timing information and we are very glad that we included it. Shah, Evens, Michael, and Rovick (2002) used this information to detect long pauses and identify tutor responses (mostly offering explicit help).

Our SGML markup has been even more cumbersome but also extraordinarily worthwhile. It has helped us to study several kinds of high level phenomena such as tutoring methods, student initiatives, and tutor responses. It has helped us to study surface phenomena like discourse markers and anaphora and politeness formulas. Our original markup was intended solely to support collaboration between researchers at distant locations. It does indeed support the collaboration between experimenters, but it has turned out to be valuable for other reasons. It also gives us an electronic record of our work. It has turned out to be extraordinarily helpful in carrying out counts and developing statistics. It also provided us with a data in a form that we could input into a machine learning program. The availability of free software to support SGML, check it for correctness, and count things for us, has been a real inducement to use markup (McKelvie et al., 1997).

If we were starting now, we would probably design our markup in the XML style instead of SGML, especially because Michael Glass has written a really elegant and usable markup tool that assumes XML (the Extensible Markup Language, Glass & Di Eugenio, 2002a,

2002b). We would most certainly use some kind of markup tool to lighten the load, if we were starting again. We would also design our markup with machine learning in mind from the start. As it is, we have sometimes had to rethink our markup to make the data convenient for the machine learning program to read.

4

The Language Used by Tutors and Students

In this chapter, we describe the tools that we used to analyze the language in our tutoring session transcripts, and discuss some of the differences between the language used in face-to-face tutoring and that used in keyboard tutoring. Next we look at the differences between tutor and student language. Then we describe tutor use of dialogue markers, because they are especially important in understanding how the dialogue changes course.

4.0 THE SUBLANGUAGE OF CARDIOVASCULAR PHYSIOLOGY

Before we could build a natural-language based tutor, we needed to study how both tutors and students use language. Obviously, we needed to study the student language in order to build a module to understand the student input and we needed to study the tutor language in order to generate the tutor's contributions to the tutorial dialogue. But a dialogue is much more than two monologues. Everything that the tutor or the student types is affected by the history of the dialogue (what was said, what worked), with the most recent history having the most immediate effect. We needed to study human dialogue processes.

One problem that we faced immediately is that educational dialogue is really different from other types of conversational interaction (Wells, 1999). Our favorite example of these differences comes from Astrid Lindgren's (1999) *Pippi Goes to School.* In this story, Pippi goes to school with her friends for the first time. The teacher decides to ask her some questions to figure out how to place her. She starts by asking Pippi what seven plus five is. Pippi, operating by the rules of ordinary conversation, is astonished and dismayed at the thought that the teacher does not know this simple sum and responds: "Well, if you don't know that yourself, you needn't think I'm going to tell you" (Lindgren, 1999, p. 15). The teacher, still playing the education game, tells her that seven plus five is twelve. Pippi is even more confused. "See that!" said Pippi. "You knew it yourself. Why are you asking then?" (Lindgren, 1999, p. 17) The teacher decides that it is hopeless to try to teach Pippi arithmetic.

The problems in this dialogue are created because Pippi assumes that she is participating in an ordinary conversation, whereas the teacher is using the special rules of educational dialogue.

Tutoring dialogue is definitely cooperative, and so it satisfies the requirement that Grice (1975) placed at the top of his hierarchy of his well-known rules for conversation. The problem is that the most helpful, cooperative tutoring dialogue breaks several of Grice's lower-level rules. Grice's maxims expressly forbid speakers to ask questions to which they know the answer. They also prohibit ambiguity of all kinds, especially hinting. But questions and hints are the tutor's most valuable tools. Person, Kreuz, Zwaan, and Graesser (1995) have discovered and documented a number of other ways in which good tutoring conflicts with Grice's maxims. For example, it is generally not helpful for the tutor to ask, "Did you understand?"

Historically, most tutoring has been carried out face-to-face and this is the kind of tutoring that the expert tutors, Michael and Rovick, were familiar with from their years of experience before this project began. Because we were planning to construct keyboard dialogues, instead, it was important for us to understand the differences between keyboard-to-keyboard and face-to-face dialogues.

There is yet another important motive for our language studies, although it was a rather nebulous long-range interest, not a well-founded plan. Our tutoring dialogues demonstrate that Michael and Rovick spend a considerable amount of time attempting to teach the language of physiology along with the content. Sometimes they comment on language issues explicitly, but more often they do it implicitly, by rephrasing what the student says in more accurate and scientific terms. It would be most satisfying and useful if we could show that student language grows closer to tutor language as the student uses our system. So we are very interested in the differences between student language and tutor language.

For all these reasons, it became clear to us (the implementers) that the first step in building a natural language based tutor was to study the sublanguage of cardiovascular physiology in detail, or at least those parts of it involved in tutorial dialogues focused on using qualitative causal reasoning to solve baroreceptor reflex problems.

Naomi Sager (1986, p. 2) defined a sublanguage as "the language used by a particular community of speakers, say those concerned with a particular subject matter or those engaged in a specialized occupation." Sublanguages typically differ, at least somewhat, from the everyday language of the speakers (English in our case) in vocabulary and in grammar.

4.1 TOOLS FOR SUBLANGUAGE ANALYSIS

The first step in any statistical study of language samples is to count words and sentences and turns. As we see, there are wide differences between student and tutor language and between keyboard language and spoken language that appear just with raw counts. Our second step was to build a Keyword-in-Context (KWIC) index, which reveals how each word is used in the sublanguage. Third, we studied differences in sentence complexity to find out what kinds of sentences we needed to parse and generate.

The labeling and numbering programs described in the previous chapter divide the dialogue into student turns and tutor turns, and then divide the turns into sentences. We needed to do some post-editing because the numbering program is sometimes fooled by abbreviations with terminal periods into thinking that there are two sentences where there is really only one. Our counting programs took the labeled and numbered sessions as input and then counted turn length and sentence length and numbers of turns and sentences. Although the CIRCSIM-Tutor system itself is written in Lisp, these programs were written in C or Icon (Griswold & Griswold, 1997), because Lisp is not especially convenient for doing arithmetic.

The KWIC Index, by definition, contains every word in its original context. Many studies use an arbitrary number of words (sometimes five or seven) on either side of the word. Because we were interested in building a lexicon and case frames and further syntactic analysis, we used the entire sentence as the context. This is easier to do in a dialogue situation like ours, because sentences tend to be shorter than in formal written text. To keep the KWIC index down to a manageable size, we made a list of "stop words," words that we excluded from the KWIC index. The original list consisted of the following:

a an and at I in it of on or the to

But we soon realized that "I" behaves in a number of peculiar ways in our sublanguage, and that it indicates "increase" more often than a first person pronoun, so we decided that we had better index it too.

A KWIC index is a kind of concordance that contains a record for each word in each sentence that is not on the stopword list and an identifier that makes it possible to find the source in the original documents. There are a number of concordance packages that can be used, but it is easy to write a program for the job. The first step is to devise the identifiers and add them to the source file. The second step is to create a file with a record for each word in each sentence (dropping the words on the stop-word list). The record includes the context and a label of some kind. Then the system sort function can be used to create the actual index.

Because we wanted to use the entire sentence as context and the sentence labels that we had already concocted, Michael Glass wrote an Icon program to produce a KWIC index whenever we needed one. Table 4.1 displays a small piece of the index that we created for sessions K1-K8, F1, and F2. Just a quick look shows that "about" occurs as a preposition rather often. It also appears as an adverb meaning "approximately" both by itself and as part of the phrasal adverb "just about." It appears as part of the phrasal verb "to bring about," and as part of the idioms "What about X?" and "How about X?" This kind of information is crucial to building the lexicon and case tables used by the parser and generator.

Physiology uses many multiword phrases. For example, all the parameters in the prediction table have multiword names. The contiguous phrases were apparent in the KWIC Index. To extract noncontiguous collocations, we followed Frank Smadja's (1993) ap-

TABLE 4.1
Fragment of a Keyword-in-Context Index From Dialogues F1-2 and K1-K8

Word	*Context*
about	Well, I think that ... the numbers that come to my mind are between a third and a sixth, and what comes to my mind is that when the heart rate is very fast, it's just {*} a sixth of the time. (F2-st-32-1)
about	An increase in heart rate, which ultimately brings {*}an increase in cardiac output, which ultimately brings back an increase in mean arterial pressure. (F2-tu-265-1)
about	I have a question {*} HR. (K4-st-72-2)
about	{*} that. (F1-tu-49-1)
about	What {*} the other variables? (K8-ti-0-2)
about	How {*} yet another variable. (K5-tu-43-3)

{*} indicates an occurrence of the word being indexed.

proach and looked for words that appeared in more than one of the KWIC contexts for any given word.

When we turned to the study of the sentence structure of individual sentences, we used Jai Seu's (1992) parser, an updated version of the parser initially developed by Yoon Hee Lee (Y. H. Lee & Evens, 1998), which developed into the parser used in our early experiments with Version 2 of the CIRCSIM-Tutor (see Table 11.1). Because Seu was still developing the parser, there were many times when it could not handle ill-formed input from students or especially complex structures from the tutors. As a result, we did a lot of hand analysis of sentence structure. Much of this work was done by Ru-Charn Chang (Chang, 1992; Chang, Evens, Michael, & Rovick, 1994), who was starting to work on the sentence generation program and wanted to find out what range of structures her module needed to be able to produce. We were startled to discover what complex sentences the tutors generated as they typed.

4.2 DIFFERENCES BETWEEN FACE-TO-FACE AND KEYBOARD TUTORING

The earliest studies of keyboard-to-keyboard communications in natural language (Grosz, 1978; Thompson, 1980) showed that keyboard language is terser and more elliptical than face-to-face language. These experiments involved natural language interfaces to databases, but the findings appear to hold for tutoring sessions; Gamoran (1991) reported three times as many words in face-to-face tutoring sessions as in remote sessions over a given amount of time.

Our most detailed studies examined 10 hour-long sessions, two of them conducted face-to-face and eight of them using the keyboard system (CDS). We chose these samples because the two sets of sessions contained roughly the same number of words. The two face-to-face sessions contained a total of 6,410 running words (tokens) divided into 489 turns, whereas the eight keyboard-to-keyboard sessions contained a total of 7,303 words divided into 699 turns. Some of these results are summarized in Table 4.2. Simple arithmetic shows that the number of words per turn fell from 13.1 in the face-to-face sessions to 10.1 in the keyboard-to-keyboard sessions. The students reacted to the change in communication medium much more strongly than the tutors, with the result that the tutor took an even larger role in the keyboard sessions. In the face-to-face sessions, the tutor spoke 4,094 (62.8%) of the 6,410 words and the student spoke 2,386 (37.2%). In the keyboard sessions, the tutor typed 5,462 (74.7%) of the 7,303 words, whereas the student typed only 1,851 (25.3%).

We had assumed that we would find a wider range of lexical items in the face-to-face sessions, on the grounds that both tutors and students would feel less constrained when talking face-to-face. The data showed that this assumption was incorrect. There are 740 types (different individual words) in the face-to-face sessions and 915 types in the keyboard sessions. Since there were 6,410 tokens (total words) in the face-to-face sessions, the type-to-token ratio is 740/6410 = 0.115. Because there were 7,303 tokens in the keyboard sessions, the keyboard type-to-token ratio is 915/7303 = 0.125.

Lexicographers often count the *hapax legomena,* the words used only once, as a step toward understanding word usage. Of the 740 types in the face-to-face sessions, 432 were used only once; 308 were used more often. Of the 915 types in the keyboard-to-keyboard sessions, 573 were used only once; 342 were more popular. Differences in word use between face-to-face and keyboard-to-keyboard sessions are shown in Table 4.3.

When we looked at the number and distribution of the sentences, we saw that the number of sentences per turn dropped only slightly

TABLE 4.2
Turn Length and Sentence Length in Face-to-Face (F1-F2) Versus Keyboard-to-Keyboard (K1-K8) Sessions

	Face-to-Face	*Keyboard-to-Keyboard*
Tutor	***F1-F2***	***K1-K8***
Number of words	4094 (62.8%)	5452 (74.7%)
Number of turns	245	350
Average words per turn	16.3	15.6
Number of sentences	497	814
Average words per sentence	8.2	6.7
Average sentences per turn	2.0	2.3
Student		
Number of words	2386 (37.2%)	1851 (25.3%)
Number of turns	244	349
Average words per turn	9.8	5.3
Number of sentences	412	403
Average words per sentence	5.8	4.3
Average sentences per turn	1.7	1.2
Combined		
Number of words	6410 (100%)	7303 (100%)
Number of turns	489	699
Average words per turn	13.1	10.1
Number of sentences	909	1217
Average words per sentence	7.1	6.0
Average sentences per turn	1.9	1.7

from 1.86 sentences per turn to 1.74 sentences per turn. The big change is in the number of words per sentence as both tutor and student sentences got terser. The average sentence length for the tutors dropped from eight words to six The average sentence length for the students dropped from five words to four

With the drop in sentence length came a significant drop in sentence complexity. We counted the number of subordinate clauses

TABLE 4.3

Distribution of Word Types in Face-to-Face (F1-F2) Versus Keyboard-to-Keyboard (K1-K8) Sessions (Adapted From Table 6 in Seu et al., 1991, p. 578)

	Face-to-Face		*Keyboard-to-Keyboard*	
Frequency of Use	*No. of Words*	*Percentage of Types*	*No. of Words*	*Percentage of Types*
Used once	432	58.4%	573	62.67%
Used more often	308	41.6%	342	37.4%
Used by tutor	611	62.4%	770	66.6%
Used by student	368	37.6%	386	33.4%
Used by both	239	32.3%	241	26.3%
Total types	740		915	

because we were convinced that they presented the greatest challenge for both the parser and the generator. We found large numbers of sentential complements ("I hope that you're keeping track of your predictions"), adverbial clauses ("And when the pressure goes up, what structures are affected by the reflex and how?"), and relative clauses ("Could you write an equation that showed how HR and MAP were related?"). These results for subordinate clauses are shown in Table 4.4. The results convinced us that it was essential for the natural language components of CIRCSIM-Tutor to handle a wide variety of subordinate clauses, although much of the student input was very brief.

As we move from face-to-face to keyboard-to-keyboard dialogues, the percentage of sentences that contain sentential complements is cut in half, along with the percentage that contain relative clauses. The percentage of adverbial clauses shows a much smaller drop and the raw number actually increases. We conjecture that this occurs because adverbial clauses are so often used to express the causal relationships that are the focus of the dialogues. These counts were made by Chang (1992), who built the sentence generator, and Seu (Seu et al., 1991), who produced the Macintosh version of the parser. Chang concluded that it was necessary for the sentence generation program to be able to construct all three types of subordinate clauses. Seu (1992) made sure that his parser could also handle them.

TABLE 4.4

Subordinate Clauses in Face-to-Face Versus Keyboard-to-Keyboard Sessions (Sessions F1-F2 Versus K1-K8, Adapted From Table 4 in Seu et al., 1991, p. 578)

	Face-to-Face		*Keyboard-to-Keyboard*	
Clause Type	*No. of Clauses*	*Percentage of Total Sentences*	*No. of Clauses*	*Percentage of Total Sentences*
Sentential complements	96	10.6%	57	4.7%
Adverbial clauses	81	8.9%	86	7.1%
Relative clauses	48	5.3%	32	2.6%
No. of sentences	909		1217	

The tutors expressed a feeling of loss of control after the first keyboard sessions. We suspect that this may explain why the tutors uttered only 10 imperative sentences out of the 909 sentences in the face-to-face-session (3 in one and 7 in the other), but they typed in 90 imperative sentences out of 1,217 in the keyboard-to-keyboard sessions. The tutors asked many more explicit questions in the keyboard sessions (217) than in the face-to-face sessions (129). They explained this as a conscious attempt to get students to respond, something that they could accomplish nonverbally in face-to-face sessions. They also sought consciously to express verbally in the keyboard-to-keyboard sessions the enthusiasm and approval that they could express nonverbally face to face. They typed in words like "super," and "excellent," which both appear four times in K1-K8, but not at all in the two face-to-face sessions. They also softened disconfirmations (cf. Fox 1988a, 1989, 1993a) by changing "No" to "Not exactly" or "Not quite."

The expert tutors (Michael and Rovick) responded to Fox's (1988b) description of exchanges involving conversational repair with great interest as their own experience had sensitized them to this issue. Analysis of problems requiring repair in our sessions showed that the most common cause of repair was the tutor's use of "How" questions. The tutors therefore took care to replace these questions with more specific questions, such as "By what mechanism ..." or "In which direction ..." The second most common cause of repair was the tutor's failure to understand a student initiative. Michael and Rovick generally welcome student initiatives (see Shah, Evens, Michael, & Rovick, 2002, for an analysis of this phenomenon) as a particularly promising sign of active involvement on the part of the student. This analysis, however, convinced them that it is sometimes wiser to avoid responding to an initiative, and just change the subject politely, if it is not clear what the student wants or how it is related to the current problem.

4.3 DIFFERENCES BETWEEN TUTOR AND STUDENT LANGUAGE

As we have seen, the tutors produce more words than the students in all of our sessions, and as we move from the face-to-face to the keyboard mode, this tendency becomes more pronounced. Tutors not only use more tokens, they use more word types, that is, they make use of a larger vocabulary. In the face-to-face sessions, the tutors use 611 (82.5%) of the 740 different words (types), whereas the students use approximately half (368 or 49.7%). In the keyboard sessions, the tutors use 770 of the 915 tokens or different words (84.2%) and the students use 386 (42.2%). A number of the words used by the tutor and not the student, as you might expect, are technical terms in physiology, like *innervation, myocardial,* and *pharmacologic blockade.* The biggest difference, however, appears in the distribution of sentence lengths, shown in Table 4.5.

As you can see from Table 4.5, the students manage to provide really short answers to tutor questions. Yanofsky (1978) found many questions answered by noun phrases, and so did we. The names of the seven cardiovascular parameters in the Prediction Table occur all the time, often abbreviated. So we see "Cardiac Output" or "CO" in answer to the tutor question "Next?"—which itself is short for "Now, predict the next parameter to change." But we also find questions that yield adverbs, adjectives, and verbs as one-word answers. Because the tutor and student are talking about these parameters and how they change, we find the adverbs "up" and "down" occurring all the time, as one-sentence answers to questions about how a particular parameter changed. The students also answer the same kind of question with a single verb "increase" or "decrease." These two words are often abbreviated "I" or "D."

TABLE 4.5

Distribution of Sentence Lengths in Tutor Versus Student Turns in F1-F2 Versus K1-K8 (Adapted From Table 3 in Seu et al., 1991, p. 578)

	Face-to-Face		*Keyboard-to-Keyboard*	
Tutor	***No. of Sentences***	***Percentage of Total Tutor Sentences***	***No. of Sentences***	***Percentage of Total Tutor Sentences***
1 to 3 words	187	37.6%	266	32.7%
4 to 10 words	155	31.1%	355	43.6%
Above 10 words	155	31.1%	193	23.7%
Total	497		814	
Student	***No. of Sentences***	***Percentage of Total Student Sentences***	***No. of Sentences***	***Percentage of Total Student Sentences***
1 to 3 words	186	45.1%	273	67.3%
4 to 10 words	155	37.6%	69	17.1%
Above 10 words	71	17.2%	61	15.1%
Total	412			
Combined	***No. of Sentences***	***Percentage of Total***	***No. of Sentences***	***Percentage of Total***
1 to 3 words	373	41.0%	539	44.2%
4 to 10 words	310	34.1%	424	34.8%
Above 10 words	226	24.9%	254	20.9%
Total	909		1217	

Adjectives are rarer, but we do see single word answers that consist of an adjective. The adjective “neural” appears often as an answer to the question, “What mechanism controls TPR?” but the noun phrase “nervous system” is still more common.

Students often answer questions about the nature of a relationship with “Direct” or “Inverse.” These words are also abbreviated “D” and “I” and the tutors had no problem understanding “I” as “inverse” in some contexts and "increased" in others. The student will sometimes insert an apology, such as "Sorry," as a separate sentence, before correcting an answer. The appearance of adjectives and adverbs as comments on the contribution of the other party has been documented elsewhere (Fox, 1993b), but, as far as we know, the appearance of content answers consisting of single adjectives and adverbs makes our dialogues unique.

The medical students in our transcripts were not only remarkably inventive in producing answers with a minimal number of words, they also managed to abbreviate those words in highly creative ways. They often stop typing whenever they believe that the tutor will be able to figure out what they mean to say, and their tutors almost always justify this faith in their ability to decode innovative abbreviations. So "sympathetic" is written as "sympa" or "symp" and "parasympathetic" turns up as "para" or "ps."

We often see complete two-word sentences such as "CO I." Here we have a subject noun phrase "CO" and a verb phrase "I" for "increased." The tutors also use a number of two-word sentences: "Still stuck?" and "Need help?" are the most common. They also use single adjectives as comments or acknowledgments: "Good," "Right," "Correct," and "Wrong" all turn up fairly frequently. We discuss acknowledgments further in Chapter 7.

Like Grosz (1978), we found both sides using "OK" very frequently. Kristina Hollingshead (2003), working with Peter Heeman at the Oregon Graduate Institute, examined occurrences of "OK" in spoken dialogues and found evidence of four different meanings or discourse functions:

1. Acknowledgment.
2. Stalling function (e.g., "Give me a moment to think").
3. Structuring signal indicating closure (e.g., "I am done with this last topic").
4. Structuring signal indicating a start (e.g., "I am ready to move on to the next topic"), with numbers 3 and 4 sometimes blending into each other.

We have seen some of the same phenomena in keyboard-to-keyboard dialogues. The tutor often types "ok" as an acknowledgment and sometimes to serve some combination of functions 3 and 4. The use of "ok" as an acknowledgment caused some of the few misunderstandings we see in our dialogues—the tutors, sometimes at least, intended it as a neutral acknowledgment, but the students took it as a positive one. In fact, we believe that the only acknowledgment that the students recognized as neutral was "go on."

We do not see "ok" used as a stalling mechanism in keyboard-to-keyboard dialogues, probably because both the tutor and the student can just pause without penalty, because they are in different rooms, but we do hear it on the student side in our face-to-face dialogues. The students in the face-to-face sessions preferred, however, to stall by repeating the question. Rosalind Horowitz (2004) suggested that students who repeat the question are attempting to signal that they are concentrating on the task. Indeed, Michael and Rovick seem to find this tactic relatively acceptable.

Gregory Sanders (personal communication, August 30, 2004) has told us that the Linguistic Data Consortium annotation specification for the DARPA EARS project agrees with the Hollingshead analysis, at least in part. The DARPA EARS project classifies "ok" as a "discourse response" blend and the description seems to combine elements of Hollingshead's functions 3 and 4. The specification describes "ok" as conveying something like "I'm responding to what you're saying and I'm also going to say something beyond that."

Bangerter and Clark (2003; Bangerter, Clark, & Katz, 2004) studied several different types of spoken dialogues involving joint actions and found that "okay" was used primarily for vertical transitions, that is, where the speakers are entering or exiting a joint task. Tutoring is certainly a "joint action" as H. H. Clark (1996) defined it and transitions from one tutoring topic to another typically occur when the student gives a correct answer and the tutor can drop the current topic and go on to the next (Brandle, 1998). This makes it very easy to blend the use of "ok" for stops and starts into its use as a positive acknowledgment.

Seu et al. (1991) examined the use of subordinate clauses by students with an eye to improving the parser's ability to understand student input. They found wide differences between students, as shown in Table 4.6. Three of the eight students abandoned subordinate clauses completely. Two students produced a majority (28) of the 37 subordinate clauses in the eight keyboard sessions. The tutors, on the other hand, were fairly consistent with each other and across sessions, so we have lumped them together.

TABLE 4.6
Student and Tutor Use of Subordinate Clauses in Keyboard Sessions

Clause Type	*S1*	*S2*	*S3*	*S4*	*S5*	*S6*	*S7*	*S8*	*Student Total*	*Tutor Total*
Sentential Complements	1	4	0	3	3	0	0	0	11	46
Adverbial	0	3	1	12	8	0	0	0	24	72
Relative	0	0	0	2	0	0	0	0	2	30
Totals	1	7	1	17	11	0	0	0	38	148

(Adapted From Table 5 in Seu et al., 1991, p. 578)

4.4 HOW TUTORS USE DISCOURSE MARKERS

One important focus of our work with machine learning is discovery of the rules governing the use of discourse markers in tutoring dialogues (J. H. Kim, Glass, Freedman, & Evens, 2000). We were motivated both by theoretical interests and practical needs. Discourse markers have played an important role in dialogue analysis. Moreover, the current version of CIRCSIM-Tutor does not use discourse markers, and this is one factor in the occasional awkwardness of the system output.

Halliday and Hasan (1976) described the role of discourse markers in creating cohesion in dialogue. Grosz and Sidner (1986) discussed how discourse markers signal change in the intentional state. Discourse markers also play an important role in Rhetorical Structure Theory (Mann & Thompson, 1986, 1987), especially in expressing rhetorical relations between segments. Schiffrin (1987) analyzed the behavior of a large number of discourse markers, including the ones that we have found in our data. Studies of discourse markers and the ways in which they express coherence relations in a variety of text have also been carried out by Bateman and Rondhuis (1997), by Oversteegen (1997), and by T. J. M. Sanders (1997; T. J. M. Sanders & Noordman, 2000). Studies of discourse markers in tutoring dialogues were carried out by Moser and Moore (1995) and by Di Eugenio, Moore, and Paolucci (1997). Forbes and Webber (2002) made a useful distinction between discourse adverbials and classical adverbials. The adverbials that we have studied are discourse adverbials, but their work makes it clear that we need to study, recognize, and generate classical adverbials as well. Members of the Autotutor team (Louwerse & Mitchell, 2003) have investigated an even larger collection of discourse markers. T. J. M. Sanders and Noordman (2000) have shown that students find it significantly easier to understand text with discourse markers than that same text with the discourse markers removed. We believe that discourse markers are just as important in making a dialogue easy to understand.

We began our study by locating and labeling the discourse markers in the tutor turns in dialogues that we had previously marked up with tutorial goals and topics, as described in Chapter 3 (J. H. Kim, Freedman, & Evens, 1998a, 1998b). In the process, we discovered that "now," "and," and "so" are the most frequent discourse markers in our human tutoring dialogues and we decided to concentrate on them. We also decided to restrict ourselves to discourse markers occurring at a topic boundary, because this made it easy to see which segments are related by a given marker.

Once a column in the Prediction Table has been filled in, the majority of the dialogue consists of tutor questions and student responses, so a typical tutor turn contains several steps (Freedman & Evens, 1996).

- An optional acknowledgment of the student turn.
- Possibly an elaboration of that answer.
- Possibly some new information.
- A question or instruction to the student.

Freedman (1996a) also characterized each student response as a correct answer, a near miss (correct but not the expected answer), a grain-of-truth answer (Woolf, 1984), a totally wrong answer, or an "I don't understand" response.

We put together 60 instances containing the context around each example occurring at a topic boundary. The data for each instance included:

- Category of the student answer.
- Presence or absence of an explicit acknowledgment.
- Discourse marker (one of " now," "and," or "so").

- Position within the sequence of topic goals (introduce, initial, middle, final).
- Presentation of the topic following the discourse marker: inform or elicit.

Using this scheme, the segment "and the reflex hasn't started to operate yet" from the third turn in Table 4.7 is coded as follows:

- Student answer category = "near miss."
- Acknowledgment = "present."
- Position in sequence = "middle."
- Discourse marker = "and."
- Type = "inform."

Running C4.5 on these 60 instances gave rise to the following rules:

- If the topic position is introduce then use "now."
- If the topic position is middle then use "and."
- If the topic position is final then use "so."
- If the topic position is initial, and if the presentation is inform, then use "so," else use "and."

These rules misclassified 8 of the 60 cases, which gave us an error rate of 13.3%. We were relieved to discover that existing theory seems to be consistent with these rules. The rule for "now" agrees with Schiffrin's (1987) analysis. She said (Schiffrin, 1987, p. 50) that "'now' marks a speaker's progression through discourse time by displaying attention to an upcoming idea unit." Grosz and Sidner (1986) said that "now" is used to mark a change to a new focus space. The misclassified cases of "now" occur when the introduction is unmarked and "now" is used to mark the initial topic.

Schiffrin (1987, p. 152) said that "and" usually appears with medial topics to "coordinate and continue" the flow. This description fits our second rule just beautifully. The misclassified examples occur with the strategy that we have named "move forward." This strategy is used when the student has corrected one prediction and the tutor is asking for a prediction for the next variable in a logical sequence. Our tutors also use "And?" to signal that the student has just given a correct but incomplete answer and the tutor wants the rest.

TABLE 4.7

Discourse Markers in Annotated Dialogue (Adapted From J. H. Kim, Glass, Freedman, & Evens, 2000, p. 267)

Turn	***Text***	***Tutoring Goal***	***Other Features***
1. T	Now let's look at your prediction for TPR.	Introduce Inform	Discourse Marker = Now
	Can you tell me how it is controlled?	Initial Elicit	
2. S	Parasympathetics.		Answer Category = Near Miss
3. T	Correct, TPR is neurally controlled.		Acknowledgment = Correct
	And the reflex hasn't started to operate yet.	Middle Inform	Discourse Marker = And
	So what is the value of TPR?	Final Elicit	Discourse Marker = So
4. S	Unchanged.		Answer Category = Correct
5. T	Great!		Acknowledgment = Great
	What other variables are neurally controlled?	Introduce Elicit	

As you can see, we have two kinds of "so." When it appears with the final topic, the tutor is asking the student to supply the logical conclusion. The other kind of "so" comes attached to an initial topic in a tutoring strategy that presents a student with an anomaly connected with the equation CO = HR × SV and asks for an explanation, as seen in Example 4.1.

Example 4.1: Use of the Discourse Marker "so" by a Human Tutor

K27-tu-72-1: So, we have hr down, sv up and co down.

K27-tu-72-2: How is this possible?

The hope is that the student will explain that HR has a larger effect than SV in this case—so the student is being asked for a logical explanation here as well. This again is consistent with Schiffrin's (1987) conclusion that the discourse marker "so" is used to mark a logical result. In our dialogues, the tutor is sometimes giving a result himself, but more often asking the student for a logical result.

4.5 TAKE-HOME MESSAGE

Our studies of the language used by students and by human tutors have been of great help in building the Input Understander and Text Generator for CIRCSIM-Tutor. We need to carry out more studies of this kind as we explore the possibility of answering open questions and recognizing student initiatives. Jung Hee Kim has recently done a study of student initiatives in face-to-face versus keyboard-to-keyboard sessions and found more initiatives in the face-to-face sessions (Zhao, J. H. Kim, & Evens, 2003). Lulis and Evens (2003) found more analogies in face-to-face sessions as well. It seems as if we may have much to learn from these sessions about how to get students to express themselves more freely to the tutoring system. We hope to see more studies of the effect of different media on tutoring as spoken tutoring systems emerge (B. Z. Clark, Bratt, Schultz, Peters, & Evens, 2003; Litman et al., 2004).

At the urging of Ramzan Ali Khuwaja, Michael and Rovick carried out a set of nine 2-hr sessions in which two different problems were solved; the goal was to identify possible changes in student language over this period of time. We became so engrossed in looking at the remarkable changes in protocol in these sessions (described in Chapter 7) that we have never done the necessary studies of possible changes in the student language. Perhaps, also, we have been afraid to look. This is one of the next items on our agenda. Two hours seems like a short time, so we will be happily surprised if we find any significant changes in student language over this period.

5

Domain Knowledge for Problem Solving and for Tutoring

In this chapter, we look at some of the knowledge required to solve problems in Section 5.0 and the much larger fund of knowledge required to tutor students in the process of solving these same problems in Section 5.1. We did not realize just how much knowledge we employed in tutoring until we tried to make it explicit for the implementers; we describe two different approaches to the discovery process in Sections 5.2 and 5.3, and then summarize what we have learned in Section 5.4.

5.0 WHAT DOES ONE NEED TO KNOW TO *SOLVE* A BARORECEPTOR PREDICTION PROBLEM?

We initially assumed that to solve a CIRCSIM problem, students only need to "know" the basic causal concept map (Fig. 5.1) and the algorithm for running such a model (Table 5.1). Both of these kinds of knowledge are presented in the cardiovascular syllabus and the scheduled lectures. Furthermore, visual representations of the baroreceptor reflex like those seen in Fig. 5.1 are referred to frequently in the problem solving sessions that are an integral part of the course.

What we discovered is that this assumption is correct although only in a limited way. Given only the causal concept map and the algorithm, it is possible to solve any CIRCSIM problem correctly as long as the description of the disturbance directly points to the initial parameter that is changed. Nakhoon Kim, one of the first graduate students to participate in this project (see Section 11.3), was able to solve all the CIRCSIM problems we used, although he had little or no knowledge or understanding of the cardiovascular system.

It is clear, however, that our students use a great deal more knowledge when they are solving some problems and when they are being tutored. Identifying the primary variable, the first parameter to undergo a change as a result of the disturbance acting on the system, requires an understanding of cardiovascular relationships that extends beyond the immediate causal concept map. For example, the procedure called "denervate the baroreceptors" requires an understanding of the anatomy and function of the nervous system components of the system. Furthermore, responding to the tutoring strategies employed by our expert tutors requires deeper levels of knowledge.

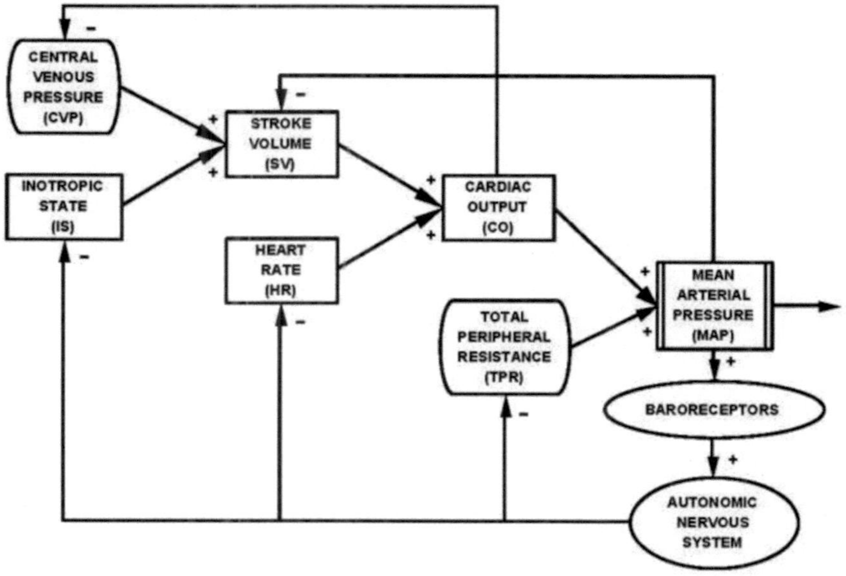

FIG. 5.1. The top level of the causal concept map describing the baroreceptor reflex.

5.1 WHAT KNOWLEDGE DOES ONE USE TO *TUTOR* A STUDENT SOLVING A BARORECEPTOR PREDICTION PROBLEM?

Here too, we assumed that the tutor used only the basic causal concept map (Fig. 5.1), the algorithm (Table 5.1), and a "generic" student model. This latter knowledge was viewed as a kind of pedagogical content knowledge (Berliner, 1986; Leinhardt & Greeno, 1986; McEwan & Bull, 1991; Shulman, 1986a, 1986b) derived from years of experience helping students solve baroreceptor reflex problems, whether in the computer classroom or in other learning venues (Ohlsson, 1987). We assumed that this generic student model consisted of statements describing those topics or steps in the solution

TABLE 5.1

Rules for Using the Baroreceptor Causal Concept Map

1. Start with the disturbance and propagate the changes to determine the change in MAP that occurs (the Direct Response).
   a. A variable can change (increase/decrease) only once during any phase of the response (DR, RR, SS). As the disturbance is propagated to each unchanged cell, the "first" change that occurs determines the new state of the variable ("later" changes that arrive at a cell that has already changed can only affect the magnitude of the initial change, not its direction). This rule applies to each of the three phases of the response.
2. The reflex response generated by BR-CNS will compensate for the original change in MAP (see Rule 1) by changing the values of TPR, HR, and IS.
   a. Changing HR changes CO (remember, changes in CO are most often the result of changes in HR).
   b. Any change in CO will result in an opposite change in CVP (and hence a change in SV).
   c. The reflex change in IS minimizes the change in SV but does not reverse the direction of change (see Rule 1a).
   d. The reflex response will return MAP towards its initial, pre-disturbance level, but will not fully compensate.
3. The new Steady State that is achieved will be the "sum" of the DR and the RR responses.

Note. MAP = Mean Arterial Pressure; DR = Direct Response; RR = Reflex Response; SS = Steady State; BR-CNS = Baroreceptor Reflex-Central Nervous System; TRP = Total Peripheral Response; HR = Heart Rate; IS = Inotropic State; CO = Cardiac Output; CVP = Central Venous Pressure; SV = Stroke Volume.

process that students found difficult and that were the source of frequent errors.

Student errors may be of several different kinds. We label some errors as "bugs," using this term loosely in the same sense that J. S. Brown and Burton (1978) used it to refer to algorithmic errors that students made in doing arithmetic, as distinguished from errors about arithmetic facts or slips in the calculation. We also distinguish "gaps," knowledge that the expert has but the student lacks, from "misconceptions," defined by Michael (1998) as a faulty mental model. VanLehn (1988, p. 62) defined a misconception as "an item that the student has but the expert does not." In other words, a misconception is a conviction that something is true when it is actually false. In any case, the result is a faulty mental model. Students seem to be ready to accept knowledge to fill a gap, but they find it much harder to correct a misconception. Michael and Rovick told the system developers to assume that a gap was successfully filled if the student used the new material correctly three times or more, but to be much more doubtful of changes in misconceptions.

Close analysis of tutoring transcripts (as described in Chapter 3) made it clear that much more knowledge was being used by the tutors than we had realized; our initial assumption here was incorrect. We discuss what this knowledge consists of, after first explaining how we identified our knowledge requirements.

5.2 ANALYSIS OF KNOWLEDGE REQUIREMENTS

We used several different techniques to identify different kinds of knowledge used by our tutors. Early in the CIRCSIM-Tutor project, Michael prepared and delivered a lecture on the physiology of the baroreceptor reflex to the graduate students and Evens. He also provided some carefully selected readings from standard textbooks. The implementation team then read and reread several early transcripts to identify the knowledge that was being used by the tutor and the student being tutored. Nakhoon Kim expressed this knowledge in Prolog rules (N. Kim, Evens, Michael, & Rovick, 1989). A year later, Yuemei Zhang and Chong Woo produced frames for the knowledge base of CIRCSIM-Tutor Version 2.0, which continue in use today (Zhang, Evens, Michael, & Rovick, 1990). These analyses confirmed the use of the knowledge contained in the causal concept map seen in Fig. 5.1 and added some knowledge of anatomy.

We were just getting Version 2 to work (with the frames built by Woo and Zhang) when Ramzan Ali Khuwaja began working on the project. He was disturbed by our interviewing techniques. He read Ericsson and Simon (1993) and other work on collecting and analyzing user protocols and decided it was time to begin a more systematic analysis of our knowledge requirements. One of his first moves was to institute a methodology for working with Michael and Rovick in think-aloud sessions to recover and represent their knowledge more systematically. These sessions not only involved the experts in the knowledge engineering process more directly, they resulted in the identification of holes in the knowledge base, and they demonstrated that student modeling, as practiced by the human tutors, was very different from the single-level process employed by the system.

Table 5.2 shows the initial portion of the third think-aloud session (T3) on January 14, 1993. Khuwaja begins by asking Rovick to talk about the procedure (problem) named "Increase Intrathoracic Pressure (PIT) from –2 to 0 mm Hg." Rovick gave a definition of PIT

TABLE 5.2

Excerpt from Think-Aloud Session T3 With Allen Rovick As the Thinker

T3-1:	The intrathoracic pressure is the pressure on the outside of everything inside the chest.
T3-2:	And the things that are most affected by it are the things that have the least support and the things like the veins, the large veins as they enter the heart and the atria as well.
T3-3:	An increasing PIT compresses all of these structures.
T3-4:	And as a result of compressing all of these structures, it increases the pressure inside these structures.
T3-5	So when you increase PIT you increase the pressure inside the atria and you increase the pressure inside the ventricle also.
T3-6:	So that the gradient for the movement of the blood between the atrium and the ventricle is not changing but the pressure is going up in the atrium.
T3-7:	So that one of the problems the student has is: if the pressure is going up in the atrium, why does that not mean increased filling pressure?
T3-8:	And the answer is because the pressure is also going up in the ventricle and therefore there is not this increased gradient for flow between the atrium and the ventricle.

Note. PIT = Intrathoracic Pressure.

(which is now stored in our knowledge base), told why it is important, and then explained the major student misconception that arises in connection with this problem. During the rest of this session, he discussed the solution to this problem. Khuwaja audiotaped these think-aloud sessions and then immediately transcribed them himself. The thinker was then asked to edit them, so the knowledge obtained was highly accurate.

Khuwaja's think-aloud sessions led to two important developments. First, a medical student was hired to spend the summer of 1993 working with Rovick on the identification of the knowledge being used by tutor and student. The student went through the transcripts underlining each appearance of a new concept and then he and Rovick made a list of the concepts and the features mentioned. Rovick and Khuwaja then worked together to make sure that all of these concepts appeared in the Domain Knowledge Base (Khuwaja, 1994).

The second development was even more fruitful. In the summer of 1993, we (Hume and Evens) had a long discussion with Kurt VanLehn at the Cognitive Science Conference, in which he gave a great many helpful pointers and references. VanLehn was, at that point, trying to figure out what the students did during the tutoring process that made it so valuable for them. Following this discussion, VanLehn agreed to visit Rush Medical College and interview medical students while Michael was tutoring them. The results of VanLehn's visit are described in Chapter 6.

5.3 WHAT DO THE TRANSCRIPTS TELL US ABOUT OTHER KNOWLEDGE USED IN TUTORING?

To teach or tutor any subject successfully, the teacher needs three quite different kinds of knowledge (Berliner, 1986; Leinhardt & Greeno, 1986; McEwan & Bull, 1991; Shulman, 1986a, 1986b): content knowledge, pedagogical content knowledge, and general pedagogical knowledge. The first of these, content knowledge, is knowledge about the discipline or phenomenon in question; in our case, knowledge about the physiology of the baroreceptor reflex. Everyone recognizes that one needs to know something about a subject to teach that subject. But having an expert's knowledge of the subject matter is not sufficient to succeed in teaching a novice about that subject. In fact, it is likely that domain expertise can contribute to a difficulty in presenting information in ways that are intelligible to the learner (Nathan & Petrosino, 2003). In addition, the teacher must understand how to best help the novice, the student, acquire that same knowledge. The expert must know what parts of the subject are particularly difficult for the student to master (and why), what teaching (or tutoring) strategies are most often helpful, and what kinds of misconceptions students have that will affect their ability to master the subject. All of this, and more, is what is meant by pedagogical content knowledge. Finally, every teacher or tutor needs to have some knowledge about general principles and practices of teaching (how to motivate students and keep them on task, how to respond in an effective manner to their questions and their answers).

5.3.1 Anatomy of the Cardiovascular System

The causal concept map seen in Fig. 5.1 does not directly represent the anatomy of the cardiovascular system in any visual sense. (The version of the map seen here does include some coding for anatomy to assist the reader, but we were not, at the time, using this version of the map with the students). However, reading the tutoring transcripts made it clear that tutors did refer to some anatomy in discussing the baroreceptor reflex. This anatomy focused on only a few critically important areas of the system: the relationship between the central venous compartment and the right atrium, the anatomy of the arterial compartment, and the anatomy of the neural elements of the baroreceptor reflex (the baroreceptors, their nerves, the central nervous system, and the sympathetic and parasympathetic innervation of the heart and blood vessels). This information is now available to CIRCSIM-Tutor in the Domain Knowledge Base.

5.3.2 Qualitative, Causal Relationships (The Causal Concept Maps)

One outcome of Khuwaja's work was the understanding that the tutor not only used the top level causal concept map (Fig. 5.1) but also used a great deal of knowledge that represented the mechanisms that explain the relationships in the top level map. For example, increased sympathetic nervous system activity causes increased inotropic state (Fig. 5.1). The mechanism by which this is accomplished involves increased calcium concentration inside cardiac muscle cells (see Figure 5.2). After analyzing a set of similar "expansions" of the top level concept map, Khuwaja drew two additional levels of causal maps (Figs. 5.2 and 5.3). The contents of the intermediate and lower level maps are used by the tutor in formulating hints and explanations. We discuss more fully how these concept maps are used in Chapter 8.

5.3.3 General Models

There are a number of simple general models, or recurring themes, that describe functions in a large number of different physiological systems (Modell, 2002). Two examples of such general models are the "pressure/flow/resistance" model and the "reservoir model." These models are in some ways similar to the "p-prims" described by diSessa (1983).

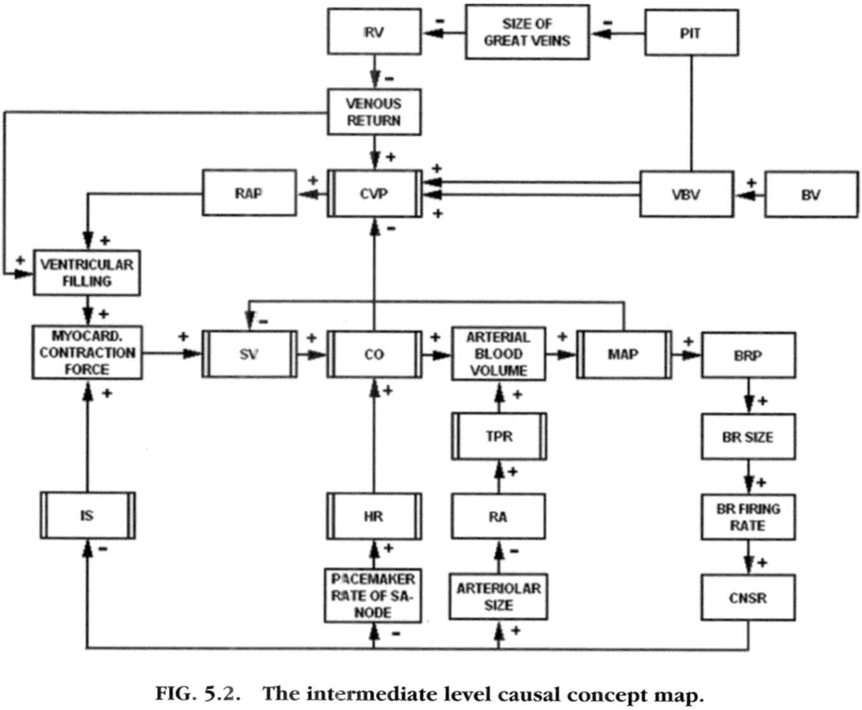

FIG. 5.2. The intermediate level causal concept map.

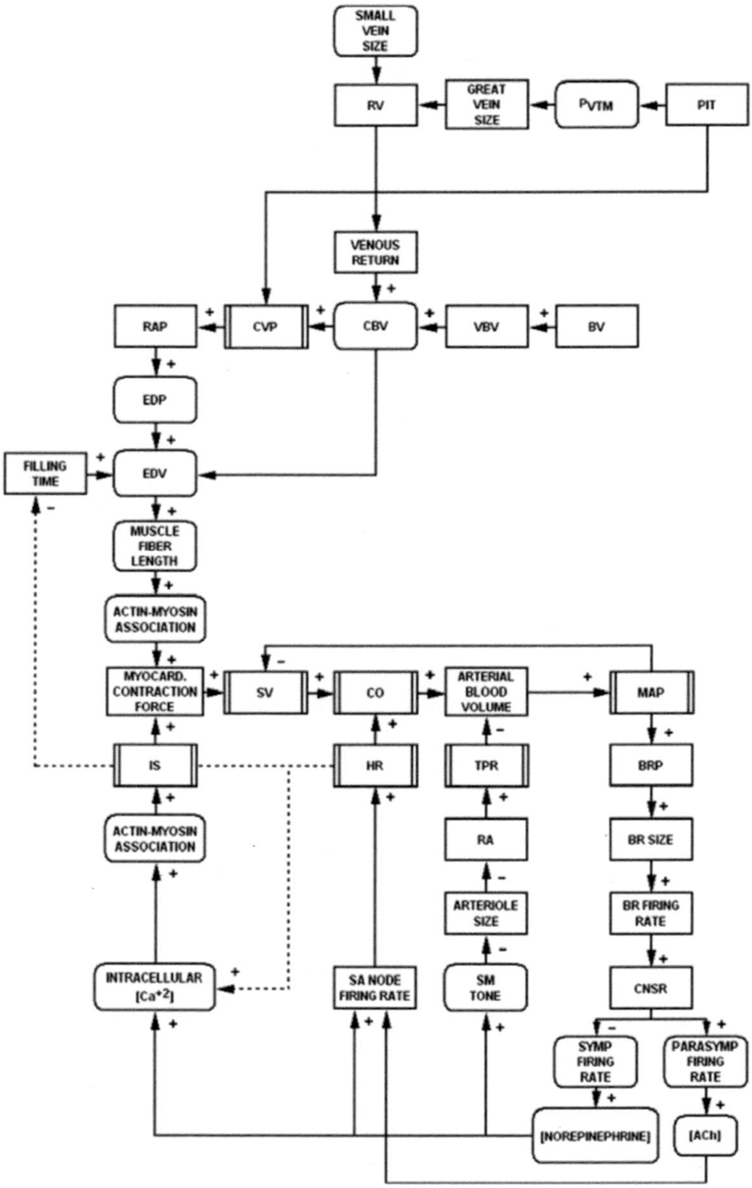

FIG. 5.3. The deep level causal concept map (adapted from Khuwaja, Rovick, Michael, & Evens, 1992).

The "pressure/flow/resistance" model describes the fact that the movement of anything (blood flow in arteries, air flow in the respiratory system, movement of ions across membranes, or the flow of electrons in a wire) occurs from a locus of high energy to one of lower energy. The magnitude of the flow is directly determined by the magnitude of the energy gradient and inversely determined by the opposition to flow (the resistance) that is present. This is, of course, a statement of Ohm's law for electron flow ($V = I \times R$). It is also a statement of the basic law of hemodynamics, which describes the flow of blood in a vessel: $Q = \Delta P/R$ (where Q is the flow, ΔP the pressure gradient, and R the resistance to flow). Another version of this equation is one of the two fundamental equations we try to teach our students: $MAP = TPR \times CO$. Here, MAP (mean arterial pressure) represents the pressure gradient, TPR (total peripheral resistance) is the resistance, and CO (cardiac output) is the flow.

The "reservoir" model is simply one representation of the law of the conservation of matter. It states that the amount of "stuff" in a reservoir or compartment is determined by the rate at which that "stuff" enters the reservoir and the rate at which "stuff" leaves it. A bathtub being filled from the faucet with an open drain is a commonly cited example of this model. This model has an important application in explaining how changes in cardiac output determine central venous pressure (see Fig. 5.1).

5.3.4 The Language of the Domain

The tutor knows the language of the domain, and how that language is used to communicate meaning about the objects and relationships making up the domain (Frawley, 1988). This language contains both common, everyday terms and specialized terms used only in talking about physiology (G. Jacobs, 1989). It is the tutor's mastery of this language that makes it possible to understand the questions and answers generated by the students, and makes it possible to generate questions, answers, and explanations for the student.

It is also important to note that the tutor knows the problems that students have in using the language of the domain. For example, there are similar sounding terms that mean quite different things. "Contractility," which is synonymous with "inotropic state," sounds like "contraction." Although both terms refer to the behavior of (cardiac) muscle, and hence have some relationship to each other, they refer to quite different phenomena. The adjectives "atrial" (as in "right atrial pressure") and "arterial" sound similar but point to different locations in the cardiovascular system. An understanding of these common language errors assists the tutor in making sense of the questions and answers generated by the students.

Another common problem faced by students learning any science is the use in the language of the domain of words that have both common, everyday meanings and precise technical meanings. Students often think they understand the technical meaning of a word while actually using the everyday meaning of the term (G. Jacobs, 1989). When those two meanings are diametrically opposed, the resulting misconception can be a serious detriment to student understanding. For example, to a physicist, an object that is very "elastic" has a high restoring force (and is hence difficult to deform or stretch), but in everyday use, the term means "easily stretched."

There is another domain language issue that deserves discussion. It is common for students to discuss or explain physiological phenomena using words that sound as if the student is arguing teleologically (reasoning based on assumptions about the "purpose" of the system; Tamir & Zohar, 1991). Thus, students commonly explain the increase in blood flows to exercising muscles as due to the fact that the "muscles need more oxygen" or they "want more oxygen." Such explanations do not provide a description of the "mechanism" by which blood flow to exercising muscle is caused to change. Teachers generally attempt to stop students from using such language precisely because it seems to lead students to avoid considerations of the causal mechanisms involved. However, it is also important for teachers to recognize that students using teleological language are not always actually anthropomorphizing the organs of the body (Tamir & Zohar, 1991); their ability to correctly articulate their understanding of the phenomenon often lags behind their understanding of the mechanisms involved.

There is, however, one kind of phenomenon for which language that sounds teleological is, in fact, quite correct. The baroreceptor reflex, like all reflexes, is a purposeful, goal-directed mechanism; it attempts to change blood pressure back to its regulated (set-point) level (Berne & Levy, 1998; L. Sherwood, 2001). Thus, in discussing the baroreceptor reflex, it is appropriate to refer to it as "wanting" blood pressure to increase or decrease. The transcripts of tutoring sessions reveal that the tutors sometimes accept student descriptions of the baroreceptor reflex "wanting" to accomplish something, but on other occasions attempt to correct the students' language. The basis for this decision is not clear, even to the tutors.

5.3.5 The Generic Student Model

Students have been using MacMan, Heartsim, and CIRCSIM for many years, and the tutors (Michael and Rovick) developed a generic student model (Ohlsson, 1987) based on their accumulated experience. Certain relationships are more difficult for students as a group to understand and apply than others (the relationship between CO and CVP is difficult, but the relationship between CO and MAP is less difficult; see Chapter 2). Some parameters are especially difficult for students to correctly predict (SV, because its changes are often quite counterintuitive; that is, it changes in a different direction than would be expected given the change in MAP that is to be produced), whereas others are relatively easy to predict (Ra, arterial resistance, rarely causes students any problem). Certain rules for running the algorithm always pose a problem for students (the fact that the "first" change that occurs determines the final direction of change that will be present although not the actual magnitude of that change is difficult for students to understand).

This generic student model also seems to contain a set of rubrics for helping correct student misunderstandings or misconceptions. These include tactics and strategies that are most likely to help correct the problem as well as actual pieces of text that seem most readily understood by the average student.

This model of a generic student thus serves as the starting point for any tutor attempt to diagnose the problem that a particular student is having. It also provides the tutor with a set of possible tools to use in helping students correct whatever problem they are encountering. We have more to say about the generic student model in Chapter 6.

5.3.6 Tutoring Strategies and Tactics

Years of interacting with students in all teaching venues had convinced the tutors (Michael and Rovick) that it is better to "ask" rather than "tell" (Cawsey, 1992, 1993; Michael & Modell, 2003). Students will develop an understanding of the behavior of the baroreceptor reflex more quickly if, faced with a decision of what to predict next, they are asked "why did you predict SV next?" rather than being told to "predict CO after you predict HR." Asking students questions and requiring them to generate answers more fully engages their thinking than does telling them answers to questions.

Equally important, it had become clear to the tutors that the students' answers to thought-provoking questions provided considerable insight to the mental model that the students were using in attempting to predict the behavior of the baroreceptor reflex. This insight then made it possible to help students repair or correct their faulty mental models more effectively, which, in turn, helped them to make more accurate predictions. In a sense, then, student answers to carefully selected questions enable the tutor to refine the generic student model into a model of the particular student at that particular time.

In an effort to engage the students in the process of repairing their mental model of the baroreceptor reflex, tutors frequently provide the students with hints. This was not initially a consciously intended strategy, but seems to have been a natural approach to interacting with students needing assistance to solve a problem. We discuss this particular strategy more fully in Chapter 8.

Finally, both tutors have available a number of different strategies that they can employ, so if one particular approach to helping a student does not work, it can be abandoned and another strategy attempted. These strategies and tactics to support them are described in more detail in Chapter 7.

5.4 TAKE-HOME MESSAGE

The content knowledge required to solve problems involving the baroreceptor reflex amounts to nothing more than the top-level causal concept map and an algorithm to run that model. However, the amount of additional knowledge needed to explain the responses of the system proved to be a surprise to the expert human tutors. This content knowledge must, of course, be available to the computer tutor if it is to succeed in aiding the students to solve the problems and understand the behavior of the system. The implementation of intermediate and deep level casual concept maps (shown in Figures 5.2 and 5.3) provides that knowledge.

The pedagogical content knowledge, the knowledge about how to teach students to understand the system, is also extensive, and here too the expert human tutors were surprised by how much knowledge is required. Generating hints requires not only content knowledge, but also an understanding of how to guide the students' solution to a problem without telling them the answer. When one approach does not succeed with a student another approach must be generated.

A great deal of knowledge of pedagogy is also required to help a student solve a CIRCSIM problem. For example, when to stop hinting, when to provide an answer, and how to deal with unproductive student initiatives, all require some general teaching skills.

Perhaps the most important message here, however, is that a great deal of this knowledge is tacit and often difficult for the tutor to explicate spontaneously. It took hours of poring over transcripts for many of the most important tutoring tactics and strategies to become evident.

6

Planning for Tutoring: What Is the Task to Be Accomplished?

6.0 INTRODUCTION

When a teacher interacts with a student on a one-to-one basis, there is inevitably a set of decisions that have to be made. First, there is a set of plans that have to be generated *before* the interaction begins: these include decisions about what the tutoring is intended to accomplish, what approach is to be used to accomplish this task, and what tutoring protocol is to be used. Second, there is a set of plans about the lesson content and the issues that will give the most help to this particular student. Then during the tutoring process, there are many more decisions to be made about appropriate ways to ask questions, how to respond to student errors as they occur, and how to help the student remedy suspected misconceptions. Whatever the case, what the expert tutors do is a product of their experience tutoring in this domain.

One-on-one tutoring is typically carried out to accomplish one of three different tasks: (a) teaching the student a new subject, (b) remedying a student's failures in understanding something, or (c) helping the student acquire a new skill.

Whatever task is to be accomplished, the tutor must make some decisions about how to reach the intended goal. There is, of course, a variety of possible ways to get there. These include delivering a lecture or in some other way conveying information, providing the student with repeated opportunities to solve problems, observing the student practicing the particular skill of interest while providing coaching (commenting only when the student signals a need for help) or giving minimal feedback ("right" or "wrong"), and entering into an interactive dialogue with the student. CIRCSIM- Tutor was designed to be a tutor that carries out a dialogue with a student while a problem is being solved.

The descriptions of how our tutors function to be found in this and the next three chapters are based on a number of sources: (a) Joel Michael was one of two people doing the tutoring, and he has spent a great deal of time reflecting on what he was doing as he did it; (b) there were extensive discussions between the two tutors about their tutoring experiences; (c) there were extensive discussions between the tutors and other participants in the CIRCSIM-Tutor project; (d) transcripts of the tutoring sessions have been read and analyzed from many different perspectives; (e) as implementation of CIRCSIM-Tutor proceeded, tutoring rules were extracted from the transcripts and formalized so they could be converted to computer code; and (f) we carried out extensive markup of about 5,000 turns.

In this chapter, we consider the issues that arise before tutoring actually begins. In Chapter 7, we discuss the decisions that the tutor must make while actually implementing a tutoring session with a student. In Chapter 8, we discuss the techniques of hinting that the tutor employs to keep the student actively involved in the learning process. Finally, in Chapter 9, we analyze, essentially line by line, an episode from a tutoring transcript.

6.1 DEFINING THE TASK

The first step was to define the task to be accomplished by our expert tutors, Joel Michael and Allen Rovick, and thus, the task that we wanted CIRCSIM-Tutor to emulate, if only partially. CIRCSIM-Tutor, like its predecessor CIRCSIM, assumes that students have acquired the facts about the baroreceptor reflex. The goal of both programs is to help students integrate these facts into a coherent mental model and learn to use this model to solve problems about the reflex using qualitative, causal reasoning. Although it is true that students do learn facts from their interaction with the computer tutor that were not learned before, neither program is meant to be a vehicle for the delivery of information. Both programs are designed to help students repair whatever faults may appear in their mental model of blood pressure regulation, by solving well-defined problems.

The task for the human tutors was, therefore, to help students solve a CIRCSIM problem (make predictions about the responses of the cardiovascular system to a disturbance, a change, in blood pressure). To do this requires the students to (a) recall the facts that they have accumulated through class attendance (lectures, computer laboratories, small group problem-solving sessions) and through reading the textbook, (b) integrate these facts into a useful mental model of the baroreceptor reflex, and (c) learn to run their mental models to make predictions and solve problems. The tutor's job was to help the student accomplish these things, and, when necessary, to provide the student with relevant pieces of information that had not been previously acquired.

6.2 DEFINING THE FRAMEWORK FOR TUTORING

6.2.1 Pursue an Active Learning Approach

Simon (2001, p. 210) pointed out what should be obvious: "learning takes place inside the learner and only inside the learner." As a consequence, the job of the teacher or tutor is to help the learner learn (Michael & Modell, 2003). Meaningful learning, the acquisition of knowledge that can be used in solving problems or carrying out appropriate tasks, is most likely to occur in an active learning environment (Michael, 2001), in which students are encouraged to build, test, and refine their mental models (Michael & Modell, 2003).

We assert that a necessary condition for one-on-one tutoring to succeed, whether the goal is acquisition of new knowledge, remediation, or problem-solving skills, is that the learner be engaged in active learning. Human tutors encourage this through the medium of natural language dialogue. However, the ultimate success of a tutoring session depends on what the student does.

The global approach adopted by the expert tutors (Michael and Rovick) for the one-on-one tutoring session that we captured and analyzed was the establishment of an active learning environment.

6.2.2 Tutor Opportunistically and Scaffold Student Learning

To implement this approach, the tutors present a problem to be solved to the student. As this problem is solved, the tutor's interactions with the student are largely determined by what the student does; that is, what the tutor says depends on how the student proceeds to solve the problem, whether the steps in the solution (the predictions) are correct, and whether the explanations that the student generates for his or her predictions when challenged by the tutor are appropriate. This approach to tutoring is opportunistic in that the tutor is always reacting to the student (Freedman, 2000a, 2000b, 2001; Young & Moore, 1994a, 1994b; Young, Moore, & Pollack, 1994).

It is clear, however, that the tutors have an agenda of their own. Their experience assisting students who are using CIRCSIM in the computer laboratory has led them to identify a set of common sources of confusion and common misconceptions that need to be corrected before the student can become successful at predicting the behavior of the negative reflex system that regulates the blood pressure. Thus, they are alert to situations that will allow them to help students remedy these problems whenever there is evidence from the student's responses that the problem is present. The tutors scaffold the students' learning (Anderson, Corbett, Koedinger, & Pelletier, 1995; Heffernan & Koedinger, 2000a, 2000b; Katz, Lesgold, Eggan, & Gordin, 1993, Katz, Lesgold, Eggan, & Greenberg,1996; Merrill & Reiser, 1994; Moore, 1995; Moore, Lemaire, & Rosenblum, 1996; Pea, 2004; Reiser, 2004; Sherin, Reiser, & Edelson, 2004), assisting them when assistance is needed, allowing the students to proceed on their own when no assistance is required.

6.2.3 Generate a Model of the Student

To tutor in the manner being described, the tutor must have some expectations about student behavior in this problem domain. This knowledge about what students find difficult and what they find easy constitutes a generic student model (Ohlsson, 1987). It clearly does not describe all students all of the time, but where the tutor's experience is extensive, it is likely to fit most students most of the time. Such a generic student model is one component of the pedagogical content knowledge (Berliner, 1986; Leinhardt & Greeno, 1986; McEwan & Bull, 1991; Ohlsson, 1987; Shulman, 1986a, 1986b) that experienced teachers develop. Table 6.1 lists a set of "bugs" that make up the generic student model.

TABLE 6.1
Bugs Catalogued in the Generic Student Model

Bugs That Appear in All Three Columns
CO = SV × HR error
MAP = CO × TPR error
RAP (or CVP) not proportional to 1/CO
SV not proportional to RAP (or CVP)
TPR is determined by CO
The effects or preload (filling) and IS are the same
Predictions not made in causal sequence (CO before SV and HR predicted)
Argues that parameter changes more than once during a phase of the response
Distinction between SV and CO not understood
DR-Only Bug
Neural variables are not all 0s (no change)
RR-Only Bugs
MAP-RR not the inverse of MAP-DR
CC(IS)/HR/TPR-RR not the inverse of MAP-DR
All RR parameters either increase or decrease
SS-Only Bugs
MAP-SS is 0 (no change); disturbance completely corrected
DR and RR "summed" incorrectly

Note. CO = cardiac output; HR = heart rate; MAP = mean arterial pressure; TPR = total peripheral resistance; RAP = right atrial pressure; CVP = central venous pressure; IS = inotropic state; CC = cardiac contractibility; DR = direct response; RR = reflex response; SS = steady state.

As the session progresses, however, the tutors immediately begin to build a model of the specific student being tutored based on the predictions being made, answers to tutor questions, and student initiatives. It appears that this model being generated on the fly has the generic student model as its starting point. That is, the tutor personalizes the generic student model by noting that (a) certain expected difficulties are not present in this student, (b) certain difficulties are present that most students do not exhibit, and (c) some of expected difficulties are, in fact, present. The individual student model that evolves as the tutoring proceeds is, in turn, used by the tutor in generating questions and explanations as the tutorial dialogue evolves.

The contents of the individual student model are limited by the working memory of the tutor. Thus, it is clear that the most recent predictions and answers have a greater weight than earlier ones because they are more likely to be remembered (see Chapter 14 for a description of the way in which CIRCSIM-Tutor models the student). It is also clear that some features present in the individual student model are forgotten as tutoring proceeds and hence no tutoring about these issues occurs. A computer tutor need not be subject to such memory limitations. One other factor that often limits how many items in the student model actually get tutored is the limited time available for tutoring in the sessions that were scheduled; the tutor may decide that some things are more important than others in a situation in which not everything can be fixed.

6.2.4 Ask, Don't Tell

The tutors' belief in the importance of establishing the tutoring session as an active learning environment and the need for information about the student to build a specific student model has led them to adopt a principle of "ask, don't tell." Questions and the answers that they elicit from the students are more valuable for both the tutor and the student than are expositions about the problem domain. Questions are frequently a component of hints (discussed later or see Chapter 8) intended to stimulate student problem solving, thus making the student as active as possible while solving the problem. At the same time the student responses to questions (and hints) provide information with which to build the most robust student model possible. Cawsey (1992, 1993) described experienced tutors asking questions where she expected explanations and in this way producing "interactive explanations." Wells (1999) described similar question-asking behavior in experienced classroom teachers.

6.3 FIGURING OUT WHERE THE STUDENTS NEED HELP

Before we start to tutor, we need to identify what kind of help students need and what they are not learning from reading and lectures and workshops.

6.3.1 Students Need Help Integrating the Facts Into Useful Models

Medical students are generally quite good at memorizing individual pieces of information. But an unorganized list of facts about the cardiovascular system can only be regurgitated from memory; a "laundry list" is of no use in solving problems. It is true, of course, that students do not literally attempt to commit to rote memory the facts that they are being asked to accumulate. Rather, they build mental models of the things that they are learning (Lesh & Kelly, 1997). However, when learning is occurring in a more or less passive environment, the model being built is likely to be fragmentary, inconsistent, built of components that are poorly interconnected, and likely to exist in relative isolation from everything else that the learner already knows. Even when the learning has occurred in a more active learning environment, it is still difficult for students to build models that will be appropriate and usable for problem solving. Thus, one of the tasks of the tutors is to help students organize or integrate the facts that they have accumulated into the most useful model for the domain.

6.3.2 Students Need Help Learning to Do Qualitative, Causal Reasoning

Physiology is a discipline that seeks to understand the mechanisms of the living organism. It seeks to establish the cause-and-effect relationships between the variables that are a part of the particular mechanism under study. The first goal, then, is to establish the qualitative, causal relationships between the important parameters.

Only after this has been established can the quantitative relationships be determined.

Qualitative, causal reasoning is difficult for students to master. Particularly in dealing with living systems, it is easier for them to reason teleologically ("the body wants blood pressure to increase ...") than it is to reason mechanistically ("blood pressure increases because cardiac output and total peripheral resistance increased"; Tamir & Zohar, 1991). However, even when students have become facile at reasoning about linear chains of causal relationships, they find it challenging to reason about systems in which there is negative feedback. The baroreceptor reflex, like all reflexes, is just such a system. One problem for students is the circularity intrinsic to a negative feedback system, which makes it difficult to determine when to stop attempting to propagate changes through the system. Even when students have a robust mental model of the reflex, using that model to predict the responses of the system to a disturbance is difficult. Thus, students need to learn how to apply qualitative, causal reasoning to the baroreceptor reflex. They need to learn a solution algorithm for using their model.

One goal of the tutor is therefore to help students learn to reason about baroreceptor reflex responses, hopefully in a way they will be able to generalize to other similar reflex responses that they will encounter in their study of physiology (e.g., chemical control of ventilation).

6.3.3 Students Need Help Learning the Language of Physiology

Students studying physiology generally have little trouble learning the new words in the specialized vocabulary of the discipline, although in some cases, associating the correct definition of a term or label with the correct mental model is challenging. For example, students may be able to define inotropic state (IS) while having a quite incorrect model of that concept. It is generally more difficult for students to deal with terms that have one meaning in everyday conversation and a very specialized meaning in talking physiology (G. Jacobs, 1989; Michael et al., 2002). For example, the term *elastic* in everyday conversation means "very stretchy" or easily stretched, that is, has a low recoil force. However, in physics (and hence in physiology), the term elastic means having a high restoring force when stretched, the exact opposite of its everyday meaning.

But speaking the language of physiology, being able to discuss or explain physiological phenomena, requires more than a list of memorized terms. It requires the ability to organize these terms into language structures that correctly communicate this speaker's meaning. This is, in general, a much greater challenge for students. One problem is that students find the language of teleology ("the exercising muscles need more oxygen so blood flow increases") more natural than the language of causal mechanisms ("blood flow to the exercising muscles increases because the resistance to flow decreases"), even when their thinking is not really teleological (Tamir & Zohar, 1991). Thus, students need practice in talking physiology and corrective feedback about their attempts to use this new language.

One task for the tutors, therefore, is modeling the language of physiology. Thus, it is not uncommon for the tutor to restate something the student just said in more acceptable scientific language. Although not the primary goal of tutoring, this attention to language usage, and the correction of incorrect usage, is frequently seen in the transcripts.

6.4 DEFINING THE CURRICULUM

The tutors' agenda in a one-on-one tutoring session is based on their choice of problems for the student to solve, and on their generic student model, which describes what students are likely to know and understand, and where they are likely to experience difficulties and develop misconceptions. For both CIRCSIM and CIRCSIM-Tutor, the curriculum is essentially a list of problems and also a list of rules that determine which to present to the current student. Lesgold also developed rules of this kind for Sherlock II (Katz, Lesgold, Eggan, Gordin, & Greenberg, 1992; Lesgold, 1988).

The eight problems representing different disturbances to the blood pressure made available to the student by CIRCSIM were listed in Chapter 2 (Table 2.4). These eight baroreceptor Prediction Table problems were picked because they force students to confront most of the major difficulties about cardiovascular function that the tutors have encountered in working with students. In CIRCSIM, students are encouraged to do these problems in the indicated sequence because this order serves to introduce new physiological issues in a helpful way and because the problems become increasingly difficult. Reiser (2004) argued that the choice of problems and the order of presentation are vitally important to learning and suggests that these processes can be viewed as a kind of scaffolding. The current version of CIRCSIM-Tutor (Version 2) presents the same set of problems as CIRCSIM.

When we were planning the one-on-one tutoring sessions, we wanted to use a problem that the students would not do in CIRCSIM (or in CIRCSIM-Tutor), because we could not be sure that they would not have used the program before the scheduled computer laboratory. (Both programs are always available on the computer-center machines.) We also wanted to use a problem that would not be too difficult because this would probably be the students' first experience solving a Prediction Table problem of this kind. The problem that has been used most frequently is one in which a patient has an electronic pacemaker that is the sole determinant of his heart rate (the physiological mechanisms that do this in a normal individual are damaged). This patient experiences a pacemaker malfunction that causes HR either to increase (from a normal of 70/min to 120/min) or decrease (from a normal of 70/min to 50/min).

Because we rarely tutored more than one problem in a session, we have not had to deal with large sets of problems. However, we have given considerable thought to this issue for future implementations of CIRCSIM-Tutor. Khuwaja (1994), working with the tutors, generated a set of problems of varying degrees of difficulty (largely determined by the number of steps of causal reasoning are required to get from the description of the disturbance to the identification of the primary variable) that could be used in a dynamic problem assignment as student performance changed over time (as the students get better the problems get harder). More recently, Byung-In Cho (2000; Cho, Michael, Rovick, & Evens, 1999) developed a total curriculum with rules for displaying appropriate collections of problems to the students and asking them to make a choice. The complete list of problems and the rules for displaying them can be found on the CD-ROM that accompanies this book.

6.5 TAKE-HOME MESSAGE

Casual observation of a tutor interacting with a student, whether in the laboratory, computer laboratory, or the teacher's office, can leave the impression that the interaction is entirely spontaneous, with little more than a vague agenda guiding the interaction. For experienced teachers and expert tutors, this is clearly not the case. Long before they interact with a student they have thought about their domain, how to teach it, and how to help individual students master it. This reflection results in decisions being made, plans being formulated, that determine the problems presented, what the tutor does and says, and how. These plans include an agenda to be pursued, identification of a plan for the nature of the interaction to be produced, and a generic model of students and the difficulties that we can expect them to experience within the domain.

7

Carrying Out the Tutoring Task

The tutors' overall goal is helping the student repair flaws in his or her mental model of the baroreceptor reflex. The approach that has been selected to accomplish this goal is to create a problem-solving environment in which the student is as active a participant in the solution as possible. The tutor accomplishes this goal by generating a dialogue with the student in which the tutor endeavors to help the student do as much of the work of solving a baroreceptor prediction problem, and in the process tries to repair any errors that were made. To accomplish these goals, the tutors must model the state of the student's understanding in order to individualize their interactions with the student and to scaffold the problem-solving process for the student. In keeping the student as active as possible, they almost always choose to ask the student something rather than tell the student something.

Our tutors make a number of decisions that provide the framework for the things they do in their interaction with the student before the beginning of the session. These decisions were described in the preceding chapter.

In this chapter, we describe the hierarchy of decisions that the expert tutor must make in carrying out a tutoring session designed to help the student learn how to solve a problem using causal reasoning. We begin with the choice of a protocol or high-level tutoring policy that is most appropriate for this problem and this student. The protocol defines when the tutor intervenes during the students' problem-solving process (see Section 7.1). Next, the tutor must choose the strategies to be used (see Section 7.2) and the topics to be discussed (see Section 7.3) to address any student errors in the problem-solving process. The final step is to choose the tactics necessary to carry out those strategies. Among these tactics are a number of ways to keep the student playing an active role in the session, asking questions, using a directed line of reasoning, giving appropriate acknowledgments and making other choices of appropriate language carefully, and especially hinting. Hinting is such a complex process and so important in tutoring that we have given it a whole chapter of its own (Chapter 8).

7.0 ALTERNATIVE VIEWS OF THE TUTORING PROCESS

Graesser, Person, and Magliano (1995) identified a five-step frame as basic to tutoring:

Step 1. Tutor asks question.
Step 2. Student answers question.
Step 3. Tutor gives short feedback.
Step 4. Tutor improves quality of answer.
Step 5. Tutor assesses student's understanding.

Chi, Siler, Jeong, Yamauchi, and Hausmann (2001) use the same basic framework in their landmark study of tutoring sessions. They give Step 4 a rather more detailed and explanatory description (p. 473): "Tutor scaffolds to improve or elaborate the student's answer in a successive series of exchanges." We sometimes see expert tutors initiating a whole new strategy during Step 4, when the student's answer totally misses the point. A new strategy tried after the first has failed is called *a nested method* by J. H. Kim, Freedman, Glass, and Evens (2002).

Our own analysis has led us to this same framework, but we differ in some important details that reflect the differences between the novice tutors studied by Graesser and by Chi and expert tutors like

Michael and Rovick and those studied by Cawsey (1992) and Lepper (Lepper, Woolverton, Mumme, & Gurtner, 1993).

The most obvious difference appears in Step 5. Chi et al. (2001) report comprehension-gauging questions like "Are you following?" or "Do you understand?" but Michael and Rovick almost never use such questions. This was one of the major differences between novice and expert tutors found by Glass, J. H. Kim, Evens, Michael, and Rovick (1999). Michael and Rovick proclaimed when we began to design CIRCSIM-Tutor that the system should never ask such "Do you understand?" questions because they are a worthless waste of time. Instead, they told the implementers, the system should ask a follow-up question that assesses whether the student understands the issue and is capable of acting on it.

This intuition on the part of Michael and Rovick has since been given a scientific basis. Graesser (1993a, 1993b) has demonstrated that most students are incapable of assessing their own understanding. This study shows that, at least when it comes to undergraduate students in Psychology, only the D students (who realize that they are lost) and the A students (who pursue whatever they do not understand until they conquer it) can accurately assess their knowledge; the majority, the B and C students, have no idea what they understood and what they had missed. Our examples also show that expert tutors blend Steps 3 and 4 in subtle ways, often providing feedback via hints and prompts that allow students to correct their own errors. Fox (1989, 1993b) also gave examples in which tutors combine acknowledgments, hints, and questions and follow-up questions.

Other studies by Fox (1993b) and by Graesser and his collaborators (Graesser, 1988; Graesser, Lang, & Horgan, 1988; Graesser & Person, 1994; Graesser, Person, & Huber, 1993) have identified some of the ways that tutors structure questions at different steps of this cycle to push students into more thought and action. This tutoring cycle differentiates tutoring from other kinds of dialogue, but tutoring dialogues apparently make use of the same kind of underlying dialogue structures that support everyday conversation. In particular, the structures posited by Schiffrin (1987) and by H. H. Clark (1996) seem to throw particular light on the tutors' use of acknowledgments (to be described in Section 7.4).

Schiffrin (1987) proposed a five-level model of discourse: the information framework supports the exchange structure, which supports the ideational structure, which supports the participation framework that structures the dialogue. The action structure organizes the speech acts into their linear sequence in time.

H. H. Clark (1996) described language use in dialogue as a series of joint actions that involve four levels of processing as shown in Table 7.1; each level is necessary to enable the level above it. At the lowest level, the speaker presents a signal and the listener attends to that signal. At the second level, the speaker signals something and the listener identifies that signal. At the third level, the speaker signals proposition "p" and the listener recognizes that the speaker means "p." At the top level, the speaker proposes a joint action and the listener accepts or rejects that proposal.

In a ladder of actions, evidence that action at one level is complete is evidence that the actions at lower levels have completed. H. H. Clark's (1996) emphasis on closure seems to be especially useful in helping us understand how tutors signal a change of topic.

When it comes to trying to understand special features of tutoring dialogues, we paid particular attention to the eight components of effective tutoring, identified in the literature by Graesser et al. (1995, p. 497):

1. Active student learning.
2. Sophisticated pedagogical strategies.
3. Anchored learning in specific examples and cases.
4. Collaborative problem solving and question answering.
5. Deep explanatory reasoning.
6. Convergence toward shared meanings.
7. Feedback, error diagnosis, and remediation.
8. Affect and motivation.

TABLE 7.1

H. H. Clark's (1996) Ladder of Joint Actions in Dialogue

Level	*Speaker*	*Listener*
4	Proposes joint action	Takes up proposal
3	Signals that "p"	Recognizes that speaker means "p"
2	Signals something	Identifies that signal
1	Presents signal	Attends to that signal

View of H. H. Clark's Ladder of Joint Actions in Dialogue (copied with permission from p. 26 of Brandle, 1998).

They commented that they have seen only items 3, 4, and 5 in the novice tutoring dialogues that they collected. As we show, all eight of these components of effective tutoring appear among the examples in this chapter and the two that follow it.

7.1 DEFINING THE PROTOCOL

We started to use the term *protocol* as a name for the overall plan for the structure of the interaction, because this is the term commonly used in medical context to define the structure of any experimental interaction. The first decision that the tutor must make as the session begins is the choice of protocol, the choice about how to structure the problem-solving process. In the Computer-Aided Instruction program CIRCSIM (Rovick & Michael, 1986), students are required to fill in all 21 predictions (seven parameters in each of three phases) before receiving any feedback about errors that they have made. In choosing a protocol for CIRCSIM-Tutor, Michael and Rovick decided that the new system should intervene more often. But the question was, when should this intervention occur.

7.1.1 The Argument for Immediate Feedback About Errors

There is a widespread understanding that corrective feedback to the learner is an essential element in promoting learning (Bransford, Brown, & Cocking, 1999; Kulik & Kulik, 1988; Pellegrino, Chudowsky, & Glaser, 2001). There are also reasons to believe that immediate feedback when an error is made is more effective than delayed feedback (Kulik & Kulik, 1988). However, when the student is learning about complex systems (made up of many interacting components), immediate feedback about an error may make it difficult for the learner to see and understand the overall behavior of the system (Schooler & Anderson, 1990).

7.1.2 The Need for Diagnostic Information Supersedes the Possible Desirability of Immediate Feedback

In classroom settings and in one-on-one tutoring situations, most teachers endeavor to provide immediate feedback to correct student errors, and our expert tutors (Michael and Rovick) are no different. However, as they were writing CIRCSIM, it became clear that immediate feedback for each individual prediction error made it impossible to adequately diagnose the state of the student's knowledge, and hence impossible to help the student correct errors in his or her mental model of the baroreceptor reflex. What was needed was a complete picture of the student's solution to the problem at hand (all the predictions for a single column). With this information, it is possible to generate a model of the student on which to base the tutoring that needs to be generated (Michael, Rovick, Evens, Shim, Woo, & Kim, 1992).

7.1.3 The "Column by Column" Protocol

The tutoring protocol that was eventually adopted for CIRCSIM-Tutor proceeds in the following way. The problem of predicting the response of the cardiovascular system to a disturbance (the baroreceptor prediction problem) is solved in three phases: the DR or the Direct Response phase (the effect of the disturbance before any reflex occurs), the RR or the Reflex Response phase (the changes produced by the baroreceptor reflex responding to the change in blood pressure that results from the DR), and the SS or the Steady State phase (the new state of the cardiovascular system; the "sum" of DR and RR). These correspond to the three columns in the Prediction Table (see Chapter 2). The student makes predictions for an entire column and then the tutoring commences.

The only exception to this column by column approach occurs when the student enters the first prediction in the first (DR) column. Here it is essential that the primary variable, the first variable to have its value changed by the disturbance during the DR phase, be correctly identified and correctly predicted. If this is not the case, if the students begin with the wrong variable, or with the wrong prediction for the correct variable, it is impossible for the tutor to make sense of the subsequent prediction errors that the student makes. Are they the result of a faulty mental model of the baroreceptor reflex? Are they the result of a faulty algorithm for solving the problem? Or, are they simply the result of the initial error in predicting the primary variable? To avoid this dilemma, the student is tutored on the primary value until the correct variable is chosen and assigned the correct value.

When Khuwaja (Khuwaja, Rovick, Michael, & Evens, 1994) carried out a thorough analysis of the first 28 tutoring sessions, he discovered three different protocols in use over the period from 1989 to 1992. (The third was the closest to the protocol that we call Protocol 1 here.) Michael and Rovick undertook to use the new Protocol 1 defined for CIRCSIM-Tutor in their human tutoring sessions in November 1993 to generate the most useful examples for the development of our intelligent tutoring system. These sessions also represented a departure because they involved two problems presented to the student, not just one.

When Cho (2000) analyzed the protocols actually used by the tutors in the nine 2-hr sessions that ensued (K30-K38), we were amazed. Although Michael and Rovick started using the column by column protocol (Protocol 1 in Table 7.2) in all of these sessions, they abandoned it, at least temporarily, in five of the nine sessions (Cho, Michael, Rovick, & Evens, 2000). If the student being tutored made many errors and started to respond to tutor questions and hints with signs of confusion, the tutors adopted a different protocol in which they tutored the student one variable at a time (Protocol 2 in Table 7.2). In Protocol 2, they attempt to guide the student through a stepwise solution to demonstrate the importance of following a path of causal relationships to arrive at a complete set of predictions for each column. As a result, Protocol 2 provides more immediate feedback to the student. Use of this protocol basically amounts to an assumption that the student requires the maximum intervention by the tutor to learn.

Cho (2000) observed that the first switch takes place when the student is doing poorly (makes a number of errors or makes predictions suggesting the presence of an important misconception). The tutor switches back at the beginning of the next phase or procedure, if the student begins to do really well. One reason for this amount of protocol switching may have been the fact that the tutors had not previous tutored the two procedures done in this set (increase Rv to 200% of normal and administer a drug that increases Ra). Whatever the reason, it is clear that our tutors make use of alternative protocols to help students solve the problems on which they are working.

At Cho's (2000) suggestion, we added a question about immediate feedback to the questionnaire that the students filled out after using CIRCSIM-Tutor in a trial with the whole class in November 1999 (see Table 18.4). When Cho analyzed the results, he discovered that

TABLE 7.2
Protocol Switching in Sessions K30 to K38 (1 = Predict Column, Then Receive Feedback; 2 = Predict Variable, Then Receive Feedback)

Tutor	*Session*	*DR*	*RR*	*SS*	*DR*	*RR*	*SS*
AAR	K30	1	1	1	1	1	1
AAR	K31	1	2	2	2	1	1
AAR	K32	1	1	1	1	1	1
AAR	K33	1	1	1	1	1	1
AAR	K34	1	2	2	2	1	1
JAM	K35	1	1	2	2	2	2
JAM	K36	2	2	2	2	1	1
JAM	K37	1	1	1	1	1	1
JAM	K38	1	2	2	2	1	1

Note. DR = Direct Response; RR = Reflex Response; SS = Steady State.

the students with lower assessment scores wanted more immediate feedback, but those with higher scores were comfortable with the present protocol (Cho et al., 2000).

7.2 TUTORING STRATEGIES AND TACTICS

Although the choice of a protocol for the tutoring sessions is a relatively global decision, so long as the student is responding well, the choice of strategies and the tactics used to implement them seems to be very dynamic (Elsom-Cook, 1988). The tutors apparently wait to choose a strategy until it is time to use it. The tutors use a variety of strategies to help the student move toward a correct solution to the problem and a more correct mental model of the baroreceptor reflex. Which strategy is used to advance the problem solution, or to correct a diagnosed misconception, is very much dependent on the context. The most frequent strategies are listed in Table 7.3. Some strategies are very simple and straightforward; others require several tactical steps. The most common tactic, hinting, is so very important in tutoring that we devote an entire chapter to it (Chapter 8). We mention some of these tactics as we discuss these strategies and give

TABLE 7.3
Tutoring Strategies Used by Our Expert Tutors

Tutor via causality—focus on the cause
Tutor via causality—focus on the result
Show contradiction
Explore anomaly
Tutor via deeper concepts
Push the student to answer the original question
Tutor via analogy
Tutor via algebra
Tutor via additive logic
Summarize
Ask for an explanation

examples of them. Although these strategies or similar ones are used in tutoring other domains that involve qualitative, causal reasoning, the topics that the tutors talk about are definitely domain dependent. These topics were reviewed briefly in Chapter 2. In this chapter, we look at effective ways of asking students about these topics. A list of typical questions about the major topics (items of domain knowledge) is given in Table 7.4.

Although the tutors use a variety of strategies and tactics, it is important to recognize that there are only two "primitive" actions that the tutor can take: (a) the tutor can *elicit* a response from the student by asking a question or requesting that the student make a prediction, and (b) the tutor can *inform* the student about something (provide hints, acknowledge answers, provide answers, explain, etc.). All of the strategies to be discussed are implemented by using some combination of these actions (see Chapter 9) that address a particular topic. We describe some common strategies here.

7.2.1 Tutor via Causality—Reasoning Backward

The baroreceptor reflex is a mechanism by which the behavior of a number of effectors (tissues or organs) is controlled to determine the value of a set of variables (HR, IS, and TPR). This mechanism con-

TABLE 7.4
Questions About Topics in the Cardiovascular Domain

What are the determinants of X (or what variable determines X)?
What are the consequences if X increases?
What is the nature of the relationship between variables X and Y?
What is the value of X (increase, decrease or no change)?
What is the definition of some variable or phase of the response?
What is the mechanism that controls this variable?
Which parameter(s) is (are) in the table?
What is the equation that relates X and Y?

tains a negative-feedback loop that causes the process to attempt to actively hold the value of one variable, mean arterial pressure (MAP), more or less constant. The baroreceptor reflex can be usefully represented by a set of causal concept maps at varying levels of detail (Figs. 5.1, 5.3, 5.4).

Because one of the major goals of the tutor is to help the student build a correct causal concept map of this process, and learn to use it to solve problems, the tutors pay a great deal of attention to the broad issue of causality. There are typically four steps involved in this backward reasoning strategy. The tutor asks (a) What variables are the determinants of the variable that has been mispredicted? (b) Which variable is the dominant one in this situation? (c) Whether the relationship between the two variables is direct or inverse, and (d) What is the correct prediction is (cf. Example 7.1)? As in the following example, if the student makes an error along the way the tutor stops to correct it and sometimes completes a step himself. As the session proceeds and the student internalizes this prediction algorithm, the student sometimes shortcuts the process by producing the answers to two or more questions in one turn.

Example 7.1 Tutoring Via Causality—Reasoning Backward

K52-tu-17-3: Now, tell me what are the determinants of SV?
{{*Step 1: what are the determinants?*}}

K52-st-18-1:	The determinates of SV are CVP, IS and HR (only if the heart rate is really really high, then there would be not enough time for the pre-fill)
K52-tu-19-1:	All correct.
K52-tu-19-2:	But you left one determinant out.
K52-tu-19-3:	Afterload is an important determinant of SV.
K52-tu-19-4:	Which variable in the table represents afterload?
K52-st-20-1:	MAP?
K52-tu-21-1:	Yes.
K52-tu-21-2:	Good. So 2 important variables that affect SV Did change in the DR response: CVP and MAP.
K52-tu-21-3:	Which do you think will have the more important effect on SV in this case? {{*Step 2: which variable is dominant?*}}
K52-st-22-1:	I was under the impression that CVP would play a more significant role in determining SV.
K52-st-22-2:	Am I correct?
K52-tu-23-1:	Yes.
K52-tu-23-2:	So what would happen to SV in DR? {{*Step 4: what change in the variable occurs?*}}
K52-st-24-1:	Well, the SV would decrease if CVP decreased, but I still don't think it is a direct response to the change in heart rate.
K52-tu-25-1:	If CVP changes, it does influence SV directly (Starling's Law of the Heart) without the intervention of a reflex.
K52-tu-25-2:	Therefore, a change in SV is direct. {{*Step 3: is relationship direct or inverse?*}}

{{*Commentary added to the example to clarify what is happening in the dialogue*}}

7.2.2 Tutor Via Causality—Reasoning Forward

In this strategy, the tutor is again prompting the student to look at causal relationships, but instead of reasoning backward from the variable that has been predicted incorrectly, the tutor invites the student to reason forward. That is, the tutor wants the student to figure out what variable will be affected next, to look at the relationships where the variable in question is the determinant, not the determined variable. Another difference between this strategy and the previous strategy is that the tutor does not typically ask the student about the nature of the relationship until the student makes a mistake. The tutor is giving the student a chance to correct his or her own errors, and, at the same time, collecting more information about the student's mental model. In Example 7.2 the tutor corrects SV and then explores the question of what happens to other variables if SV changes. We have a number of other examples in which the tutor just asks "Next?"—a neat, shorthand way of asking the student a series of questions: what variables are determined by the variable in focus, whether the relationship is direct or inverse, and what the value should be.

Example 7.2: Tutor Uses Causality—Reasoning Forward

K8-tu-61-2:	CC is one of the main determinants of SV.
K8-tu-61-3:	CC has been reflexly decreased in this experiment.
K8-tu-61-4:	What would happen to SV? {{*what is the causal relationship between CC and SV?*}}
K8-st-62-1:	Decrease
K8-tu-63-1:	Yes.
K8-tu-63-2:	So what would that do to CO? {{*what does the change in SV cause to happen?*}}
K8-st-64-1:	D

7.2.3 Show a Contradiction

Student answers or predictions are often inconsistent with the accepted model of the baroreceptor reflex or inconsistent with their own previous answers or predictions. By bringing such a contradiction to the students' attention, as in Example 7.3, the tutor expects that they will be prompted to reexamine their current answers or predictions, applying what they already know to correcting any error that might be present.

Example 7.3: Tutor Shows a Contradiction

K10-tu-39-2:	What other variable is under neural control—primarily
K10-tu-40-1:	CC?

K10-tu-41-1: Yes.
K10-tu-41-2: You predicted that it would go up.
K10-tu-41-3: Still feel that way?
K10-st-42-1: Yes.
K10-tu-43-1: But remember that we're dealing with the period before there can be any neural changes.
K10-tu-43-2: How can CC go up if it's under neural control? {{*Prediction contradicts the definition of DR*}}

7.2.4 Explore an Anomaly

One of the features of the baroreceptor reflex that makes it difficult for students to master is the fact that some of the responses that occur appear to be counterintuitive to the students. For example, in many situations in which the reflex decreases cardiac output (CO), the value of stroke volume (SV), one of the two determinants of CO, actually increases. Calling the student's attention to this seeming "anomaly" (see Example 7.4), or others like it, can be a useful way to prompt the student to think more deeply about the phenomenon.

Example 7.4: Tutor Explores an Apparent Anomaly

K26-tu-76-2: So, co decreases even though SV increases.
K26-tu-76-3: How can you explain this? {{*since CO= HR * SV, how can CO decrease when SV increases*}}

7.2.5 Tutor Via Deeper Concepts

As we pointed out earlier (Section 1.3), physiology can be difficult for students, in part, because it requires them to understand mechanisms operating simultaneously at many different organizational levels (from the cell membrane to the whole organism). It is not uncommon for a student to understand a phenomenon at one particular level but not be able to connect that level to other levels of interest. For example, at the level of the individual muscle cell, our understanding of the mechanism of contraction is quite far advanced. So the student may understand the sliding-filament model of cardiac muscle contraction but not be able to incorporate this understanding into an understanding of the operation of the whole heart (the Frank-Starling mechanism).

One tutoring strategy, therefore, attempts to prompt students to reexamine an answer or prediction by referring them to the mechanism operating at a lower level of organization ("deeper" concepts). Sometimes, as illustrated in Example 7.5, the tutor employs this strategy by following up on an explanation raised by the student:

Example 7.5: Tutor Uses Deeper Concepts

K72-st-40-1:	you would need to work at the cellular level by increasing the concentration of calcium within the heart muscle {{*student invokes a mechanism at a deeper level in the concept maps*}}
K72-tu-41-1:	absolutely right.
K72-tu-41-2:	How is a change in Ca concentration made to occur in the heart? {{*tutor continues at this deeper level*}}
K72-st-42-1:	hmmm ... by not taking up as much Ca concentration into the sarcoplasmic reticulum
K72-tu-43-1:	A plausible guess but ... actually, sympathetic stimulation of the myocardium opens Ca channels and allows more Ca to enter the cell from the extracellular space. {{*tutor offers explanation at deeper level*}}

7.2.6 Push the Student to Return to the Original Question

The tutor often finds it necessary to bring the student back to the original problem being discussed, after they have stopped to elucidate a particular issue. This happens particularly often after a student initiative, as in Example 7.6.

Example 7.6: The Tutor Returns to the Original Question

K3-tu-65-4:	Are there no other neurally controlled variables that would change at the same time?
K3-st-66-1:	Cc?
K3-tu-67-1:	How would it change?

K3-st-68-1:	Parasympathetic reflex would decrease CC.
K3-tu-69-1:	CC is determined by sympathetic input to the myocardium.
K3-tu-69-2:	The parasympathetics have very little effect.
K3-tu-69-3:	How would the sympathetic stimulation of the myocardium be affected by the reflex?
K3-st-70-1:	An increase in HR would cause a decrease in sympathetic response? {{*student is wandering from the question regarding a change in CC*}}
K3-tu-71-1:	OK except for a the point that the increase in HR causes MAP to go up and this is what triggers the reflex.
K3-tu-71-2:	But correct, the sympathetic stimulation of the myocardium decreases.
K3-tu-71-3:	What does this do to CC? {{*tutor returns to the original question*}}
K3-st-72-1:	CC d.

7.2.7 Tutor Via Analogy

Another strategy that the tutors employ to keep the student as active as possible is the use of analogy (Lulis & Evens, 2003; Lulis, Evens, & Michael, 2003). This is a commonly used strategy in teaching almost every subject (Gentner, 1983, 1998; Gentner, Holyoak, & Kokinov, 2001; Goldblum, 2001; Hofstadter, 2001), although it appears to be particularly common in the sciences. The teaching of physics, in particular, emphasizes analogy. Gentner (1998, p. 108) has defined analogies as "partial similarities between different situations that support further inferences." Analogies are used by the tutor to foster further inferences by the student.

Lulis (Lulis, Michael, & Evens, 2004a, 2004b, 2004c) analyzed the analogies in our 75 keyboard tutoring sessions as well as our 6 face-to-face sessions and discovered that analogies are not very common but that those that occur are very effective.

In using analogies, the tutor begins by referring the student to something the student already knows (the base) and then requires the student to draw a parallel between some property or response of that base system and the properties or responses of the topic being tutored (the target). So, for example, the tutor might remind the student that the big veins returning blood to the heart and the right atrium form an elastic chamber like a balloon. The expectation is that the student will be able to use that reminder to infer from his or her knowledge of the properties of elastic structures how pressures in the atrium would change if the volume in it changed. Thus, analogies serve as a kind of hint pointing the student in the direction of a correct answer or prediction without actually providing the answer or prediction as in Examples 7.7 to 7.9. Table 7.5 contains a list of analogies that were used by the tutor in the set of 81 sessions that have been analyzed for analogies, along with the number of times each base was used.

Example 7.7: Use of a Physical Analogy

K14-tu-41-1:	For a compliant structure (like a balloon filled with air) the pressure inside is a function of the compliance of the structure (how "stretchy" it is) and the volume it contains. {{*the base system*}}
K14-tu-41-2:	What parameter in the predictions table relates to the volume that will be present in the central venous compartment? {{*the target system*}}

In one important class of analogies, the base is an earlier prediction made by the student or an earlier problem already solved. The most common analogy that is used by the tutors is "another neural variable" (see Example 7.8ff). This is a reminder that the three variables in the prediction table that are determined by the output of the nervous system (IS, HR, and TPR) have certain common properties. In particular, neural variables do not change during the DR phase of the response (unless, of course, the disturbance itself causes one or more of them to change initially). So, a prediction error about a neural variable in DR is often corrected by the use of this analogy, as in Example 7.8 below. Katz (2003) has also studied this kind of reflective tutoring and found it extremely effective. In Example 7.8, the student understands the analogy and immediately makes the correct inference. There is nothing much to see in the successful cases like this one.

TABLE 7.5

Analogy Bases for Tutor Analogies

(Adapted From Table 2 in Lulis, Evens, & Michael, 2004b)

Base	***Number of Times Seen in the Corpus***
Airplane wing	1
Another algorithm	2
Another neural variable	29
Another procedure	3
Balloon	1
Balloon as a compliant structure	2
Black box	1
Bootstrap	1
Brake and accelerator	1
Compliant structure	3
Dimmer switch	1
Elastic reservoir	1
Flight or fight	1
Gravity	1
Last problem	1
Ohm's law	2
Physician	1
Pump	1
Reflex	2
Sugar or glucose	1
Summation	1
Traffic jam	2

Example 7.8: Example of Human Tutoring by Analogy Working Perfectly

K4-tu-31-2:	What other variable is also neurally controlled?
K4-st-32-1:	Cc
K4-tu-33-1:	Super.

K4-tu-33-2:	So what value do you assign to it?
K4-st-34-1:	Cc 0
K4-tu-35-1:	Great.

But when the student misses the point of the analogy or fails to make the required inference, the tutor most often proceeds to explain the analogy in some detail, as in Example 7.9.

Example 7.9 "Another Neural Variable" Analogy.

K5-tu-35-4:	What other variable is under neural control?
K5-st-36-1:	TPR. {{*the target*}}
K5-tu-37-1:	Right.
K5-tu-37-2:	So how will it be affected in DR?
K5-st-38-1:	TPR I.
K5-tu-39-1:	NO!
K5-tu-39-2:	DR is before there are any neural changes.
K5-tu-39-3:	LIKE CC! {{*the base*}}
K5-st-40-1:	TPR 0.

Sometimes the student shows signs of real confusion and the tutor needs to explain each stage in the structure mapping process as in Example 7.10.

Example 7.10 Example of Extensive Analogy Repair by a Human Tutor

K44-tu-128-1:	Do you know Ohm's Law for electrical circuits?
K44-st-129-1:	V=ir
K44-tu-130-1:	Well, the circulation is exactly analogous.
K44-tu-130-2:	That being the case, in the circulation, what does v represent?
K44-st-131-1:	I'm embarrassed. I can't remember what they mean
K44-tu-132-1:	Well, v is the potential gradient (electrical) and the equivalent hydraulic parameter is the pressure gradient
K44-st-133-1:	I've got the map =pressure part but if you tell me what i and r are I'll extrapolate to the real situation here

K44-tu-134-1: Well, i = current (flow of electrons) and r = resistance to flow.
K44-tu-134-2: Does that help?
K44-st-135-1: Isn't it hr and tpr
K44-tu-136-1: Well, it's true that tpr is the total peripheral RESISTANCE.
K44-tu-136-2: But, how can heart rate (beats/min) be a flow?
K44-st-137-1: I know it didn't make sense.
K44-st-137-2: Its got to have something to do with the fluid obviously or map.
K44-tu-132-2: Does that help to define map = ... ?
K44-tu-138-1: What do we call the amount of blood per minute that leaves the heart?
K44-st-139-1: Co
K44-tu-140-1: Sure! So we have the following relationship: map = co × tpr where co is the cardiac output ml/min) and tpr is the resistance to flow posed by the entire circulatory system.

Human tutors also understand and respond to analogies proposed by the student. Example 7.11 shows an interchange from a face-to-face tutoring session where the student proposes an analogy and the tutor responds with understanding and proposes a better analogy.

Example 7.11: Example of the Tutor Recognizing and Correcting a Student Analogy

F1-st-62-1: If I make an analogy of you try to fill a sink with water and you ...
F1-tu-63-1: Try to fill a balloon with water, since that's what we're dealing with, a distensible object.

7.2.8 Tutor Via Algebra

Two of the most fundamental relationships that are incorporated into the baroreceptor reflex mechanism are commonly expressed as simple algebraic equations:

cardiac output (CO) = stroke volume (SV) × heart rate (HR)

mean arterial pressure (MAP) = cardiac output (CO) × total peripheral resistance (TPR)

Both relationships must hold at all times and under all conditions. Given that these relationships must be true, one can never predict that SV and HR both increase but CO decreases or is unchanged. Neither can one predict that CO and TPR are both unchanged but MAP increases. Both sets of predictions violate their respective equations. The tutors often appeal to these two equations and try to ensure that their students can use them correctly, as in Example 7.12.

Example 7.12: Tutor Via Algebra

K3-tu-21-3:	Look at it again and write an equation for the determinants of CO.
K3-st-22-1:	CO=TPR*HR
K3-tu-23-1:	Still not correct.
K3-tu-23-2:	CO = HR SV.

7.2.9 Tutor Via Additive Logic

In a similar way, in thinking about the changes that are present in the new Steady State (SS phase), a kind of algebra must apply. If a parameter increases in the Direct Response (DR) and increases during the Reflex Response (RR), it cannot be correct to predict that in SS the parameter is decreased or unchanged. In Example 7.13, the tutor points out a bug in the student's use of this logic.

Example 7.13: Tutor Via Additive Logic

K25-tu-158-2:	The reflex will move the value back in the right direction but it can't get it all the way back.
K25-tu-158-3:	So, in ss what will map be?
K25-st-159-1:	Up a bit.
K25-tu-160-1:	Right.

K25-tu-160-2:	And you can start from that point in figuring out the other changes in ss.
K25-tu-160-3:	Note that in ss you can apply some simple logic.
K25-tu-160-4:	If dr is up and rr is up then ss MUST be up, etc. {{*tutor describes how the "additive logic" works*}}
K25-tu-160-5:	Only when dr and rr are different (one up one down) can you not use logic. {{*tutor indicates where this logic doesn't apply*}}
K25-tu-160-6:	In these cases ss almost always follows what happened in dr (since the reflex can't fully correct).

7.2.10 Summarize

The tutors occasionally will summarize, or ask the student to summarize, the predictions that have been made (Example 7.14). Or the tutor will summarize an argument that the tutor and student have been building together (Example 7.15). In either instance, the intention is to provide a new starting point from which to pursue a new topic about which some intervention is required.

Example 7.14: Tutor by Summarizing Predictions

K1-tu-70-2:	So where are we.
K1-tu-70-3:	Would you repeat your predictions for RR so far?
K1-st-71-1:	CC d, SV d, CO d, TPR d, MAP d
K1-tu-72-1:	Only missing one — -RAP.

Example 7.15: Tutor by Summarizing Physiology

K52-ti-45-1:	You got it.
K52-ti-45-2:	In the DR, the CVP fell first and caused SV to fall.
K52-ti-45-3:	IS didn't change at all.
K52-ti-45-4:	In RR, IS is directly under nervous control and changes first.
K52-ti-45-5:	Therefore, it drives SV.
K52-ti-45-6:	A fall in IS caused SV to decrease.

7.2.11 Ask for an Explanation

Tutors quite often ask for an explanation, as in Example 7.16. This strategy is most often used late in a session, because it is a good way to assess how much the student has learned. This strategy tends to be more successful with good students than poor ones. We put it at the end of the list partly because it is relatively infrequent, but also because this particular strategy also gets used quite often on the tactical level to support some other strategy. It is a good way to bring a misconception to light or to finish off the discussion of an anomaly.

Example 7.16: Tutor by Asking for an Explanation

K51-tu-76-1:	Now, you predicted that IS, HR and TPR would decrease.
K51-tu-76-2:	Why do think this happens? {{*tutor asks for an explanation of the student's predictions*}}

7.3 CHOOSING THE TOPIC

At this point, we need to depart from the hierarchy of tutor choices described at the beginning of this chapter (which prescribes that the strategy be chosen first before the topic), because choosing the topic and choosing the strategy often go hand in hand. Sometimes the next topic that the student needs help with is chosen first, sometimes the tutoring strategy, sometimes they are chosen together. Certain topics and certain strategies match very well. The CO-SV anomaly is one that the tutors consider especially important and so it is often addressed at the time these variables are mentioned as part of another strategy. We thought it important to separate these two steps in the tutoring process because the strategies described in Section 7.2 are largely domain independent (e.g., every domain has anomalies and analogies). The topics, on the other hand, are typically items of domain knowledge or previous student inputs, whether a pattern of predictions or an answer to a tutor question, with the possible exception of the algorithms for causal reasoning.

The choice of a strategy and topic to pursue is obviously dependent on the context in which the decision has to be made. There are many factors that make up the context. Where are we in the tutoring process? Are we at the beginning of the DR phase? Are we in the midst of discussing the RR response? Has the student been generally been successful (many correct predictions and right answers to tutor questions) or is the student struggling to successfully solve the problem? Which strategies have worked with this student and which ones have not? How well does the student respond to hints? What is the particular goal at this point in time? How much time is left in the tutoring session? Are there important topics (misconceptions) yet to be covered? In Chapter 9, we analyze a complete tutoring episode from the perspective of the tactics pursued and the basis for the various decisions that were made in that session.

To implement a strategy or one of the tactics that make up a strategy, to engage in a dialogue with the student to surmount some difficulty that the student is encountering in the problem-solving process, requires the tutor to ask questions about or tell the students about domain topics. These topics to be talked about are aspects of knowledge about the domain and the student's responses to questions and predictions. Table 7.4 lists the most common topics that the tutors discuss. To implement a strategy, the tutor pursues some set of topics until the tutor is satisfied that the student now understands the physiology being discussed or that as much has been accomplished as possible, given time limitations.

If the student has incorrectly predicted the change in stroke volume (SV) that will occur, or has answered a question about SV incorrectly, the tutor makes a decision about what strategy to pursue to help the student correct whatever difficulty is present. The tutor implements the chosen strategy by pursuing certain related topics of domain knowledge or the student's responses, either by *eliciting* a response or by *informing* the student about something. Later we describe some of these topics that are pursed in implementing a chosen strategy and give examples.

7.3.1. What Are the Determinants?

If a student has made an incorrect prediction about RAP, it is common for the tutor to use the strategy of tutor causality and to begin reasoning backward with the question, "What are the determinants of RAP?" In other words, the tutor asks the student to look for the cause of this change. In Example 7.17, the tutor asks this question three times (tu-40-1, tu-44-1, and tu-48-2). The baroreceptor mechanism is built from a complex sequence of variables serving as determinants for other variables, and this kind of question is frequently pursued.

Example 7.17: Topic Question: Determinants

K22-tu-40-1:	You are correct, but what parameter DOES produce a change in RAP? {{*i.e., what are the determinants*}}
K22-st-41-1:	End diastolic volume
K22-tu-42-1:	When you talk about EDV what structure in the heart are you referring to?
K22-st-43-1:	Oops the ventricles
K22-tu-44-1:	Right, so what does alter RAP? {{*what are the determinants*}}
K22-st-45-1:	Venous resistance and blood volume
K22-tu-46-1:	You are correct, both of these would alter rap.
K22-tu-46-2:	However, neither of these are in the prediction table.
K22-tu-46-3:	Do you remember a relationship between CO and RAP?
K22-st-47-1:	Inverse proportion
K22-tu-48-1:	Right.
K22-tu-48-2:	So, given what you predicted would happen to CO, what would you predict will happen to RAP? {{*tutor asks how the change in CO would determine the value of RAP*}}

7.3.2 What Is the Result?

When the tutor pursues the previous topic, he is invoking the cause. Here the topic has shifted to the result. An intrinsic feature of the domain is that a change in the value of any variable will cause the value of other variables to change (will have consequences for the other variables). So the tutor may pursue the consequences of a change in

RAP by asking what other variable would change, and perhaps, in what direction, as in Example 7.18.

Example 7.18: Topic Question: Results

K36-tu-170-4:	So, CO inversely determines RAP and you predicted (correctly) that CO would increase.
K36-tu-150-5:	So what happens to RAP? {{*what is the result of that increase in CO?*}}
K36-st-171-1:	RAP decreases
K36-tu-172-1:	And if RAP decreases what will happen to SV? {{*what is the result?*}}

7.3.3 What Is the Relationship?

The causal concept maps are made up of two kinds of relationships, direct and inverse ones. A direct relationship between two variables means that if A increases or decreases, then B, which is determined by A, must increase or decrease. An inverse relationship is one where a change in the determinant A causes an opposite change in the variable being determined. This can get quite complex. For example, there are two quite different relationships between cardiac output (CO) and central venous pressure (CVP). If CVP is caused to increase, then there is a direct relationship that will eventually cause CO to increase (increased CVP causes increased SV which causes increased CO). On the other hand, if CO is made to change, there is an inverse relationship that causes CVP to decrease (increased CO causes decreased CVP). The importance of the nature of the relationship, inverse or direct, between causal related variables, makes this a common topic (see Example 7.19).

Example 7.19: Topic Question: Relationship

K55-tu-71-1:	What's the relationship between CO and CVP?
K55-st-72-1:	Inverse
K55-tu-73-1:	Yes.

7.3.4 What Is the Value?

The last step in tutoring a student about some incorrect prediction is to ask the student to predict the corrected change in value of that parameter. This is usually done in a direct manner, as in Example 7.20.

Example 7.20: Topic Question: Value

K11-tu-67-2:	If the volume of blood in the central veins decreases, what would happen to central venous pressure? {{*how would its value change*}}
K11-st-68-1:	D
K11-tu-69-1:	Yes.

7.3.5 What Is the Definition?

There are a number of situations in which the tutor will begin to deal with an erroneous prediction or incorrect answer by asking the student to define something. If the student has predicted that a neural variable, say Inotropic State (IS), will change in DR, the tutor may begin by asking for a definition of DR or a definition of IS, as seen in Example 7.21. In many cases, this serves as a hint, reminding the students of something they already know but failed to use correctly in solving the problem.

Example 7.21: Topic Question: Definition

K47-tu-56-4:	However, I want to pursue IS with you.
K47-tu-56-5:	Can you tell me what you think that IS means?

7.3.6 By What Mechanism?

The values of the seven variables in the prediction table are determined either by neural inputs to the respective effectors (in the case of IS, HR, and TPR) or by the physical interaction of other variables (CVP, SV, CO, MAP). The tutor may ask the student about the mechanism by which a variable is determined to (a) gauge the student's level of understanding, and (b) provide a possible hint to the student to be used in correcting an error (see Example 7.22).

Example 7.22: Topic Question: Mechanism

K10-tu-29-2:	Let's take a look at some of your predictions.
K10-tu-29-3:	Take the last one first.
K10-tu-29-4:	Can you tell me how TPR is controlled? {{*by what mechanism*}}
K10-st-30-1:	Autonomic nervous system
K10-tu-31-1:	Yes.

7.3.7 What Parameter(s)?

When tutoring the DR phase of the response, the tutors often inquire about which parameters in the prediction are neurally controlled rather than ask about individual members of that class. Or, again in DR, the tutor might ask which parameter represents what is called *preload*. As with many other subjects that are pursued by the tutor, the intent is both to acquire information about the student's understanding and to provide hints. In Example 7.23, the tutor asks the parameter question five times.

Example 7.23: Topic Question: Parameter

K67-tu-29-1:	What are the determinants of SV? {{*what parameter*}}
K67-st-30-1:	End diastolic volume.
K67-tu-31-1:	Yes that's certainly one of them.
K67-tu-31-2:	We also call it preload.
K67-tu-31-3:	Which variable in the table represents a major determinant of EDV? {{*what parameter*}}
K67-st-32-1:	CVP?
K67-tu-33-1:	Absolutely correct.
K67-tu-33-2:	And if CVP went up what effect would that have on SV?
K67-st-34-1:	SV would also go up.
K67-tu-35-1:	Yes.

K67-tu-35-2:	Now let's try to get at the other determinants of SV. {{*what parameter*}}
K67-tu-35-3:	Any ideas yet before I try to help?
K67-st-36-1:	The contractility?
K67-tu-37-1:	Sure.
K67-tu-37-2:	Which variable in the table is contractility? {{*what parameter*}}
K67-st-38-1:	IS.
K67-tu-39-1:	Right again.
K67-tu-39-2:	And it does not change here.
K67-tu-39-3:	How about afterload?
K67-st-40-1:	I do not know how afterload plays into it.
K67-tu-41-1:	Afterload is the pressure against which the ventricle must pump.
K67-tu-41-2:	The higher the afterload, the lower the SV.
K67-tu-41-3:	Which variable in the table represents afterload? {{*what parameter*}}

7.3.8 What Equation?

There are two sets of three parameters that are related to one another by simple equations:

$$\mathbf{CO = SV \times HR}$$

$$\mathbf{MAP = CO \times TPR}$$

Errors in predicting CO or MAP may therefore elicit a request that the student write down the relevant equation, as in Example 7.24.

Example 7.24: Topic Question: Equation

K24-tu-96-1:	Your last statement is absolutely correct ...
K24-tu-96-2:	Reflexes never fully compensate for a disturbance.
K24-tu-96-3:	However, I disturbed by something else that you said.
K24-tu-96-4:	Can you write the equation relating MAP, CO, and TPR?
K24-st-97-1:	MAP=CO × TPR
K24-tu-98-1:	Right.

7.4 NEGATIVE ACKNOWLEDGMENTS: TELLING STUDENTS WHEN THEY ARE WRONG

Learners need feedback about the relative success or failure of their attempt to learn something or do something. They need to know whether they have successfully demonstrated that they understand something. Feedback can be provided in a variety of ways (e.g., answers to problems posted in the back of the book, experiments that are seen to fail because the results do not conform to what the student knows to be the expected outcome). In a face-to-face tutoring session, feedback can be provided by the facial expression, voice quality, and by what the tutor says in response to a student utterance. In a keyboard-to-keyboard tutoring session, the only feedback that is available arrives via the words used by the tutor. We carefully examined how our tutors delivered both negative and positive acknowledgments, in part to understand tutor behavior, and in part to be able to implement effective negative and positive acknowledgments in CIRCSIM-Tutor. In this section, we discuss negative acknowledgments, or correction in tutoring, as Fox (1989) termed it; we discuss positive acknowledgments in Section 7.5.

What should a tutor say when a student's answer to a question is incorrect? In the original design of CIRCSIM-Tutor, the tutor responds with "Right" to every correct answer and "Wrong" to every wrong one. We did not even think about this issue until Susan Chipman came on a site visit just before the 1991 Cognitive Science Conference at the University of Chicago, tried out the very new and shaky system, and commented that real tutors are not likely to tell students that they are wrong.

Chipman's comments were based on the work of Barbara Fox (1989, 1993a) and reflect the findings of the Human Tutoring Project at the University of Colorado. Fox's tutors try hard to avoid giving a directly negative response; they provide additional information when the student seems to be heading into difficulty, they ask leading questions, and they generate a variety of hints.

An examination of our tutoring transcripts, however, reveals that Michael and Rovick seem to be much less reluctant to give an explicit negative response than Fox's tutors, but they only do this about a quarter of the time. They certainly do not say "Wrong" every time. To understand how our tutors generate negative acknowledgments, and as a first step toward making the tutor sound more human, we

(Evens, Spitkovsky, Boyle, Michael, & Rovick, 1993) studied the negative acknowledgments in our tutoring transcripts. We found that our expert tutors use a number of different ways of bringing the student to a realization that a prediction or an answer is wrong. These vary from very direct and explicit to quite indirect and only implied.

7.4.1 Direct Negative Response

Tutor responses of this kind are the most direct and explicit; they contain an unmistakable negative key word, such as "Wrong," "No," "Nope," or "Incorrect." The acknowledgment is often followed by an explanation, as in Example 7.25.

Example 7.25: Direct Negative Acknowledgment

K1-tu-52-2:	What nerves are affected and in what way?
K1-st-53-1:	Sympathetic cholinergic nerves.
K1-tu-54-1:	No.
K1-tu-54-2:	They're not part of the baroceptor reflex.
K1-tu-54-3:	The sympathetic adrenergic vasoconstrictor nerves are.

7.4.2 Indirect Negative Response

Sometimes the tutor flatly contradicts the student but does not use a negative key word. A response like this clearly communicates to the student the fact that the prediction or answer is incorrect. In Example 7.26, the tutor explains that the "parasympathetics have very little effect" and suggests that the student think about the sympathetics instead.

Example 7.26: Indirect Negative Acknowledgment

K3-tu-67-1:	How would it change?
K3-st-68-1:	Parasympathetic reflex would decrease CC.
K3-tu-69-1:	CC is determined by sympathetic input to the myocardium.

K3-tu-69-2:	The parasympathetics have very little effect. {{*the implication is that the student answer was wrong*}}
K3-tu-69-3:	How would the sympathetic stimulation of the myocardium be affected by the reflex?

7.4.3 Challenge the Student's Answer

There are several different ways in which the tutor directly challenges the student's answer as a way of conveying to the student the fact that the prediction or answer was wrong without using any overtly negative language.

A definite challenge without an abrupt change in the course of the conversation can be conveyed by restating the student's answer, often with a question mark, as in Example 7.27.

Example 7.27: Challenge Answer (1)

F5-tu-113-1:	What does cardiac output do to the volume of blood in the central venous compartment?
F5-st-114-1:	It's increasing it.
F5-tu-115-1:	It's increasing it? ... {{*tutor repeats answer but never says it is wrong*}}
F5-tu-115-2:	It seems to me that every time the heart beats, it's pulling a stroke volume of blood out of the central venous compartment.

Here is another way in which the tutor can challenge the student's answer. This kind of response and the ones following it all give the student an opportunity for self-correction with a minimum of embarrassment. The request to "Try again" is the most negative thing about Example 7.28.

Example 7.28: Challenge Answer (2)

K1-tu-46-2:	What change in MAP is triggering this reflex?
K1-st-47-1:	MAP i

K1-tu-48-1:	If the reflex caused TPR to go up, it could not correct the change in MAP. {{*tutor points out a contradiction*}}
K1-tu-48-2:	But that's what reflexes do.
K1-tu-48-3:	Try again.

In Example 7.29, the tutor's question, "Still feel that way?" although intended to be negative, was apparently too gentle and the tutor had to get more explicit to get the negative message across:

Example 7.29: Challenge Answer (3)

K10-tu-41-2:	You predicted that it would go up.
K10-tu-41-3:	Still feel that way? {{*causes student to question answer*}}
K10-st-42-1:	Yes.
K10-tu-43-1:	But remember that we`re dealing with the period before there can be any neural changes.
K10-tu-43-2:	How can CC go up if it's under neural control?

7.4.4 Ambiguous Acknowledgments

We have finally arrived at a category where the student may not be immediately sure whether he or she has made an error. In fact, the tutor uses very much the same language when asking the student to justify an answer. In Example 7.30, the student's prediction for CO is wrong.

Example 7.30: Ambiguous Acknowledgment (1)

K33-tu-122-1:	Now look at your predictions: MAP D, TPR I, CO 0.
K33-tu-122-2:	Is this possible? {{*tutor does not tell the student that answer is right or wrong and tutor has undoubtedly challenged correct answers earlier in session*}}

But in Example 7.31, the student's predictions are actually correct and the student goes on to explain the apparent anomaly successfully.

Example 7.31: Ambiguous Acknowledgment (2)

K25-tu-62-1:	So, in DR HR is up, CO is up, but SV is down.
K25-tu-62-2:	How is this possible? {{*if HR is up more than SV is down this is possible; student has to decide whether predictions were correct*}}

Finally, Example 7.32 displays a case in which the student has made an incorrect prediction for TPR and the tutor leads the student to correct it.

Example 7.32: Ambiguous Acknowledgment (3)

K1-tu-28-1:	We're dealing now with the DR period.
K1-tu-28-2:	That's before there are any neural, reflex changes.
K1-tu-28-3:	The TPR is neurally controlled.
K1-tu-28-4:	So what do you think would happen to it? {{*tutor does not say that prediction is incorrect*}}
K1-st-29-1:	During the DR period it would remain unchanged.
K1-tu-30-1:	Correct.

7.4.5 Signal That an Answer Is Incomplete

There are situations in which a student's answer to a question is correct but incomplete, and the tutor responds in a way that tells the student this without suggesting that the student has made a mistake. The single word "And?" that is used by the tutor in Example 7.33 seems to get this point across very effectively.

Example 7.33: Response to an Incomplete Answer

K33-st-189-1:	The baroreceptor reflex measure MAP and tries to maintain the MAP by altering the other parameters.
K33-tu-190-1:	What parameters does it ordinarily affect?
K33-tu-190-2:	List them.
K33-st-191-1:	HR, TPR

K33-tu-192-1: And? {{*implies that something is missing*}}
K33-st-193-1: CONTRACTILITY

It is clear that these different ways of telling students that something is wrong with their answer fall along some sort of scale of explicitness or severity. Sometimes the tutor delivers negative acknowledgments indirectly or by implication, and other times the negative acknowledgment is frank and explicit. We are continuing to examine the rules that determine which kind of negative acknowledgment should be used at different points in the dialogue generated by CIRCISM-Tutor.

There is clearly a difference in behavior between Michael and Rovick, on the one hand, and the tutors studied by Barbara Fox, on the other. Michael and Rovick give explicit negative acknowledgments at least 25% of the time, whereas Fox's tutors apparently use such negative acknowledgments much more rarely (Fox, 1989, 1993a, 1993b). The social and economic relationships involved are certainly different: Michael and Rovick are professors tutoring their own students and paying them to participate in the experiment. Fox's tutors are graduate students hired by undergraduates to help them succeed in examinations. Michael and Rovick are both men; Fox's tutors are all women. Do these differences matter? We do not know.

The subject matter and the context for the tutoring may play a part. Person, Kreuz, Zwaan, and Graesser (1995) suggested that it is easier for tutors to give explicit negative acknowledgments in solving algebra problems than problems in the design of experiments, because the difference between right and wrong answers is more clearly defined. Physiology would seem to be more like algebra problem solving, or physics, than like experimental design in that there are clear differences between right and wrong answers. However, the differences in context between the tutoring that occurred in the Fox studies (students seeking help to do well on an exam) and the tutoring that we conducted (as part of an experiment where the domain knowledge is known to be important by the students) may contribute to it being harder for the Fox tutors to say "no" as often as our tutors do.

There is another less tangible factor about which we can only speculate. The medical students are generally five to ten years older and involved in learning something they know they need to know to be successful in the course and ultimately to function as physicians; Michael and Rovick feel that it is important for them to learn this material and it is a stated objective of the course. However, Michael and Rovick were tutoring the solution to a single problem. Fox's tutors, on the other hand, had to deal with a much wider array of possible problems brought to them by the students, and may well have felt that improving their students' morale was as important as debugging their problem-solving skills for a more open-ended set of possible problems.

7.5 POSITIVE ACKNOWLEDGMENTS, BANDWIDTH, AND STUDENT AFFECT

7.5.1 Implicit and Explicit Positive Acknowledgments

How does the tutor tell his students that their predictions or answers to questions are correct? In reading the transcripts, it is clear that much of the time the tutor uses quite explicit terms or phases to communicate a positive acknowledgment: "yes," "good," "right," "correct," "OK," "sure," "great," "absolutely," "excellent," and "exactly" all appear often. Table 7.6 contains a list of the positive acknowledgments in the last set of 25 human tutoring sessions from November 1999. We can see from this table that Michael gives fewer explicit positive acknowledgments than Rovick (an average of 10.2 per session vs. 13.0). Michael is more likely to combine positive acknowledgments with one another and with domain material and he also produces more evaluative sentences at the end of the session. Some examples are as follows: (a) "You seem to understand this one quite well," and (b) "I think you did a pretty good job with this problem." This seems to be a feature that we should add to CIRCSIM-Tutor.

Careful examination of the transcripts show that the tutor does not always communicate a positive acknowledgment in this same direct fashion. Brandle (1998) noticed that H. H. Clark's discussion of closure (1996) could explain our observations that the tutor can leave many acknowledgments implicit without confusing the student. In fact, the student can infer that, if the tutor is ready to go on to a new topic, then the student's last contribution to the old topic must be satisfactory. Example 7.34 contains an example of an implicit positive acknowledgment illustrating this phenomenon.

TABLE 7.6
Explicit Positive Acknowledgments in Human Tutoring Sessions K52 to K76 (November 1999)

Acknowledgment	***Joel Michael***	***Allen Rovick***	***Combined***
Yes/Yes again	12	62	74
Good	16	29	45
Right/Right again	23	7	30
Correct/Correct again	34	26	30
OK	15	10	25
Sure	0	15	15
Great	2	7	9
Absolutely	3	4	7
Excellent	0	6	6
Absolutely correct	2	0	5
Exactly	5	3	5
Very good	3	2	5
All correct	0	3	3
Great job	3	0	3
You are correct	3	0	3
You got it	0	2	2
Absolutely right	1	0	1
Basically correct	1	0	1
Good job	1	0	1
Good thinking	1	0	1
Outstanding	0	1	1
True	1	0	1
Total explicit positive acknowledgments	112	182	294
Combined	49	16	65
Embedded in sentences	12	7	18

Example 7.34 Implicit Positive Acknowledgment

K5-tu-23-3:	Now what's affected next?
K5-st-24-1:	Map
K5-tu-25-1:	And how is it affected?
K5-st-26-1:	MAP I.

Here the tutor's decision to move on has indeed communicated an implicit positive acknowledgment. The student often continues this line of reasoning still further and figures that if the tutor does not move on but continues to discuss the same topic, then there is a tacit negative acknowledgment attached. This may be why students often assume that they must be wrong, even when they are perfectly correct, whenever the tutor tries to probe their level of understanding in more detail. Emphatic positive acknowledgments like the one in Example 7.35 most often occur when the student corrects a previous error.

Example 7.35: Emphatic Positive Acknowledgment

K34-tu-60-3:	We're talking about what happens before that.
K34-tu-60-4:	Now what do you say?
K34-st-61-1:	Obviously, heart rate would not change in the immediate response.
K34-tu-62-1:	Absolutely correct. {{*an emphatic positive acknowledgment*}}
K34-tu-62-2:	Are there any other parameters in the table that are controlled by the ANS?

7.5.2 Bandwidth and Positive Acknowledgments

Many of our most emphatic positive acknowledgments come from the first keyboard-to-keyboard tutoring sessions recorded in the fall of 1989, in which Allen Rovick is serving as tutor. In the first session K1, he typed the following positive acknowledgments: "Good," "Excellent," "Super," "Couldn't do better myself," "Correct" (three times), "Again correct," "Right on," "Couldn't be better," "Certainly," "That's right," "Right," "OK."

In face-to-face tutoring, both parties, the tutor and the student being tutored, have available a great many nonlinguistic clues that each party uses in generating its contribution to the dialogue. These include facial expressions such as raised eyebrows, furrowed brows, frowns or smiles, and changes in tone of voice. For the tutor, these clues provide information about the extent to which the student understands the topic currently under discussion or the degree of confusion that is present. For the student, these clues provide feedback about how he or she is doing without the need for, or even before, any verbal feedback is provided.

Both tutors (Michael and Rovick) have had extensive experience with face-to-face tutoring and they initially had some concerns about keyboard-to-keyboard tutoring in which the bandwidth of communications was severely limited by the lack all clues except the linguistic ones. Rovick decided that, in the absence of positive feedback from facial expressions and other nonverbal channels, he needed to express some of his enthusiasm verbally in his positive acknowledgments, and became somewhat more effusive than he had been in face-to-face sessions. This lasted until he discovered from post-session feedback that a number of students felt that his frequent use of superlatives was patronizing! He, of course, immediately stopped. Lepper (Lepper & Chabay, 1985, 1988) reported similar responses in elementary school students and suggested the need for tact in computer tutors, even when expressing empathy.

During the following year, Rovick and Jun Li did a series of experiments with a more conventional Computer-Aided Instruction system that they were building called ABASE (Li, Seu, Evens, Michael, & Rovick, 1992) and discovered that students really appreciated enthusiastic feedback when they had been having serious difficulties with a problem but finally managed to solve it.

7.5.3 Positive Acknowledgments and Student Affect

This episode with positive acknowledgments is just one reflection of Michael and Rovick's deep concern about questions of student affect. We saw in Section 7.1 how they change the protocol when students become confused or discouraged. They argue that protocol change, like other responses to distress signals from students, is a matter of good tutoring—there is no point in tutoring material that students are not prepared to learn. Here, we have room for only a couple of examples of the tutor's concern for student distress, but you can find many more on the accompanying CD-ROM. In Example 7.36, the tutor tells the student that the topic is really "tough" before giving a partial explanation and asking a question. Lepper, Woolverton, Mumme, and Gurtner (1993) labeled this tactic as setting the student up to win.

Example 7.36: The Tutor Sets the Student up to Win

K73-tu-63-1:	It's a really tough, but an important question.
K73-tu-63-2:	IS was directly altered by the reflex—sympathetic nerves innervating the myocardium.
K73-tu-63-3:	So its effect on SV occurred early.

Fox (1993b) described the way that her tutors avoid saying "No" to students. Michael and Rovick give direct negative acknowledgments more than Fox's tutors do, but they still do so only about 25% of the time (Evens, Spitkovsky, Boyle, Michael, & Rovick, 1993). When the student seems especially confused, they try particularly hard to avoid a direct confrontation. In Example 7.37, the tutor describes a correction as a rephrase of the student's answer.

Example 7.37: Tactful Rephrase from the Tutor

K71-tu-17-2:	Central venous pressure is determined by the volume of blood in the central veins.
K71-tu-17-3:	Is there a variable in the table whose change would cause a change in CVBV?
K71-st-18-1:	Stroke volume elevation would lower the cvbv.
K71-tu-19-1:	Not bad, but I would say that changes in CO (sv × hr) will change CVBV and hence change CVP.

In Example 7.38, the tutor provides tactful reassurance when the student expresses distress. We have seen here that expert tutors can and do intervene when students seem distressed. We suspect, however, that the cumulative effect of their constant insistence that the student can solve the problem, their modification of the problem on hand to make sure that the student can indeed solve it, and their determination to ask questions, rather than telling the student the answer, have a greater effect on the emotional state of the student than any kind words. Lepper et al. (1993) mentioned that compliments to students, even elementary school students, require some sophistication or the students will stop believing them. On the other hand, an unshakable conviction that the student can indeed solve the problem will never seem patronizing.

Example 7.38: An Expert Tutor Reassures a Student

K49-tu-56-1:	well, if the volume of blood on the venous side decreases (since it was just pumped to the arterial side) what happens to CVP?
K49-st-57-1:	ok, i feel like a moron.
K49-st-57-2:	it decreases
K49-tu-58-1:	There was nothing moronic about your mistake ...
K49-tu-58-2:	it's probably the most common mistake people make initially when solving this kind of problem.

7.6 STUDENT HEDGING

During the first eight tutoring sessions in 1989, Michael and Rovick often commented on student hedges. In their discussion and debriefing after those eight sessions were completed, they decided to stop doing so because they felt that hedging was not a good clue to student knowledge but instead a matter of student style and self-presentation, so commenting on hedges is a waste of tutor time. They did, however, continue to respond to those few hedges that seemed to indicate real student distress.

Because questions about hedging have been raised at several recent Office of Naval Research Grantees Meetings and at workshops of the Special Interest Group on Discourse and Dialogue, and because we had spent a considerable amount of time agonizing over the problems of parsing hedged input (Glass, 1999), we decided that we should try to study hedging in our human tutoring sessions. We have recently (Bhatt, 2004; Bhatt, Evens, & Argamon, 2004) done a preliminary study of hedges in the 25 most recent expert human tutoring sessions, K52 to K76, carried out in November 1999. We found that all 25 of the students hedged, but in widely varying amounts. One student hedged only twice in an hour; another hedged 22 times. There were 188 hedged turns in the 25 sessions, 151 of which involved hedged answers, whereas 37 were hedged initiatives. The mean number of hedges per session was 6.04 (some turns contained multiple hedges), the variance was 14.92, and the standard deviation was 3.77. Hedged answers to tutor questions are more likely to be wrong than unhedged answers; nevertheless, hedged answers are more likely to be right than wrong. This seems to confirm Michael and Rovick's belief that hedging is not a good clue to student confusion, but we need to count the hedges in the other 50 expert tutoring sessions before we come to any firm conclusions.

Our only previous study of hedging was confined to hedging in student initiatives. In this study, Shah, Evens, Michael, and Rovick (2002) found that women hedged significantly more than men in raising initiatives (almost twice as much). This result motivated us to look for gender effects in Bhatt's (2004) study as well. We found that there was no significant difference between hedging in men and women, when it comes to hedged answers. This appears to be consistent with Robin Lakoff's reports (1975) of hedging by women. She said that hedging is often used to express deference and politeness. It seems reasonable that a woman student may wish to express deference in proposing to take over the control of the conversation, but may feel no need to do so when giving an answer to a question.

7.7 COMPOSITE STRATEGIES FOR REMEDYING MISCONCEPTIONS AND HANDLING OTHER COMPLEX ISSUES

We have already discussed a number of sophisticated tutoring strategies, most of which seem to be applied in a highly spontaneous manner. But there are some especially complex issues for which the expert tutors have constructed rather detailed plans, tested them with students, and shared the successful ones with each other. These plans tend to involve not just one strategy but a series of strategies and tactics. Several of these stored plans are aimed at misconceptions, a central concern for our tutors.

As we mentioned in Chapter 1, one of the major stimuli for launching the CIRCSIM-Tutor project was Michael and Rovick's realization that regardless of how effective CIRCSIM was, it was not very helpful at correcting student misconceptions because it could not diagnose them.

In a typical tutoring dialogue, expert tutors spend a significant amount of the time probing for misconceptions, and, once they are detected, attempting to remedy them. The fundamental method of diagnosing these faulty mental models is to ask probing questions and then recognize particular wrong answers or patterns of prediction errors (see Table 6.1; Michael & Modell, 2003). In Example 7.39, we can see the tutor carrying out the diagnostic process followed by a series of remediation steps. This misconception here is a very common one, a confusion between the Frank-Starling effect and the concept of Cardiac Contractility, also known as IS. The underlying remediation plan is as follows:

1. Elicit or explain the Frank-Starling effect.
2. Elicit or explain the definition of Cardiac Contractility.
3. Elicit or explain how these two concepts are related.

Example 7.39: Diagnose and Remedy Misconceptions

K38-tu-26-4: How will a change in vasc. smooth muscle cause a change in CC?

K38-st-27-1: BY VASOCONSTRICTION, MORE BLOOD WILL BE SENT BACK TO THE HEART, INCR. VENOUS RETURN, INCR.END-DIASTOLIC VOL AND ACCORDING TO STARLING, INCR CONTRACTILITY

K38-tu-28-1: No, you have it slightly (but importantly) wrong. {{*the tutor has asked a question and the student's answer reveals a misconception about cardiac contractility*}}

K38-tu-28-2: What f&s said was that increasing the filling of the ventricles caused them to contract more strongly (dev. a higher pressure or pump a larger vol.), BUT THAT'S NOT WHAT WE M EAN BY CONTRACTILITY.

K38-tu-28-5: Can you give me a definition of contractility?

K38-st-29-1: I THINK SO.

K38-st-29-2:	CONTRACTILITY INVOLVES THE OVERLAP OF ACTIN AND MYOSIN.
K38-st-29-3:	BY INCR EASING CONTRACTILITY, WE INCREASE THE INTERDIGITATION OF THE FILAMENTS?.
K38-tu-30-1:	No.
K38-tu-30-2:	What you have described is the length-tension relationship that characterizes cardiac (and all other) muscle.
K38-tu-30-3:	Contractility refers to the cardiac muscle's ability to generate force at any given degree of overlap of the A and M filaments.
K38-tu-30-4:	So, with the same overlap varying cc causes different outputs from the heart. {{*in an interactive manner the tutor attempts to help the student correct the misconception*}}
K38-tu-30-5:	Does this sound familiar?

The tutors sometimes carry out this process even when the student's predictions are correct, if the topic is one known to be particularly problematic for students, as is this one. It is well known that students can generate correct answers for quite incorrect reasons (Michael & Modell, 2003).

7.8 FOLLOW-UP QUESTIONS

When tutors complete an interaction about some particular topic, it is natural for them to want to determine whether they have been successful in helping the student to "understand" this topic. One common practice, at least among novice tutors (Graesser et al., 1993, 1995; Chi et al., 2001), is to ask the student the following question: Do you understand? The problem with asking this question is that students' assessments of their own understanding are notoriously inaccurate. Chi et al. (2001) acknowledged that this is a problem. Thus, it is not clear how to evaluate whatever answer the student produces.

An examination of our tutoring transcripts reveals that our expert tutors almost never ask this question and ask a related question (Does this help?) only slightly more frequently. In conversations with members of the CIRCSIM-Tutor team, both tutors emphatically stated that such questions are a waste of time because they do not know whether the student's answer is correct.

On the other hand, examining the transcripts of tutoring sessions conducted during our novice tutor experiments, it is obvious that novice tutors ask "do you understand" questions with great frequency (confirming the results reported by Grasesser et al., 1995). An analysis of 14 novice tutor transcripts and a comparison set of 22 transcripts from sessions with our expert tutors show that the novice tutors asked "do you understand" questions an average of 4.4 times per session, whereas the experts asked this kind of question only 0.7 times per session, a difference that is statistically significant at the 0.001 level.

How do our tutors gauge the level of understanding achieved by the students they are tutoring? Presumably the student model that they generate for each student as they are tutoring provides a measure of the students' probable level of understanding (at the level of the immediately concluded exchange, and at a more global level). There is, however, another tactic available to them, which is the open-ended question. An open-ended question is unconstrained, so the content of the student's answer may be difficult to predict, as in Example 7.40.

Example 7.40: Follow-Up Question

K62-tu-51-1:	Great.
K62-tu-51-2:	All correct.
K62-tu-51-3:	Even so.
K62-tu-51-4:	Tell me how you arrived at CVP +? {{*even though the student's prediction was correct, the tutor is probing the student's understanding of this phenomenon*}}
K62-st-52-1:	well, it initially increased due to decreased LV output.
K62-st-52-2:	Its decrease via the RR was due to the increase in SV.
K62-st-52-3:	You know, actually—I know from class that these reflexes aren't capable of returning these elements back to their original levels.
K62-st-52-4:	Also, we've learned that HR tends to have a greater effect than SV—but is that due to greater range or actual greater potency?

K62-st-52-5:	So I used these two thoughts to guess well (I guess) at the right answer—but I'm having a hard time with why CVP can't actually return to it's original level.
K62-tu-53-1:	You've got a lot of things in that statement.

Here the student's predictions were correct, but the tutor nevertheless asks a quite open-ended question seeking to determine whether the student's understanding is as robust as his predictions suggest. The student's answer is long and complex, containing statements about a number of causal relationships. This answer provides the tutor with information about what aspects of the response were misunderstood and require further tutoring.

This use of open-ended questions to gauge student understanding is something that the tutors do often in their role as classroom teachers. These are commonly "how" or "why" questions, although it is clear that students sometimes have a problem correctly interpreting what the tutor is asking. Regardless of how much experience they have acquired, the tutors often have a real problem with understanding what the student is saying in response to an open-ended question. This problem is, of course, harder to solve for an intelligent tutoring system like CIRCSIM-Tutor, and we are still working on tutoring routines that can deal with the answer to such open-ended questions.

7.9 LEXICAL CHOICE

The language used by the tutor in generating the dialogue has to serve two functions: It must, as clearly and understandably as possible, communicate the tutor's message to the student. At the same time, it must serve as a model for how language should be used to talk about the baroreceptor reflex, causal models, and, more generally, cardiovascular physiology (Frawley, 1988; Lemke, 1990).

Students today are increasingly heterogeneous in ethnic and language backgrounds (Michael & Modell, 2003). Goldman and Durán (1988) have shown that college students who are not native speakers of English sometimes fail in reading comprehension tasks because they do not understand the significance of discourse markers in English text. Furthermore, today's students have grown up in a world in which language changes rapidly, potentially creating a gap between the language used by the tutor and that used by the students. As a consequence, there is usually some need for the tutor to find a language style that is understood by the student while remaining correct in its communication of the discipline.

Kumar Ramachandran (1994; Ramachandran & Evens, 1995) has shown that the expert tutors typically pick up and make use of the student's language so long as that language is appropriate for the task. Susan Brennan has identified a similar phenomenon in task-assistance dialogues and named it "lexical entrainment" (Brennan & Clark, 1996). P. Brown and Levinson (1987) classified this behavior as a kind of politeness, and Portele (2002) described it as an element of style. For example, there are a number of different verb pairs that describe parameter change; "go up–down," "increase–decrease," "rise–fall" are the most common ones. The tutor typically continues the discussion using whichever pair the student has most recently used. Ramachandran gave this process the name "user-driven lexical choice" and implemented it for our system with other kinds of lexical choice (which are described in Chapter 16).

7.10 TAKE-HOME MESSAGE

The expert tutors (Michael and Rovick) whose work we studied carry out all the sophisticated kinds of tutoring that Graesser et al. (1995) described. They constantly push the student to be more active. They use a variety of sophisticated pedagogical strategies. They anchor learning in a specific problem. They collaborate with the student in the problem-solving process. They explain deep reasoning—but first, they ask the student to explain. They probe what the student says to assure "convergence toward shared meanings." They do sophisticated diagnosis of errors and then provide feedback and remediation. They are very concerned about the student's affect and motivation and do everything that they can to improve both, not so much by kind words as by insisting that the student can solve the problem and structuring the solution process so that the student can succeed. One significant difference between novice and expert tutors is that the experts constantly ask the student questions, they do not explain, instead they ask the student for explanations. Another difference is that novice tutors frequently ask "Do you understand?" but experts almost never do this.

8

Hinting As a Technique to Keep Students Active

We have already discussed the tutors' determination that the student be kept as active a participant in the problem-solving process as possible. The primary means by which the tutors attempt to accomplish this is the use of hinting. It is not clear whether hinting should be classified as a tactic or a delivery mode—a way of carrying on a dialogue that pushes the student into greater activity—that can be combined with almost any other teaching tactic. In this chapter we define hints, tell how we identified them in the tutoring sessions, describe the different kinds of hints that we found, look at the rules governing when tutors give hints and when they stop hinting, and give some information about numbers of hints.

8.0 WHAT IS A HINT?

Expert tutors spend most of their time pushing their students to take a more active part in the dialogue by posing problems, asking questions, and hinting at the answers. Hints, speech acts designed to help students figure out the answers for themselves, are among the tutors' most important verbal tools.

When we looked for previous work on hinting, we found so little that we felt compelled to produce a definition of our own as a basis for collecting examples. We (Hume, Evens, Rovick, & Michael, 1993) defined a hint as

> a rhetorical device that is intended to either: (1) provide the student with a piece of information that the tutor hopes will stimulate the student's recall of the facts needed to answer a question, or (2) provide a piece of information that can facilitate the student's making an inference that is needed to arrive at an answer to a question or a prediction of system behavior. (p. 564)

We are not the only ones to discover that hints are extremely important in tutoring, especially expert tutoring. McArthur, Stasz, and Zmuidzinas (1990), Merrill and Reiser (1994), and Merrill, Reiser, Ranney, and Trafton (1992) have all commented on tutors' use of hints. Hints are often used in scaffolding; they are an excellent way to provide the student with unobtrusive support during the problem-solving process (Pea, 2004; Reiser, 2004; Reiser et al., 2001). Some other designers of computer teaching systems, whether conventional CAI systems or intelligent tutoring systems, also use hints, at least occasionally. However, the hints used have tended to be rather simple ones. But we believe that we are the first to carry out a systematic study of hinting (see Hume, Michael, Rovick, & Evens, 1996a) and to try to use hinting in a computer tutor in a systematic, principled way to help students master the subject at hand (see Zhou et al., 1999b).

8.1 WHAT LED US TO LOOK FOR HINTS?

From the very beginning of the CIRCSIM-Tutor project, Michael and Rovick told the implementers that hints are of great importance in tutoring. They provided a rule of thumb: hint twice and then give the student the answer. With their help, this was decoded into a series of plans that were rewritten so that the Discourse Planner (Chapters 11 and 16) could execute them. The problem was that the implementers did not fully understand what the expert tutors meant by the word *hint*. They assumed that a hint was an explicit reminder of something the student should know, so they collected some samples from the first group of eight keyboard-to-keyboard sessions in

November 1989, and used them as models for generating hints. The first examples that they noticed, like this one in Example 8.1, involved the key word *remember:*

Example 8.1: Use of "Remember" as a Hint

K3-tu-27-3:	How would TPR change in the DR?
K3-st-28-1:	TPR would decrease
K3-tu-29-1:	Remember two things.
K3-tu-29-2:	1-the DR is the period in which only physical or hemodynamic changes occur.
K3-tu-29-3:	2-TPR is neurally determined.
K3-st-30-1:	TPR would not change.
K3-tu-31-1:	Great.

Turn K3-tu-29 in Example 8.1 is clearly a hint and it prompted a successful prediction from the student. It seemed like an ideal model to copy. In Example 8.2 the tutor needed to provide two hints to get the correct prediction; this is a perfect example of the rule of thumb: hint once, hint again more broadly, and then tell the student the answer—or at least part of it.

Example 8.2: Two Hints Needed to Get Student to Correct Answer

K7-tu-37-4:	Remember the vascular function curve?
K7-st-38-1:	No
K7-tu-39-1:	Let me remind you then.
K7-tu-39-2:	CO represents a process of taking blood from the central blood compartment and putting it into the arterial system.
K7-tu-39-3:	That decreases central blood volume.
K7-tu-39-4:	Now do you remember?
K7-st-40-1:	Sort of
K7-tu-41-1:	Well, that means that central blood volume and therefore central blood pressure is inversely related to CO.
K7-st-42-1:	Ok
K7-tu-43-1:	So how does RAP change when CO I?
K7-st-44-1:	RAP D
K7-tu-45-1:	Yes.

These hints were the examples that Chong Woo and Yuemei Zhang followed when they built the first complete working version of CIRCSIM-Tutor (see Table 11.1). When Michael and Rovick were asked to try out this version, their first comments about the system were mostly polite surprise that it worked at all. However, after trying the system several times, they identified two major problems: (a) The hints were poorly worded and therefore not helpful, and (b) the system repeatedly reused a tutoring strategy that had just failed to teach the same topic to the same student. In retrospect, it is clear that the tutors had failed to communicate effectively (probably because at that point they had not yet reflected deeply enough on how they hinted) and the implementers had not fully understood what the tutors were trying to say.

However, it was immediately clear that to fix the second objection, we needed more tutoring strategies and a way to store the tutoring history in terms of plans that failed or succeeded. Because we still did not really understand the scope of hinting, we assumed that what we needed to improve the hints was more domain knowledge. It is certainly true that hints are knowledge-intensive. Ramzan Ali Khuwaja (Khuwaja, Rovick, Michael, & Evens, 1992) was starting to carry out think-aloud sessions with the experts and he worked on obtaining more information about both tutoring strategies and domain knowledge.

Kurt VanLehn played a major role in our struggle to understand hinting. Gregory Hume and Martha Evens were lucky enough to have a long talk with VanLehn about common research interests at the Cognitive Science Conference in Boulder, CO, that summer (1993). VanLehn was trying to determine what students were doing during tutoring sessions that made their participation so valuable to them. When we told Joel Michael about this, he recalled memories of a very productive conversation with VanLehn at an ONR Grantees Meeting and invited him to interview Rush Medical College students while he was tutoring them. The actual visit took place in November 1993.

While Michael sat in his office and tutored a student in keyboard-to-keyboard fashion, VanLehn sat with the student in another room and asked a series of questions. In response to urging from Khuwaja, Rovick and Michael had already agreed to carry out tutoring sessions lasting 2 hr using two new perturbations. They scheduled sessions lasting 2 hr for the work with VanLehn as well, because it was clear that the interview process would slow down the sessions. Gregory Hume sat next to Joel Michael throughout this process and then asked questions himself during the pauses when the student was talking to VanLehn. Those of us who were listening in on Kurt VanLehn's discussion with the student learned a great deal about student modeling and about interviewing techniques, but Hume's discussion with Michael totally revolutionized our understanding of hints.

Michael described the first student being tutored as a "really live one." When Hume asked what he meant, he explained that the student seemed to respond readily to hints. By contrast, he decided that another student was confused by hints; he then resolved to stop hinting—and indeed stopped for the rest of the session. During these sessions, we discovered that hints were even more important and far more consciously chosen than we had ever realized. We also discovered that we had recognized and labeled as hints only about half of the utterances that the experts thought of as hints. Essentially, we had recognized only those that involved some explicit reminder, whereas the experts also classified as hints exchanges where they gave part of the answer to a question and thus laid the groundwork for the student to figure out the rest of the answer. Hume resolved at that point to make hints the focus of his thesis research (Hume, 1995).

8.2 HOW WE FOUND THEM

Hume and Michael went through the transcript of one of the nine new 2-hr sessions identifying hints together. Then they each went through the other eight sessions and marked the hints in the transcripts. Finally, they got back together and agreed on a list. Next, Hume tried to categorize the hints, and he and Michael met again to agree on the hint categories. In this process, Hume did our first sustained electronic markup (see Chapter 3). He marked the beginning of each hint with the hint category, and then sent it to Michael electronically. It took us some time to realize that this was a revolutionary process. We had hitherto marked up paper transcripts with pens in every color of the rainbow, but never produced an electronic record (cf. Section 3.3).

8.3 WHAT WE FOUND

In his analysis of transcripts, Hume found two major types of hints: Convey Information or CI hints and Point-To or PT hints (Hume,

1995; Hume, Michael, Rovick, & Evens, 1995, 1996a, 1996b). Convey Information (CI) hints actually convey a piece of missing information and thus enable the student to come up with the next step in the process. Some hints prompt students to recall what they know; we call these hints that merely point to the information required to produce the answer Point To (PT) hints. Within these main categories, Hume found a number of different subtypes of hints appropriate to different discourse contexts.

8.3.1 Convey Information or CI Hints

Hints are rhetorical devices intended to help students proceed with the problem-solving process. The major categories are determined by the kind of help that is provided. If the tutor feels that the student needs more information to solve the problem, he uses a CI hint. If the tutor thinks that the student just needs a pointer in the right direction, he uses a PT hint.

Hume et al. (1993) found three general types of CI hints: (a) Type A hints (shown in Example 8.3) consist of a summary followed by a question, (b) Type B hints (shown in Example 8.4) contain an explanation followed by a question, and (c) Type C hints (shown in Example 8.5) are made up of some combination of a summary and an explanation followed by a question. The questions in hints of Type A, B, and C are usually explicit but are sometimes left implicit. The examples that follow contain explicit questions because this is the pattern that we have followed in generating hints in CIRCSIM-Tutor (Zhou, 2000; Zhou et al., 1999b). We did this because, although students who are carrying on a conversation with Rovick or Michael, whether face-to-face or keyboard-to-keyboard, will always respond to a hint in some way, students conversing with a program really need explicit questions.

Example 8.3: Summary Followed by a Question (CI Hint Type A)

K38-tu-144-1: Right, so the first change that occurs in the system is that RAP is decreased.
K38-tu-144-2: What do you w ant to predict next?

Example 8.4: Explanation Followed by a Question (CI Hint Type B)

K33-tu-132-1:	This drug acts on alpha adrenergic receptors.
K33-tu-132-2:	Do you know what cardiovascular structure has receptors?

Example 8.5: Combination of Summary and Explanation Followed by a Question (CI Hint Type C)

K37-tu-56-1:	Let me deal briefly with your second thought.
K37-tu-56-2:	Most of the blood that is displaced to the periphery is in the veins.
K37-tu-56-3:	While it is true that they will get bigger, the veins contribute so little to TPR that we can ignore this effect.
K37-tu-56-4:	So, your first line of thinking is correct—TPR in DR is unchanged.
K37-tu-56-5:	Do you want to now think about HR and CC?

8.3.2 Point-To or PT Hints

Although CI hints are typically expressed in declarative sentences, PT hints come in all flavors: interrogative ("What are the neurally controlled variables?"), declarative ("You have not predicted RAP yet."), or imperative ("Remember the definition of DR.") Hume identified four types appropriate to different discourse contexts: (d) Type D hints (shown in Example 8.6) are questions, (e) Type E hints (shown in Example 8.7) answer a question with a question, (f) Type F hints (shown in Example 8.8) are partial acknowledgments, and (g) Type G hints (shown in Example 8.9) ask the student to consider the implications of an incorrect response. In Example 8.7, the student's "question" is "I think I'm confusing venous return with preload." We realize that this is a declarative sentence, not an interrogative one, but we treat declarative sentences like this one as questions in any circumstances. Sentences in which students say that they are confused or wondering or unsure about something are always treated as questions.

Example 8.6: A Pointed Question (PT Hint Type D)

K35-tu-80-1: Do you remember which of the CV effectors have alpha receptors?

Example 8.7: Answering a Question with a Question (PT Hint Type E)

K34-st-139-1: I think I'm confusing venous return with preload.
K34-tu-140-1: What factor in the table represents preload?

Example 8.8: Partial Acknowledgment (PT Hint Type F)

K30-tu-76-3: Now lets talk about all of the determinants of SV.
K30-tu-76-4: You have one, RAP.
K30-tu-76-5: Are there any others?

Example 8.9: Implications of an Incorrect Answer (PT Hint Type G)

K33-tu-122-1: Now look at your predictions: MAP D, TPR I, CO 0.
K33-tu-122-2: Is this possible?

8.3.3 Hinting and the Causal Concept Map

When the tutor generates a hint, whether it be a CI or PT hint, the goal is always to help the student arrive at a correct prediction or answer to a question *without telling the student the answer*. Learning is enhanced if the student does most of the work. The domain in which the student is solving problems, the baroreceptor reflex, can be represented at three different levels of complexity by causal concept maps (Figs. 5.1, 5.3, and 5.4). A hint, typically, serves to provide the student with a starting point in the domain (some variable in one of the three concept maps) with the expectation that the student will then be able to reason correctly to the requested prediction or answer.

A CI hint tells the student something—"This drug acts on adrenergic receptors"—thereby suggesting where in the causal concept map (Figs. 5.1, 5.3, or 5.4) to start thinking about the requested answer or prediction. A PT hint does not give the student some piece of information, but it does tell the student that he or she knows something that is applicable to answering the question at hand. When either a CI hint or a PT hint directs the student to somewhere in a causal concept map in close proximity to the requested answer or prediction, the hint is an obvious one. A hint that directs the student's attention to a point in the causal concept map that is further away from the answer is obviously a more difficult one for the student to decode and apply.

Table 8.1 records the hints of each type found in sessions 30 to 38. For the first five of these sessions (K30–K34), Rovick was the tutor. Michael was the tutor in the other four (K35–K38).

8.4 DIRECTED LINES OF REASONING

Gregory Sanders read Barbara Fox's (1988a, 1988b, 1990) descriptions of tutors and students collaborating to construct solutions to

TABLE 8.1

Hints in Nine 2-Hr Keyboard-to-Keyboard Sessions (K30–K38)

Session ID	***K30***	***K31***	***K32***	***K33***	***K34***	***K35***	***K36***	***K37***	***K38***	
Tutor	***AAR***	***AAR***	***AAR***	***AAR***	***AAR***	***JAM***	***JAM***	***JAM***	***JAM***	
Hint Category										***Total***
A. Sum + Q (CI)	2	3	3	0	4	1	1	3	1	18
B. Exp + Q (CI)	13	10	7	3	10	7	9	4	6	69
C. Sum + Exp + Q (CI)	0	1	3	2	1	0	1	1	0	9
D. Pointed Q(PT)	12	22	8	4	7	9	10	5	7	84
E. Answer a Q with a Q (PT)	0	0	0	0	1	0	0	1	0	2
F. Partial Ack (PT)	3	0	1	1	6	0	0	0	0	12
G. Implications of Ans (PT)	1	0	0	2	0	1	0	2	1	7
Totals	31	37	22	12	29	18	21	16	15	201

Note. Sum = summary; Q = question; CI = convey information; Exp = explanation; PT = point-to; Ack = acknowledgments; Ans = answer.

difficult problems and also Alison Cawsey's (1992) book, *Explanation and Interaction,* and set out to look for evidence of the same phenomena in our tutoring dialogues. He found that this kind of collaboration is common in our sessions, and indeed, our expert tutors work hard to achieve this kind of interaction.

When the student makes a number of mistakes in predictions for a particular stage, the process of tutoring the variables in error may take some time. If the process is long and involved, a human tutor often decides that a summary of the preceding argument would be helpful. Sometimes the tutor produces this summary himself, especially if he wants to emphasize the causal reasoning involved.

G. Sanders pointed out that many of these summaries are delivered interactively as a series of questions and answers, not as a monologue. One advantage of this approach is that if the student is missing some of the underlying material, the tutor can tutor about it in the middle of the summary. In Example 7.23, the student makes a number of predictions, which leads to a long discussion of SV. The tutor wraps up that discussion and then asks the student to summarize. G. Sanders also noted that tutors use this approach to give explanations and to correct student misconceptions, not just for summaries.

A DLR is typically a series of questions, prompts, and hints, which expert tutors use to deliver explanations and summaries and to remedy misconceptions interactively, to make the student a more active participant in the session. Instead of embarking on a monologue, the expert tutor delivers some extended material as a series of questions and hints. Again, before the tutor begins a DLR, he needs to believe that the student can participate successfully in this interactive process. If the student makes an error somewhere during the DLR, the tutor switches to some other delivery mode—either producing a monologue after all or tutoring the student to correct the error. G. Sanders (1995) was the first to recognize this phenomenon in our tutoring sessions and the first to give it the name Directed Line of Reasoning or DLR. The term DLR is now being widely used in the world of dialogue-based tutoring.

Most DLRs, like single hints, are designed to help the student work through the concept map. They start students thinking somewhere in the concept map and help them reason one step at a time to the requested answer or prediction. The further away the starting point, the more difficult it is for the students to use the assistance being provided to reach the correct answer.

As an example, consider the tutoring plan for the remediation of a common student misconception, the confusion between the Frank-Starling effect and the concept of Cardiac Contractility, also known as IS (see Chapter 2). The underlying three-step plan here was described in Chapter 7: (a) elicit or explain the Frank-Starling effect, (b) elicit or explain the definition of Cardiac Contractility, and (c) elicit or explain how the two are related. If the student is totally confused, the tutor may decide to deliver this whole schema himself or herself, as in Example 8.10, but if he or she believes that the student is able to respond, the tutor chooses to deliver this content interactively, as a DLR, as in Example 8.11.

Example 8.10: Remediation of a Misconception Using a Monologue

K10-tu-45-1:	Well, first you have two phenomena confused.
K10-tu-45-2:	Increased filling (preload) does increase ventricular contractile performance; but this is the cardiac length/tension relationship (Starling's Law), not contractility.
K10-tu-45-3:	Contractility change shifts the position of the Starling curve.
K10-tu-45-4:	CC I would shift it upwards and to the left so that a constant filling would still cause an increase in contractile force.

The interactive DLR version of the content in Example 8.10 appears in Example 8.11.

Example 8.11: Remediation of a Misconception Using a DLR

K49-tu-40-3:	what about your prediction of IS increase?
K49-st-41-1:	I thought that more blood would be entering the heart, leading to increased length-tension, leading to increased contractility.
K49-tu-42-1:	can you define what we mean by "contractility" (which, by the way is synonymous with IS)?
K49-st-43-1:	the number of actin-myosin cross bridges formed?
K49-tu-44-1:	No, you have defined (in some sense) the basis for the length-tension or Starling effect).

K49-tu-44-2:	Contractility is the ability to generate different levels of force WITH THE LENGTH OF THE VENTRICULAR FIBERS CONSTANT.
K49-tu-44-3:	HOW IS THIS BROUGHT ABOUT?
K49-st-45-1:	sympathetic stimulation?
K49-tu-46-1:	Right. This changes the level of intracellular Ca AND THUS CHANGES THE FORCE OF CONTRACTION

Occasionally, the tutor starts with a question or a hint but then produces the explanation himself, if the student fails to provide the answers expected, as in Example 8.12, which also appeared in Chapter 7 (Example 7.39).

Example 8.12: Remediation of a Misconception—DLR/Monologue Transition

K38-tu-28-5:	Can you give me a definition of contractility?
K38-st-29-1:	I THINK SO.
K38-st-29-2:	CONTRACTILITY INVOLVES THE OVERLAP OF ACTIN AND MYOSIN.
K38-st-29-3:	BY INCREASING CONTRACTILITY, WE INCREASE THE INTERDIGITATION OF THE FILAMENTS?
K38-tu-30-1:	No.
K38-tu-30-2:	What you have described is the length-tension relationship that characterizes cardiac (and all other) muscle.
K38-tu-30-3:	Contractility refers to the cardiac muscle's ability to generate force at any given degree of overlap of the A and M filaments.
K38-tu-30-4:	So, with the same overlap varying cc causes different outputs from the heart.

Hume (1995) pointed out that Joel Michael and Allen Rovick use DLRs to increase the activity on the part of the student. He described the expert tutors as pushing the student to be as active as possible in all circumstances. So whenever the student might know the answer, the tutor asks a question. If the student cannot answer, the tutor tries a hint. If the first hint does not succeed, the tutor tries a broader hint. Telling the student the answer is the last resort.

8.5 RULES DETERMINING WHEN TO HINT AND WHEN TO STOP HINTING

8.5.1 When Do Tutors Hint?

Tutors use hints when students make errors. All but 5 of the 295 hints that Hume (1995) studied occur after student errors. The tutor must also believe that the student is likely to be able to respond positively to the hint.

Both Hume's observations and the experts' think-aloud sessions suggest that tutors postpone decisions about hinting until the last minute. That is, they determine what material needs to be covered next, or figure out the next step in the problem-solving process, and then decide whether to hint and what kind of hint is most appropriate. In other words, the content is chosen first and then the delivery mode is selected. The delivery mode chosen is the most active one that the student can handle. If the tutor believes that the student will be able to produce the answer, he asks a question. If the student produces a wrong answer, the tutor tries to stimulate the student to recall the information with a hint. If this first hint is unsuccessful, the tutor will provide some information and hint again. If this second hint is unsuccessful, then the tutor will generally give the answer. The evidence for the occurrence of this pattern appears in the appendix to Hume's dissertation (1995), which presents a list of 157 hint sequences that he found in an analysis of 19 transcripts. As far as we can tell, however, the tutors do not actually count hints. Instead, they stop hinting and give the answer when they no longer expect that the student can make effective use of a hint. This usually occurs after two hints, but it may occur after a particularly confused response to a single hint. At other times, it does not happen until a third hint has been tried and found unsuccessful.

8.5.2 How Do Tutors Decide What Kinds of Hints to Use?

Hume et al. (1996a) concluded that the goal of hinting is to push the student to be as active as possible. Hume (1995) drew an "activity scale" with questions at the most active end, PT hints next, then CI hints, then explanations by the tutor. We believe that the expert tutor chooses the most active alternative that he expects the student to be able to respond to with success. So after a student fails to answer a question, the tutor will try a PT hint if he thinks that the student can handle it, otherwise, the tutor will deliver a CI hint. The tutor will only give the answer if he feels that the student cannot make use of a hint or if he recognizes that the student is becoming frustrated.

There are certain situations where the tutor typically uses a prompt instead of a hint. The most frequent is the "And?" prompt, which is used when the student has given a partially correct answer. This prompt commonly appears when the tutor asks for the determinants of the parameter under consideration and the student answers with one of the determinants when there are two or three. It seems to be a kind of shorthand for "That's correct, now give me more." We classify this tutor input as a prompt and not a hint because it does not really give the student any information except an indication that there is more to the answer than the student has delivered so far. Hume did not include prompts on his activity axis but they seem to fit neatly between questions and PT hints, because they do not require as much from the student as the original question, but they do not give as much help as a PT hint. This is consistent with the fact that the prompt seems more likely to appear when the student is doing fairly well. Otherwise, the tutor will use a more informative hint. The "So?" prompt tells the student that he or she should now be able to draw a conclusion (J. H. Kim, Glass, Freedman, & Evens, 2000).

The choice between the different kinds of PT hints seems to depend on the local dialogue context. If we consider the different alternatives for PT hints, we see immediately that Type E (tutor replies to the student's question with a question) is only feasible when the student asks a question. The partial acknowledgment prompt only works when the student has given an incomplete or partially wrong answer to a previous question. The tutor usually discusses the implications of an incorrect answer (Type G) as the first step of an attempt to tutor by contradiction. For this to work, the student's wrong answer has to lead to fairly obvious immediate consequences. Type D—a question that doubles as a hint—is the most versatile.

The choice between different varieties of CI hints is also constrained by the dialogue context. In a CI hint, the tutor begins by conveying information that provides part of the answer and then the student is expected to supply the rest. The alternatives here are between providing a summary (A), or providing an explanation (B), or providing both (C) (see Table 8.1). Summaries are only appropriate when the tutor and student have already covered a fair amount of material. Sometimes it takes a good deal of ingenuity to split an explanation into a CI hint and a question. There is even more art in choosing the right explanation for this student at this particular moment and in combining an explanation and a summary felicitously, but the dialogue context seems to dictate what kind of solution the tutor expects.

8.5.3 How Do Tutors Decide When to Stop Hinting?

Hume (1995, p. 89) noted that Michael and Rovick cease to hint when the student shows "a lack of background information or poor problem-solving skills." They stop hinting about a particular issue if repeated hints (usually two) are not successful. Hume discovered from personal observation that tutors also stop hinting if the student seems to be seriously confused by hints. When Hume was observing Michael in a keyboard-to-keyboard tutoring session, Michael noticed that the student seemed to be confused by hints, announced that he was going to stop hinting, and stopped hinting completely for the rest of that session.

8.6 HOW CONSISTENTLY DO TUTORS USE HINTS?

Expert tutors use hints all the time unless the student is made uncomfortable by hinting. Table 8.1 shows that the total number of hints in those nine 2-hr sessions was 201. This gives us an average of 11.2 hints per hour. Rovick hinted more often than Michael. Rovick produced a total of 131 hints or an average of 13.1 hints per hour, whereas Michael produced 70 for an average of 8.75 per hour. Does this mean that Rovick is more optimistic about student performance? We don't really know.

There were 96 CI hints (47.8%) and 105 PT hints (52.2%). The distribution of CI and PT hints was almost the same for both. Rovick produced 62 CI hints (47.3%) and 69 PT hints (52.7%), whereas Michael produced 34 CI hints (48.6%) and 36 PT hints (51.4%). Rovick used more implicit questions, Michael more explicit ones. We were happy to see these explicit questions because we feel that the system must be explicit.

8.7 TAKE-HOME MESSAGE

Hinting is a technique for assisting a student to solve a problem or answer a question basically by reminding the student of something already known. Hinting is a far more prevalent tactic than is generally realized and it is far more complex and subtle. It is not just replying to a question with another question. Hints require a great deal of domain content knowledge (more than is needed to solve the problem directly), as tutors search for ways to help students recall what they already know. For experienced tutors with deep expertise in the domain that they are tutoring, hinting becomes a partly unconscious tactic. It is, therefore, one that is difficult for the tutor to define without the kind of knowledge engineering process that we employed. We hope that our work will give rise to a greater emphasis on hinting strategies and their use by human and computer tutors; they are a powerful tool for promoting active learning.

9

A Tutoring Episode Analyzed

9.0 INTRODUCTION

In this chapter, we present the complete transcript for tutoring the Direct Response from one human keyboard-to-keyboard tutoring session (K72, November 14, 1999). We describe what is happening in the tutoring interaction, and how and why the tutor made each decision. The session selected was one in which Joel Michael was the tutor. It is one of the later sessions in our studies and thus exemplifies the approach to tutoring that developed over the duration of the CIRCSIM-Tutor project and which has been embodied in CIRCSIM-Tutor. An earlier transcript would undoubtedly show some significant differences in the approach to tutoring being pursued. The tutors' participation in all phases of the CIRCSIM-Tutor project demonstrably resulted in changes in their approach to tutoring. The session chosen is particularly rich in issues raised by the student's performance, and the tactics and the approaches that the tutor took in response to student errors. But no single tutoring session can ever contain examples of all of the strategies and tactics that have been described in the preceding chapters.

The transcript presented here has been stripped of extraneous turns that do not contain actual tutoring, and the timing information that CDS provides has also been removed for increased readability. As in previous chapters, we have corrected typographical and spelling errors, and expanded abbreviations to make the transcript as understandable as possible. However, neither the grammar nor the content has been changed in any way. Finally, a number has been assigned to each sentence and action (entry of predictions into the table) generated in the session for ease in identifying what parts of the transcript are being discussed. (The machine-generated labels that are added to the transcripts collected by CDS can be hard to read; see Chapter 3.) The native labeled transcript is available on the CD-ROM that accompanies this book (its numbering will differ slightly from that found in this chapter).

The student being tutored was a first-year student at Rush Medical College. The tutoring session occurred at a time when the student had completed all of the lectures, laboratory exercises, and problem--solving sessions, but he had not yet done the scheduled CIRCSIM computer laboratory. The problem to be solved by the student is shown in Table 9.1.

In brief, the patient experiences the failure of an implanted pacemaker that results in an increase in heart rate. The consequence is an increase in blood pressure (MAP). This gives rise to a baroreceptor reflex response that will lower MAP, although not to the predisturbance level. Hence, in the new steady state, MAP is elevated, although less so than initially. The relevant physiology is succinctly described in Chapter 2.

9.1 TUTORING THE PRIMARY VARIABLE (Sentences 1–15)

As described in Chapter 7, the protocol adopted both for tutoring purposes, and for implementation in CIRCSIM-Tutor, requires that

TABLE 9.1
The Problem Being Solved in Session Number K72

Mr. X has an implanted pacemaker which is the sole determinant of his heart rate. A sudden failure of the pacemaker causes his heart rate to increase from 70/min to 120/min.

the student correctly identify and correctly predict the direction of change (increase or decrease) of the primary variable, the variable in the Prediction Table that is directly affected by the described disturbance. The problem being tutored was selected precisely because the connection between the disturbance described (the malfunction of the pacemaker) and the primary variable HR, would seem to be obvious. However, as we see in Example 9.1, for this student, the connection was not so obvious.

Example 9.1: Sentences 1–15 in K72 (Tutoring the Primary Variable)

1	TU:	On the right you can see the prediction table.
2	TU:	The rows are the seven CV variables I will be asking you to predict.
3	TU:	The columns are the three phases of the response, with DR being the DIRECT RESPONSE.
4	TU:	Tell me (type) the name of the first variable in the table to be changed by what happens to the patient.
5	ST:	+ cardiac output
6	TU:	No ...
7	TU:	Please read page 2 again and tell me what changes first.
8	ST:	Well, we have an increase in the firing rate of the pacemaker
9	TU:	So, what variable is changed first?
10	ST:	Heart rate
11	TU	Exactly.
12	TU:	How does it change?
13	ST:	It nearly doubles (+)
14	TU:	Please make that prediction in the table and then press enter.
15	ST:	DR HR = + {{*student enters prediction in table*}}

There are a number of things that can be noted in this tutoring interaction. When the student incorrectly identifies CO as the primary variable, the tutor responds with a quite explicit "No" (sentence 6). This is followed by a PT hint (sentence 7) that directs the student to reread his instruction book. The student does so (sentence 8), and recognizes that the firing rate of the pacemaker has increased. The tutor then prompts him (sentence 9) to connect this to an increase in the patient's HR (which is actually stated quite explicitly in the statement of the problem). The tutor cannot know whether the student initially failed to read the notebook carefully, failed to attend to all of the words on the page, or did not understand the causal connection between the pacemaker malfunction and the change in HR. This leading of the student in a stepwise fashion (sentences 7–12) is a form of DLR. Note also that the student is asked (sentence 14) to make the change in the prediction himself, something that CIRCSIM-Tutor also requires of the student. We think that this, admittedly minimally, active response contributes to the student's learning the lesson being taught.

9.2 COMPLETING THE DIRECT RESPONSE COLUMN (Sentences 16–23)

The student is then asked (sentence 16 in Example 9.2) to fill in the remaining six predictions in the DR column and he starts to do so (line 17). However, he stops after making the first prediction, and the tutor reminds him to complete the column (sentence 18), which he does (lines 19–23).

Example 9.2: Sentences 16–23 (Completing the DR Column)

16	TU:	Now fill in the other DR predictions, doing so in the order that you think the variables will change.
17	ST:	DR CO = +
18	TU:	Please fill out the entire column and then we'll discuss your predictions.
19	ST:	DR IS = 0
20	ST:	DR CVP = 0
21	ST:	DR SV = 0
22	ST:	DR TPR = 0
23	ST:	DR MAP = +

9.3 SEEKING CONFIRMATION (Sentences 24–41)

The DR predictions made by the student contain several patterns of errors, and some correct predictions that suggest possible student misconceptions or other difficulties to the tutor. The student's prediction for the change in CVP is incorrect, although the prediction for CO is correct. This suggests that the student's understanding of the relationship between these two variables is shaky. The prediction for SV is also wrong, possibly reflecting an uncertainty about the determinants of this parameter. Finally, the student has correctly predicted that there will be no change to the neural variables (IS and TPR). The crucial decision for the tutor at this point is where to start. Which of the possible problems that the student might have should be tutored first in trying to confirm that the student suffers from the difficulties that the error patterns suggest?

The tutor begins (see Example 9.3) by pursuing the student's prediction of a particular variable, IS, although the student correctly predicted that it will not change (it is one of the neural variables that, by definition, cannot change in DR). Why did he do this?

The generic student model suggests that students commonly misunderstand the definition of the DR phase of the response, and thus it is common for the tutors to seek confirmation (in spite of correct predictions) that the student being tutored does understand this. Furthermore, the generic student model suggests that of the three neural variables, IS is the one that is most commonly misunderstood. So, the tutor's question about the IS prediction (sentence 24) is an attempt to determine what the student knows or doesn't know about IS; that is, it is aimed at refining the tutor's model of this particular student. What the tutor discovers (first part of sentence 25) is that the student seems to understand that IS is a neurally controlled variable, but at the same time has an incorrect understanding of the concept of IS (second part of sentence 25). It appears that the student confuses the IS of the ventricle with the effects of changing the filling of the ventricle (which is determined by CVP). This too is a common student misconception.

Example 9.3: Sentences 24–41 in Session K72 (Seeking Confirmation)

24	TU:	Why did you predict that IS would not change?
25	ST:	In order for IS to change, we have to stimulate the nerves supplying this area or else increase CVP
26	TU:	You are correct, to change IS you would have to change the neural inputs.

27	TU:	If CO changes (increase) is there another variable in the table that will be changed?
28	ST:	Increasing CO will cause an increase in the pressure within the aorta, thus increasing MAP
29	TU:	Of course, but there is also another variable that will change as a consequence of CO changing.
30	ST:	Would it be the baroreceptors?
31	TU:	No, because by definition the DR is a period of time BEFORE the baroreceptor reflex operates.
32	TU:	If MAP increases (and it does as you predicted) then the volume of blood in the arterial compartment is increased.
33	TU:	Where does that increased volume come from?
34	ST:	It comes from the central venous compartment
35	TU:	And if the central venous blood volume decreases, what else changes?
36	ST:	Central venous pressure.
37	TU:	And in what direction does it change?
38	ST:	It becomes negative
39	TU:	Well, it decreases (and maybe becomes actually negative).
40	TU:	Change your prediction in the table.
41	ST:	DR CVP = -

The tutor begins to deal with the issues that have been uncovered here by confirming that the prediction about IS is correct (sentence 26), and he does this by rewording the student's answer; the tutor is modeling language usage for the student. The tutor then pursues the student's prediction about CVP (which is incorrect) by reminding the student that he had predicted that CO was increased (sentence 27) and asking what consequence of this change might be visible in the Prediction Table. This question is, in fact, a PT hint in that it "points to" something that the student should know but does not convey information about it.

The student's answer to this question (sentence 28) is correct, and the tutor acknowledges this (first two words of sentence 29), but it is not the answer that the tutor expects. So the tutor repeats the hint (remainder of sentence 29), hoping that the student will identify the other variable that will change if CO changes. The student's response to this hint (sentence 30) is wrong, in at least two different ways. First, the tutor had asked for a variable in the Prediction Table and the baroreceptors and their responses do not appear in the Prediction Table. More significantly, a change in CO will not directly and immediately alter baroreceptor function.

One should also note that the student's answer here (sentence 30) is "hedged." That is, he has indicated, through his use of the question mark at the end of the answer, that he is not certain about the correctness of his reply. In this instance, the tutor does not follow up on the hedged answer, but simply informs the student (sentence 31) that his answer is wrong and tells him why (the reason it is wrong is that we are thinking about the DR phase of the response).

The tutor continues his attempt to help the student understand that there is a causal connection between the change in CO that he had (correctly) predicted and a change in the value of CVP. He does this by providing a kind of CI hint (if MAP increases then blood volume in the arterial compartment increases; sentence 32) and asks a series of questions (sentences 33, 35, and 37)—constituting a DLR—to get the student to arrive at a correct prediction for CVP. The student is successful (sentence 38), although the tutor again corrects his language (sentence 39).

9.4 TUTORING THE DIFFERENCE BETWEEN INOTROPIC STATE (IS) AND VENTRICULAR FILLING (Sentences 42–56)

Now that the student has correctly predicted that CVP will decrease (in Example 9.4) as a consequence of the increase in CO, the tutor returns to the issue of the student's understanding of the difference between IS and ventricular filling as determinants of stroke volume, a problem first revealed in sentence 25.

Example 9.4: Sentences 42–56 in Session K72 (Tutoring IS Versus Ventricular Filling)

42	TU:	If CVP decreases what else must change?
43	ST:	I would have to say that IS changes because the volume of blood filling the ventricle is less.

44	TU:	Can you define IS for me?
45	ST:	Inotropic state ... the "contractility" of the heart muscle
46	TU:	Yes, IS is synonymous with contractility.
47	TU:	Let's imagine an experiment.
48	TU:	On two successive beats of the heart I cause filling of the ventricle to be identical.
49	TU:	On the second beat I do something to the heart and the result is that at the same filling I see a bigger output.
50	TU:	What would I have to change to produce that effect on the second beat?
51	ST:	You would need to work at the cellular level by increasing the concentration of calcium within the heart muscle
52	TU:	Absolutely right.
53	TU:	How is a change in Ca concentration made to occur in the heart?
54	ST:	hmmm ... by not taking up as much Ca into the sarcoplasmic reticulum
55	TU:	A plausible guess but ... actually, sympathetic stimulation of the myocardium opens Ca channels and allows more Ca to enter the cell from the extracellular space.
56	TU:	The change in output that occurs at constant filling is a change in IS.

The tutor does this by pursuing the causal relationships visible in the causal concept map in Fig. 2.1. So he asks what else must change if CVP changes (sentence 42). And again the student reveals a fundamental misunderstanding of the difference between IS and ventricular filling (sentence 43). At this point, the tutor tries to determine if the student knows the definition of IS (sentence 44). The student responds (sentence 45) with a synonym for IS, but not an actual definition of the phenomenon for which IS is the label.

At this point, the tutor attempts to clarify the meaning of IS by describing an experiment (sentences 47–49) that results in the heart generating a bigger output and asking how the state of the system could be changed to produce the effect described (sentence 50). The student's response is absolutely correct (sentence 51) and the tutor acknowledges this quite emphatically (sentence 52). Continuing to pursue a causal chain of reasoning, the tutor then asks how the required change in the heart muscle (increasing intracellular concentration of calcium) could be made to occur (sentence 53). The tutor acknowledges that the student's answer (sentence 54) is "a plausible guess" (sentence 55) but is not, in fact, correct. The tutor does this by implication, because he never says that the guess is wrong; instead, he proposes another mechanism (remainder of sentence 55). He ends this interaction with the student about the subject of IS by offering a definition (sentence 56).

9.5 TUTORING THE CHANGE IN STROKE VOLUME (Sentences 57–68)

The tutor starts the piece of dialogue in Example 9.5 by summarizing (sentence 57) the most recent piece of the dialogue and the corrected predictions that resulted: IS does not change and CVP decreases. He then proceeds to help the student correct the prediction for SV by first determining whether the student knows the determinants of SV (sentence 58).

Example 9.5: Sentences 57–68 in Session K72 (Tutoring the Change in SV)

57	TU:	Now, you correctly predicted that IS doesn't change and that CVP would be decreased.
58	TU:	Tell me what determines the value of SV?
59	ST:	Stroke volume is determined by 3 factors: preload, and 2 other factors that I can't remember right now …
60	TU:	Well, we just discuss the next most important one, IS.
61	TU:	The greater the IS the bigger SV.
62	TU:	The third factor is afterload which is equivalent to MAP.
63	TU:	So, with no change in IS and CVP down, what would happen to SV?
64	ST:	Decrease
65	TU:	Right, please change the prediction.
66	ST:	In the dr?
67	TU:	Yes
68	ST:	DR SV = -

The student correctly remembers (sentence 59) that there are three determinants, although he confesses to only being able to remember one of them, preload (which is represented in the Prediction Table by CVP). The tutor first reminds the student (sentences 60–61) that a second determinant is IS, a parameter that they had just discussed, and then says (sentence 62) that the third determinant is afterload (represented by MAP).

Finally, the tutor reminds the student that IS is unchanged and that CVP is decreased (sentence 62) and asks what must happen to SV (sentence 63). The student correctly predicts that it will be decreased (sentence 64), and corrects the prediction in the table (sentence 68).

It is interesting to note that in asking the student to predict the change in SV, the tutor ignores the third determinant that he has just identified, MAP, which is increased. The tutor also appears to assume that the student knows that preload is represented in the Prediction Table by CVP. Finally, he also seems to assume that the student knows that preload has the largest effect (and that afterload, MAP, has a very small and usually negligible effect). The student's correct prediction of the change in SV at least suggests that the tutor's assumption may be correct.

This completes the tutoring about the DR phase of the response. The student now has a completely correct set of predictions for this phase of the response. Most important, he has correctly predicted that the effect of the perturbation is to increase MAP. This change in MAP represents a stimulus to the baroreceptor reflex and will determine the changes that occur in the RR phase of the response.

The tutor now asks the student to read the next page of the booklet in order to start the RR phase tutoring.

9.6 WHAT DID THE TUTOR DO AND HOW DID HE DO IT?

Two things should be obvious in this tutoring excerpt. Almost every question that the tutor asked was intended to help assess the conceptual understanding of the student. That is, the tutor is constantly trying to update his model of the student. At the same time, the tutor is attempting to give the student every opportunity to do the work of solving the problem. This is accomplished by asking questions that the student must answer or by providing hints that serve to advance the student toward the requested answer without telling him more than is necessary. By telling the student as little as possible, the tutor is letting the student solve the problem himself. The tutor is also giving the student an implicit affect-boosting message, that he is convinced that the student is capable of solving the problem himself.

9.7 TAKE-HOME MESSAGE

In generating a one-on-one tutoring session, the tutor has two overarching goals: (a) to make the student do as much of the work of solving the problem as possible, while (b) acquiring as deep an understanding of the student's level of understanding as possible.

Based on the evolving model of the student's understanding, the tutor makes a great many decisions about what topics to tutor, and what tactics are to be used in furthering those two goals. In any real-world situation where tutoring can only go on for a limited amount of time, not every topic can be pursued, not every piece of missing knowledge can be filled in, and not every misconception can be remedied. Tutoring requires making choices about what to do next and how to attempt to accomplish the chosen goal.

10

How Effective Are Human Tutors?

10.0 INTRODUCTION

One-on-one tutoring usually involves attempts to achieve one of three different goals:

- Remediation of some deficiency ("Johnny can't read" or at least not at grade level).
- Acquisition of new knowledge (geography, philosophy, or physics).
- Learning a new skill (reading, golf, bridge, problem solving).

Whatever the goal, an interaction between a teacher, tutor, or coach and a single student (one-on-one tutoring) is thought to be the most efficacious teaching modality. The current education policy of the U.S. government treats tutoring as the panacea for students in failing schools (U.S. Government, Department of Education, 2001). Certainly a great deal of money is spent purchasing the services of tutors or coaches. But, however widespread this support may be, we must ask whether there is actually data to support the claims that are made for one-on-one tutoring.

The interest of the CIRCSIM-Tutor project team has focused on tutoring to help students learn a skill, namely, using already acquired knowledge to solve problems. The fact that in learning to solve problems students probably also acquire new knowledge is important, but, in a sense, incidental. Another by-product of learning to solve problems is the repair of student misconceptions and faulty mental models. But this is really different from tutoring for remediation of a deficit, because the students being tutored have not demonstrated their failure to master the subject matter. We have observed, however, that many medical students have serious difficulty applying their knowledge to solve problems involving negative reflex systems, like the baroreceptor reflex.

The number of studies of one-on-one tutoring, whether by human tutors or machine tutors, is growing. These studies generally address one of three possible questions:

1. Does one-on-one tutoring (whether by human or machine tutors) work? That is, are there measurable learning gains as a consequence of the tutoring experience?
2. Does one-on-one tutoring work better than some other learning modality? For example, is one-on-one tutoring better than whatever happens in the conventional classroom? Is one-on-one tutoring by a human tutor better than one-on-one tutoring by a computer tutor?
3. Finally, there are a host of issues about how tutoring ought to be carried out to be most effective (whether by human or computer tutors) or how human tutors actually carry out one-on-one tutoring without asking whether it works or whether it works better than something else.

In this chapter, we review the literature dealing with these questions as they relate to *human tutors* with emphasis on our own experiments at Rush Medical College. In Chapter 18, we discuss a similar set of issues as they relate to one-on-one tutoring provided by *intelligent tutoring systems* (ITSs).

In looking at the literature on one-on-one tutoring, it is important to ask several critical questions about any study, regardless of which of the three questions outlined above is being addressed:

- What *student population* was studied (elementary or high school students, students at risk or high achievers, undergraduates, or adults in a job training program)?
- What was the *level of expertise* of the tutors (were they peers, older students, content experts, tutoring experts, classroom teachers, paraprofessionals)?
- What was the *goal of the tutoring* (learning a new subject or a new skill, or remediation)?
- What was the *subject matter* or domain of the tutoring (bridge, mathematics, science)?
- In what *context or setting* was the tutoring carried out (as part of an experiment, as a component of a course, or as a part of a job training program)?
- What was the *motivation of the students* participating in the study (successful performance in a school assignment, extra credit in a course, a higher course grade, a higher score on a standard exam, payment as a volunteer participant in an experiment)?
- What was the *motivation of the tutors* being studied (were they school employees worried about job performance ratings, volunteers in an experiment, members of the experimental team)?

As we see, all of these factors can vary considerably across different studies, and thus the breadth of conclusions that can be safely reached about tutoring in general may be fairly narrow.

We also need to ask questions about the nature of the outcomes that are examined. Is the measure of success the "amount learned" (as measured by locally generated examinations, or national, standardized examinations), the "amount learned per unit time on task," "retention" (short-term or long-term), or the number of problems that can be correctly solved? On the other hand, in many studies, particularly of intelligent tutoring systems, the outcome measures may relate to student attitudes (did the students "like" being tutored more or less than learning by some other modality) or teacher attitudes about tutoring.

Thus, as we have seen, there are a multitude of variables that are relevant to assessing the effectiveness of one-on-one tutoring. We are only able to touch on a few of the possible interactions here.

10.1 STUDIES OF HUMAN TUTORS: A BRIEF LITERATURE REVIEW

10.1.1 Does Tutoring Work?

Students do learn from an interaction with human tutors, whether we look at Oxford or Cambridge University students studying modern history with their tutors, a fourth grader learning probability or cartography from a "good tutor," a second grader learning reading from a peer or an older student, or an adult learning to play tennis from the local tennis pro. Learners who are tutored undoubtedly acquire knowledge and learn to use that knowledge to do something. No study that we are aware of claims that learning *does not* occur. Whether such one-on-one tutoring or coaching leads to better learning (more knowledge acquired, deeper understanding achieved, a greater facility at application of knowledge), or even possibly poorer learning, is quite another question (which we address later).

It is of considerable interest that students learn from one-on-one tutoring carried out by tutors ranging from novices (peers, older students, para-professionals) to experts (experienced teachers, trained tutors). We will have more to say about the issue of tutor training and expertise below.

The research on which these claims are based comes from a great variety of sources. The early studies of one-on-one tutoring cited by P. Cohen, Kulik, and Kulik (1982) almost all involved peer tutors (students in the same class) and cross-age tutors (older students) teaching reading or mathematics. Shanahan (1998) has pointed out that most studies of tutoring by American researchers during the period from 1970 to 1985 focused on peer and cross-age tutoring of younger children. He also pointed out that much of this research was conducted with underachieving students or "students at risk." On the other hand, the studies reported by Bloom (1984) involved elementary students learning probability or cartography from teachers. All of the studies cited by P. Cohen et al. (1982) and by Bloom (1984) focused on the question of whether tutoring works (produces learning gains), or in comparing tutoring with other teaching modalities. It must be noted, however, that in more than a few studies, the effect size was very small, even when statistically significant, and the treatments tested were of little or no value in the classroom (Shanahan, 1998). Furthermore, the effects of one-on-one tutoring are far from uniform across different student populations and under different tutoring regimes.

Later studies carried out by a great many investigators (Chi, Siler, & Jeong, 2004; Chi, Siler, Jeong, Yamauchi, & Hausmann, 2001; Fox, 1990, 1993b; Graesser et al., 1995; Merrill, Reiser, Ranney & Trafton, 1992; VanLehn, Siler, Murray, & Baggett, 1998) have also examined the consequences of tutoring carried out by peers (other students) or tutoring by graduate students of students in high school or college. Many of these studies were focused on the issue of how tutoring is carried out, and what features of the tutoring process might contribute to the outcomes observed.

Taken together, the studies that have been carried out support the claim that one-on-one tutoring works, for many different student populations (but not equally well for all students) learning many different subjects (but not equally well for all subjects), regardless of the level of expertise of the tutor.

10.1.2 Does Tutoring Work Better Than Other Methods of Instruction?

So, one-on-one tutoring does work. However, it is widely acknowledged that one-on-one tutoring by expert human tutors is a very expensive teaching modality (which is one reason for the interest in peer tutoring, and the growing interest in computer tutors). Thus, it is essential to know whether one-on-one tutoring works better than some other teaching modality (classroom lectures, mastery learning, technology-based approaches, etc.; see Shanahan, 1998).

Bloom (1984) analyzed results obtained by two of his graduate students and concluded that one-on-one tutoring produced levels of learning that were 2 standard deviations (2 sigma) greater than that achieved by the control groups (conventional classroom instruction and mastery learning). His challenge to the education community was to develop other approaches to learning that would yield as great a gain as one-on-one tutoring.

The meta-analysis conducted by P. Cohen et al. (1982) demonstrated that students experiencing one-on-one tutoring achieve at a higher level than students learning in other ways, although the effect sizes cited were never as large as 2 sigma. Furthermore, the effect sizes were considerably larger for mathematics than for reading, and larger for low ability students than for high ability students. Finally, in many cases, the effect size of tutoring was not sufficiently larger than the effect size of whatever control treatment was used to make tutoring, an "expensive" modality, economically attractive.

Shanahan (1998) has reviewed more recent studies of one-on-one tutoring of reading and concluded the following: "On the basis of this review of the literature, it seems clear that tutoring can be an effective strategy for improving student achievement" (p. 230). But he went on to caution, "While tutoring can help, educators should not expect it to automatically lead to gains in school achievement or student learning ..." (Shanahan, 1998, p. 230).

10.1.3 How Does Tutoring Work?

What accounts for the success of one-on-one tutoring? What are the features of this approach to teaching that make it so powerful?

We can identify several characteristics of one-on-one tutoring that seem to contribute to its success: (a) it encourages dialogue, interaction between the learner and the tutor; (b) it encourages the learner to articulate his or her understanding of the subject; (c) it permits the most complete diagnosis of any problems that the learner is encountering; and (d) it makes possible the most effective scaffolding of the learning process.

The interactive (Socratic) dialogue that occurs in one-on-one tutoring, in and of itself, is a powerful stimulus for learning; both historically longstanding experience and more recent research findings (see, e.g., Aleven, Koedinger, & Popescu, 2003; Rosé, Moore, VanLehn, & Allbritton, 2001) support this assertion. Socratic dialogues also have the benefit of requiring the learners to articulate their understanding of the material. Thus, the learners get practice in using the language of the discipline as well as in using the concepts being learned. Graesser et al. (1993) argued that it is the deep questions raised in Socratic tutoring that make the difference.

Encouraging the learner to use the language of the discipline also contributes to the effectiveness of one-on-one tutoring in another important way. Chi and her colleagues (Chi, de Leeuw, Chiu, & LaVancher, 1994) have demonstrated quite convincingly that one of the characteristics that distinguish good learners is their generation of "self-explanations" as they confront new material or solve problems. Our expert human tutors seem to encourage this behavior as they interact with students attempting to solve problems about blood pressure regulation (see Chapters 6–9). This can be viewed as an alternative approach to student modeling; if the student can correctly explain the prediction just made, it is likely that the student does, in fact, understand the concepts involved.

The learning sciences have come to understand the importance of student misconceptions as serious impediments to learning. A one-on-one interaction with a learner allows the tutor to diagnosis the presence of misconceptions, the first step in helping the student to repair the faulty mental model that underlies their misconceptions (Michael & Modell, 2003). An examination of the tutoring transcripts makes clear the fact that our expert human tutors spend significant time trying to understand the student misconceptions that lead to prediction errors. Only when a diagnosis is available (the student model is updated) can the tutor decide how to help students correct their predictions and repair their misconceptions.

Finally, in a one-on-one interaction, it is possible for the tutor to monitor the progress that the student is making closely, and hence, allows the tutor to offer only as much help as is needed for the student to solve the problem. This process of scaffolding student learning keeps the student continuously challenged without creating a situation in which the student is likely to fail. Such scaffolding is a powerful aid to student learning (Merrill & Reiser, 1994; Pea, 2004; Reiser, 2004; Reiser, Tabak, Sandoval, Smith, Steinmuller, & Leone, 2001).

10.2 OUR STUDIES OF HUMAN TUTORING

10.2.1 The 1993 Experiment

In 1993, we conducted our first experimental study of the effects of one-on-one tutoring by our expert tutors (Michael and Rovick). This experiment was modeled after the experiment in which Rovick and Michael (1992) examined the learning outcomes of using CIRCSIM in a number of different modes (see Section 1.3.5).

Seventeen paid volunteers were recruited for the tutoring experiment from the first-year class at Rush Medical College. Nine students were assigned to a control group (they read a selected text, but received no tutoring) and eight students were assigned to the experimental group (each student underwent one-on-one tutoring). The experiment was scheduled to occur at the end of the cardiovascular block but before students had done CIRCSIM in the regularly scheduled laboratory session.

All students took a two-part pretest. Pretest 1 presented a list of the seven variables found in the CIRCSIM Prediction Table. Students were asked to complete fill-in-the-blank questions about the relationships between variables. There were 12 correct answers and an essentially unlimited number of possible incorrect responses. Pretest 2 presented the students with a paper-and-pencil description of a perturbation of the cardiovascular system and a Prediction Table and asked them to predict the qualitative changes to seven important cardiovascular parameters (see Chapter 2). There were two versions of this problem: Version A described an increase in arterial resistance that could not be altered by the baroreceptor reflex, and Version B described a decrease in arterial resistance that could not be altered by the reflex. Another experiment showed that these two problems are of equivalent difficulty (see Section 18.2). There are 21 predictions to be made. Student predictions were analyzed for the presence of nine possible "bugs" in the students' responses (see Rovick & Michael, 1992).

After completing the pretest, the nine students in the control group then read an edited text segment (taken from Heller & Mohrman, 1981) that described the regulation of mean arterial pressure by the baroreceptor reflex. Careful reading of this text was judged to require about 1 hr. The nine students in the experimental group each underwent 1 hr of one-on-one tutoring while they solved a CIRCSIM problem in which a malfunction of an artificial pacemaker caused heart rate to change (see Chapter 3 for a description of how such tutoring sessions were conducted). Thus, both groups spent about the same amount of time thinking about the mechanisms of the regulation of blood pressure between the pretest and the posttest. Table 10.1 shows sample questions from both parts of the pretest and the posttest. Samples 18.1 and 18.2 show similar problems using a better format, devised later for the system evaluations.

Following the interventions described earlier, each student took a two-part posttest identical in format and content to the pretest. Students who had solved Problem A on the pretest were given Problem B to solve on the posttest and vice versa.

We then asked two questions: (a) Did learning take place in either of the groups, and (b) did more learning occur in the experimental

TABLE 10.1

Sample Questions from Parts 1 and 2 of the Pretest/Posttest Used in the Experiments in 1993 and 1994

Sample Questions From the Pretest and Posttest:

Answer the questions below using the variables listed below. Any variable may be used once, more than once, or not at all. What is being sought in each case is (are) the variable(s) that most immediately and closely satisfies(y) the condition that is described.

CARDIAC OUTPUT (CO)

CENTRAL VENOUS PRESSURE (CVP)

HEART RATE (HR)

INOTROPIC STATE (IS) (= CARDIAC CONTRACTILITY)

MEAN ARTERIAL PRESSURE (MAP)

STROKE VOLUME (SV)

TOTAL PERIPHERAL; RESISTANCE (TPR)

Part 1:

In each blank, enter the abbreviation for ANY AND ALL of the variables that correctly satisfy that statement.

1. An increase in __________ directly and immediately increases cardiac output.
2. An increase in the cardiac output will directly (not via any reflex) cause the value(s) of ___________ to decrease.
3. As a consequence of the baroceptor reflex, an increase in mean arterial pressure will directly result in a decrease in the value(s) of ________________ via the autonomic nervous system.
4. The baroceptor reflex regulates the value(s) of _______________.

Part 2: (which was on a separate page when the students saw it):

Answer each question with a + = increase, – = decrease, 0 = no change. Assume that the stated change is the only one that occurs.

1. If the frequency of firing of the cardiac pacemaker increases then heart rate will ____.

(tutored) group? *T* tests (one tailed, two samples with equal variance) were performed to examine the statistical significance of the differences between pretest and posttest and to determine whether there was a significant difference between the tutored students and the control group.

The results are clear (see Table 10.2 for the individual test scores and Table 10.3 for the summary statistics). For the control group, learning the isolated "facts" about the baroreceptor reflex, their knowledge of the relationships between the parameters (the number of cardiovascular relationships correct), was improved by reading the text (the prepost difference is significant; $p = .005$). Students in the control group also made more correct predictions in the posttest than in the pretest, but this difference was not significant ($p = .401$). The control students showed a significant decrease in the number of bugs ($p = .024$). Note that if a learning gain occurs, the number of bugs should decrease.

On the other hand, the posttest scores, on all three measures of performance, improved significantly following 1 hr of one-on-one tutoring by Michael and Rovick (*p* values for all three measures were less than .001).

We also calculated the gain scores (the difference between the posttest score and the pretest score) for all student participants. A comparison of the gain scores for each of the three measures between the control group and the tutored group shows that there is no significant difference ($p = .162$) between the two groups on the relationship point measure; both reading and being tutored increases the students' knowledge of the individual relationships. However, for both correct predictions and the number of bugs present, the tutored group shows a significantly greater improvement than the control group ($p = .001$ for each measure). Tutoring increases the ability to solve problems (make predictions) with one's knowledge of the relationships, and increases the depth of understanding about the behavior of the baroreceptor reflex.

Examination of the individual scores and the gains in Table 10.2 underlines the importance of the way that the expert tutors diagnose the individual student and tailor the tutoring to the needs of that individual. Every single one of the tutored students showed a gain in prediction scores and in bug scores (remember that a loss of bugs is an improvement in the score), whereas sev-

TABLE 10.2

Effects of Expert Tutoring Compared With Effects of Reading: 1993 Experiment (One-Tailed t Test Assuming Two Samples With Equal Variance)

Group	***Pre rel***	***Pre pt***	***Pre bug***	***Post rel***	***Post pt***	***Post bug***	***Gain Rel***	***Gain Pt***	***Gain Bug***
Control	7	11	3	8	10	3	1	–1 0 2	0
Control	10	16	3	11	16	3	1	0	0
Control	8	9	6	10	11	3	2	–1	–3
Control	7	14	5	8	14	3	1	–5 2 6	–2
Control	9	12	4	11	11	2	2	0	–2
Control	7	17	4	10	12	5	3	0.33	1
Control	6	15	4	10	17	3	4	2.96	–1
Control	8	9	4	8	15	3	0		–1
Control	9	11	4	12	11	4	3		0
Mean	7.89	12.67	4.11	9.78	13.00	3.22	1.89		–0.89
SD	1.27	2.96	0.93	1.48	2.55	0.83	1.27		1.27
Pre–Post									
p values	0.005	0.401	0.024						

Group	***Pre rel***	***Pre pt***	***Pre bug***	***Post rel***	***Post pt***	***Post bug***	***Gain Rel***	***Gain Pt***	***Gain B***
Tutored	5	8	6	9	13	1	4	5	–5
Tutored	7	7	7	10	15	3	3	8	–4
Tutored	9	11	5	10	16	0	1	5	–5
Tutored	6	9	3	10	12	1	4	3	–2
Tutored	7	12	3	10	15	0	3	3	–3
Tutored	7	14	3	9	18	1	2	4	–2
Tutored	7	10	5	9	15	0	2	5	–5
Tutored	8	13	1	9	18	0	1	5	–1
Mean	7.00	10.50	4.13	9.50	15.25	0.75	2.50	4.75	–3.38
SD	1.20	2.45	1.96	0.53	2.12	1.04	1.20	1.58	1.59
Pre–Post	0.00059	0.00006	0.00056						
p values	0.00005	0.00049	0.00036						

TABLE 10.3
Effects of Expert Tutoring Compared With Effects of Reading: 1993 Experiment (One-Tailed t-Test Assuming Two Samples With Equal Variance)

	Pretest Mean (SD)	*Posttest Mean (SD)*	*Gain Score*	*Pre–Post p Value*	*Effect Size*	*Control Versus Tutored Gain Score p Value*
Control (*N* = 9)						
Relationship points[a]	7.89 (1.27)	9.78 (1.48)	1.89	.005	1.49	
Correct predictions[b]	12.67 (2.96)	13.00 (2.55)	0.33	.401	0.11	
Bugs[c]	4.11 (0.93)	3.22 (0.83)	–0.89	.024	–0.70	
Tutored (*N* = 8)						
Relationship points[a]	7.00 (1.20)	9.50 (0.53)	2.50	< .001	2.09	.162
Correct predictions[b]	10.50 (2.45)	15.25 (2.12)	4.75	< .001	3.04	.001
Bugs[c]	4.13 (1.96)	0.75 (1.04)	–3.38	< .001	–2.11	.001

[a]Maximum score = 12. [b]Maximum score = 21. [c]Maximum score = 9.

eral of the individual scores for the control students show no gains in these categories.

In addition, we calculated the effect size (J. Cohen, 1988; Coe, 2000) to determine whether the learning gains were large or small using the following formula:

ES = (Posttest mean–Pretest mean)/standard deviation of the gain scores

The tutors obtained an effect size of 2.09 for the gain on relations, 3.04 for predictions, and –2.11 for the drop in bugs, indicating much better results than obtained by reading, which produced effect sizes of 1.49, 0.11, and –0.70 (see Table 10.3).

We can thus say that in this instance, tutoring worked and it worked better than reading a carefully chosen text on the topic for the same amount of time. Furthermore, tutoring was successful for students who are academic high achievers (first-year medical students) and are highly motivated (they knew they would be tested on the subject matter of the experiment and that this subject matter was highly relevant to their future goal of practicing medicine). It is worth noting that the student population studied in this experiment was quite different from the populations that have been studied in previous studies of the effects of one-on-one tutoring (Shanahan, 1998), who were mostly underachieving students in elementary and middle schools.

It is also interesting to note that in the CIRCSIM experiment (Rovick & Michael, 1992; see also Chapter 1), the control group (which was assigned nothing to do in the interval between the pretest and the posttest) showed no increase in the number of correct predictions and no decrease in the number of "bugs." The groups that used CIRCSIM all showed an increase in correct predictions and a decrease in "bugs." However, the CIRCSIM group that worked in the regularly scheduled computer lab with the instructors (Michael and Rovick) available for interaction showed the biggest decrease in bugs. One-on-one interaction in this setting with students focused on solving a realistic problem seems particularly effective in assisting students to achieve a deeper level of understanding.

10.2.2 The 1999 Experiment

In 1999, we repeated the study of the effectiveness of one-on-one tutoring by experts (Michael and Rovick), this time with a much larger number of students. Fifty-three medical students in their first year at Rush Medical College were recruited to participate in a weekend experiment. Twenty-eight students were randomly assigned to the control group (they read a text, but received no tutoring), and 25 students served in the experimental group (they received one-on-one tutoring).

The protocol was the same as was used in the 1993 experiment described earlier. All students took a pretest, then they either read a text or were tutored, and they all finished by taking a posttest. The pretest and posttest had three parts. Part 1 asked the students to identify all immediate causal relationships between the seven cardiovascular variables involved in the baroreceptor reflex (with a maximum possible score of 24). This test assessed the same knowledge that the 1993 relationship test assessed, although the format was different. Part 2 described another cardiovascular perturbation and asked the students to enter predictions in a prediction table using paper and pencil in which the primary variable (the first variable to change) was identified for the students. The maximum score was 20, because the tutor made sure that the students started out with a correct first prediction. Part 3 was a set of four multiple choice questions (MCQs) describing "clinical" scenarios involving the mechanisms of the baroreceptor reflex, so in this part the maximum score was 4.

In reading the student responses, we identified four categories of bugs: (a) errors related to the two fundamental equations, (b) errors relating CO and CVP, (c) failure to understand that neural variables not directly changed by the disturbance do not change in DR, and (d) confusion about the behavior of neural variables during RR (they must change in the opposite direction from MAP in DR).

The text read by the control students was the same as was used in 1993. The problem tutored was the pacemaker problem, which has been used in most of our studies of one-on-one tutoring (see Chapter 3). For both the control group and the experimental group, the time on task was approximately 1 hr.

Once we had completed the 1999 experiment, we had enough data to analyze the validity of our experimental design. We set out to discover whether the pretest and the posttest questions are, in fact, comparable, by comparing the scores on the individual questions. This process showed that the relation questions and the prediction questions are comparable, but we were saddened to discover that two pairs of questions among the four pairs of multiple choice questions are not comparable. We decided therefore not to report the multiple choice results.

The results obtained in this experiment (shown in Table 10.4) were similar to the results of the 1993 experiment. The control students showed gains in relationship points ($p < .001$) and in the number of correct predictions ($p = .023$), but they showed no significant decrease in the number of categories of bugs present ($p = .072$) and no significant decrease in the total number of bugs present ($p = .072$).

TABLE 10.4

Effects of Expert Tutoring Compared With Effects of Reading: 1999 Experiment (One-Tailed t Test Assuming Two Samples With Equal Variance)

	Pretest Mean (SD)	*Posttest Mean (SD)*	*Gain Score*	*(Post–Pre) p value*	*Control Versus Tutored Gain Score p value*
Control (N = 28)					
Relationship point[a]	14.07 (4.80)	19.89 (4.47)	5.82	< .001	
Correct predictions[b]	12.21 (2.99)	13.75 (2.63)	1.54	.023	
Bug categories[c]	1.93 (0.90)	1.64 (0.95)	–0.29	.072	
Bugs[d]	3.68 (1.59)	3.00 (1.83)	–0.68	.072	
Tutored (N = 25)					
Relationship points[a]	13.0 (4.47)	15.6 (5.53)	2.6	.040	.004
Correct predictions[b]	10.2 (3.09)	13.4 (3.80)	3.2	.002	.052
Bug categories[c]	2.4 (0.93)	1.6 (0.86)	–0.8	.004	.037
Bugs[d]	4.8 (1.62)	3.4 (1.63)	–1.4	.003	.079

[a]Maximum score = 24. [b]Maximum score = 20. [c]Maximum score = 4. [d]Maximum score = 9.

Students who were tutored showed significant improvements in all measures; relationship points increased ($p = .040$), as did correct predictions ($p = .002$). Bug categories decreased ($p = .004$), as did the total number of bugs ($p = .003$).

Thus, both the controls and the tutored students learned the isolated relationships from their treatment. Students who were tutored showed a significantly bigger gain in the number of correct predictions they made, and showed a larger decrease in the number of "bugs" and "bug categories" in their predictions than did the control students. A comparison of the pretest to posttest gains of the control group and the tutored group shows that the students in the *control* group increased their relationship points more than did the *tutored* group ($p = .004$). But *tutored* students showed a larger increase in the number of correct predictions than did *control* students (3.20 vs. 1.54), and that difference approached significance ($p = .052$). The decrease in the number of bugs was not significantly different at the $p = .05$ level. But *tutored* students decreased their number of bug categories more than did the *control* students ($p = .037$). Thus, the results of the two tutoring experiments described here, as well as the results from the CIRCSIM experiment described in Chapter 1, suggest that tutoring has its most important effect on helping students to correct their mental model of the baroreceptor reflex and learning to use that model to correctly predict the behavior of the system. Both of these experiments demonstrate that students who are tutored learn significantly more than students who read a carefully chosen and edited section from a standard textbook.

10.2.3 The First Novice Tutoring Experiment (1994)

Another approach to understanding what it is that expert tutors do to produce bigger learning gains than novice tutors is to examine transcripts of the tutoring sessions conducted by novice tutors and compare them with transcripts of the tutoring sessions carried out by experts. We conducted our first novice tutoring experiment in April 1994 and November 1994. We have pretest and posttest results from nine students in November 1994.

Michael and Rovick recruited four medical students who had done many hours of peer-tutoring for first-year students, but who had never been tutored by Michael or Rovick (although they had themselves taken the medical physiology course from Michael and Rovick as first-year students). All four novice tutors underwent a brief preparatory training program aimed at making them as expert in the CIRCSIM domain as possible. However, care was taken not to expose them to the tutoring behavior of Michael and Rovick. They then received minimal training in the use of our communications system, CDS (see Chapter 3).

These novice tutors then conducted tutoring sessions with first-year medical students, and a total of nine sessions were recorded, lasting from 1 to 2 hr each. (Three novice tutors each tutored two students; the fourth tutored three. The transcripts of these nine sessions appear on the CD-ROM numbered N08–N16.) The problems to be solved and the protocol for the sessions were the same as those used in the tutoring sessions conducted by our expert tutors. The actual novice tutoring sessions were held while Michael and Rovick were away from Rush Medical College attending a conference. One of the Illinois Institute of Technology students working on the project attended each session, however, to make sure that the CDS software was running properly on both computers, to administer the pretest and posttest to the student being tutored, and to prevent the novice tutor and the student from talking to each other. We had hoped to prevent the novice tutor and the student from setting eyes on each other and from finding out each other's identity, sex, and race. This was not entirely successful; the participants did not speak but they did sometimes see each other, because we were using computers in Michael's and Rovick's offices, which are on the same corridor and only a few rooms apart.

We began our study with simple word counts. We compared the novice tutor transcripts with the 47 expert tutor transcripts we had available in 1994 and with a set of transcripts of tutoring conducted by two other experts in physiology. The counts of tutor words per turn appear in Table 10.5.

Reading the novice tutor transcripts immediately revealed that the novice tutors show very little of the questioning and hinting behavior that characterizes the expert tutors. The most frequently used tutoring tactics are very expository in nature and rarely encourage active learning. This difference in approach to tutoring is reflected in the fact that the number of words per turn generated by the novice tutors (17.2) is greater than the number of words per turn generated by the expert tutors (13.2). These counts include all the turns generated during a session, although a substantial fraction of these turns do not actually involve tutoring in the material but are devoted to making sure that the student has read the directions and the procedure description.

It is interesting to note that the tutors' word counts from transcripts of tutoring by two experienced physiologists not connected in any way with the CIRCSIM-Tutor project lie between the word counts for the novice tutors and Michael and Rovick. On the other hand, the number of student words per turn is essentially the same for both the expert tutors and the nonproject expert tutors, suggest-

TABLE 10.5

Differences in Word Counts in Tutoring Transcripts From Expert and Novice Tutors (1994 Novice Tutoring Experiment)

Counts of Tutor Words Per Turn in the Keyboard-to-Keyboard Transcripts			
	Expert Tutors[a]	*Novice Tutors*	*Nonproject Expert Tutors*[b]
Number of transcripts	47	7	9
Number of tutor turns	3044	544	736
Mean words per turn	13.2	17.2	15.7
Median words per turn	7 to 8	5 to 6	11 to 12
Counts of Student Words Per Turn in the Keyboard-to-Keyboard Transcripts			
	Expert Tutors[a]	*Novice Tutors*	*Nonproject Expert Tutors*[b]
Number of transcripts	47	7	9
Number of tutor turns	3036	5464	744
Mean words per turn	5.7	8.5	5.8
Median words per turn	1 to 2	1 to 2	1

[a]Michael and Rovick. [b]Tutoring conducted by two experienced teachers of physiology not connected with the CIRCSIM-Tutor project.

ing similarities in what both groups of experts were attempting to accomplish.

We were also interested in discovering whether expert tutors produce better results than novice tutors. Unfortunately, we can only compare the results from the November 1994 novice sessions with the expert sessions from the previous year (1993). This means that we are comparing results for students from two different classes. Although the lecture and laboratory sessions that these students attended were taught by the same faculty members and involved the same exercises, we cannot be sure that these students had the same experience in class, so the validity of the results (shown in Table 10.6) is not entirely clear. Another problem is that we do not have enough information to determine the bugs from the student pretests and posttests in the novice sessions, so we can only compare the results on the basis of the relation and prediction points.

Examination of Table 10.6 shows some important differences between the results obtained by the novice tutors (shown in the top half of the table) and those obtained by the experts (shown in the bottom half of the table). The students tutored by the novice tutors did improve their relationship scores, but the difference was not significant ($p = .247$). When we turn to the prediction scores, we see that three students improved their scores but three others were apparently really confused by the novice tutors and lost points on the prediction questions, and the scores of two others did not change. As a result, the mean score on the predictions did not improve.

On the other hand, all of the students tutored by the experts improved their prediction scores. In fact, as we saw in Section 10.2, the students tutored by the experts (Michael and Rovick) showed significant gains in all categories. Analysis of these results shows that the learning outcomes obtained by the expert tutors were significantly better than those obtained by the novice tutors. Using one-tailed t tests with equal variance, we obtain $p = .036$ for the relations gains and $p < .001$ for the prediction gains. The effect sizes produced by the expert tutors, 2.09 for relations and 3.04 for predictions, were also much larger than the 0.21 and –0.13 produced by the novice tutors.

10.2.4 The Second Novice Tutoring Experiment (1996)

In 1996, we again studied one-on-one tutoring carried out by novices (Glass, Kim, Evens, Michael, & Rovick, 1999). Four 2nd-year medical students were recruited to serve as novice tutors. All had had some prior experience as tutors (either as peer tutors at Rush Medical College or as tutors prior to attending medical school). The resulting sessions appear on the CD-ROM as N17 to N31. The DR tutoring in N28 was lost due to a CDS failure, so most of the counts shown later are based on the other 14 novice sessions and on expert sessions K10 to K27 and K47, K48, K49, and K51, which all used the pacemaker procedure.

We were interested in answering the question: Do novice tutors behave differently than expert tutors, that is, do they tutor differently? To answer this question, we looked at the way in which the tu-

TABLE 10.6

Comparison of Nine Students Tutored by Novice Tutors in November 1994 With Eight Students Tutored by Expert Tutors in April 1993. (Note: t Tests on the Gain Scores Give $p = .036$ for the Relation Gains and $p < .001$ for the Predictions)

Group	***Pre rel***	***Pre pt***	***Pre bug***	***Post rel***	***Post pt***	***Post bug***	***Gain Rel***	***Gain Pt***	***Gain Bug***
Novice	7	8		4	10		–3	2	
Novice	5	11		3	7		–2 1 5	–4 0 0	
Novice	6	11		7	11		0 4 0	0	
Novice	2	12		7	12		–1 1	–1	
Novice	6	10		6	10		0.56	–1 1 1	
Novice	2	11		6	10		2.60	–0.22	
Novice	6	12		6	11			1.72	
Novice	6	11		5	12				
Novice	3	10		4	11				
Mean	4.78	10.67		5.33	10.44				
SD	1.92	1.22		1.41	1.51				
Pre–Post									
p values	0.247	0.368							
Effect size							0.21	–0.13	

Group	***Pre rel***	***Pre pt***	***Pre bug***	***Post rel***	***Post pt***	***Post bug***	***Gain Rel***	***Gain Pt***	***Gain Bug***
Expert	5	8	6	9	13	1	4	5	–5
Expert	7	7	7	10	15	3	3	8	–4
Expert	9	11	5	10	16	0	1	5	–5
Expert	6	9	3	10	12	1	4	3	–2
Expert	7	12	3	10	15	0	3	3	–3
Expert	7	14	3	9	18	1	2	4	–2
Expert	7	10	5	9	15	0	2	5	–5
Expert	8	13	1	9	18	0	1	5	–1
Mean	7.00	10.50	4.13	9.50	5.25	0.75	2.50	4.75	–3.38
SD	1.20	2.45	1.96	0.53	2.12	1.04	1.20	1.58	1.59
Pre–Post									
p values	0.00005	0.0005	0.0004						
Effect size							2.09	3.04	–2.11

tors, novice and expert, interacted with students about their predictions for two different variables, central venous pressure (CVP) and stroke volume (SV). As in our previous study of novice tutors, there were significant differences in the behavior of novice and expert tutors. As part of our analysis of these differences, we identified five "primitive dialogue acts" (four by the tutor and one by the student) and counted their occurrences in novice and expert tutor transcripts; these features are described in Table 10.7 and the counts can be seen in Tables 10.8 and 10.9.s

TABLE 10.7

Primitive Dialogue Acts Found in Transcripts From the 1996 Novice Tutor Experiment

Primitive Dialogue Act	*Description*
t-elicit	Tutor elicits information from student
t-inform	Tutor informs or asserts something
t-ack	Tutor acknowledges student answer
s-ans	Student answers
t-asks-confirmation	Tutor asks "do you understand?"

TABLE 10.8

Tutoring Counts for Central Venous Pressure

(1996 Novice Tutor Experiment; Adapted From Glass, Kim, Evens, Michael, & Rovick, 1999, Table 4, p. 46; Used by Permission of AAAI Press)

	Novice		***Expert***	
	n	***n/segment***	**n**	***n/segment***
Segments	7		5	
Turns	24	3.4	35	7.0
Elicits	12	1.7	26	5.2
Informs	40	5.7	23	4.6
Acknowledgments	12	1.7	17	3.4
Ask-confirmation	6	0.9	2	0.4
Total primitive acts	70	10.0	68	13.6
Concepts	39	5.6	31	6.2

TABLE 10.9

Tutoring Counts for Stroke Volume

(1996 Novice Tutor Experiment; Adapted From Glass, Kim, Evens, Michael, & Rovick, 1999, Table 2, p. 45; Used by Permission of AAAI Press)

	Novice		*Expert*	
	n	n/*segment*	n	n/*segment*
Segments	5		6	
Turns	26	5.2	26	4.3
Elicits	13	2.6	17	2.8
Informs	52	10.4	18	3.0
Acknowledgments	13	2.6	15	2.5
Ask-confirmation	7	1.4	0	0.0
Total primitive acts	85	11.2	50	8.3
Concepts	56	10.4	30	5.0

To narrow our search, we looked at episodes ("segments") involving the tutoring about errors in predicting two different cardiovascular variables, CVP (see Table 10.8) and SV (see Table 10.9). Table 10.10 summarizes results from all three tables.

Two differences are quite striking. Novice tutors spend a lot of time during a session telling students things ("informs") and much less time asking the students questions ("elicits"). Expert tutors, on the other hand, spend proportionately more time asking questions and less time telling students things. These differences are statistically significant (Glass et al., 1999). This difference is certainly consistent with the expert tutors' insistence that the students do as much of the work of solving the problem as possible (see Chapters 6, 7, and 8).

Another interesting difference is that the novice tutors frequently ask the students if they understand the phenomena just discussed (see "Ask-confirmation" in Tables 10.8 and 10.9), whereas the expert tutors almost never do so. The expert tutors (Michael and Rovick) have repeatedly voiced the opinion that asking "Do you understand?" and similar questions is a waste of time; they prefer to ask substantive questions that allow them to gauge the students' depth of understanding for themselves. Graesser et al. (1995) offered em-

TABLE 10.10
A Comparison of the Proportion of "Elicit" and "Inform" Acts in Novice and Expert Tutoring of Stroke Volume and Central Venous Pressure
(Data From Glass, Kim, Evens, Michael, & Rovick, 1999)

	Novice Tutors	*Expert Tutors*
Tutoring stroke volume		
Elicit	13	17
Inform	52	18
Elicit/(elicit + inform)	0.20	0.49
Tutoring central venous pressure		
Elicit	12	26
Inform	40	23
Elicit/(elicit + inform)	0.23	0.53
Combined stroke volume and central venous pressure tutoring		
Elicit	25	43
Inform	92	35
Elicit/(elicit + inform)	0.21	0.51

pirical evidence that most students do not know whether or not they understand.

There are several other marked differences. The novice tutors introduce extraneous concepts into tutoring segments. A count of the number of concepts introduced by the novice tutors versus the expert tutors shows that the novice tutors consistently use more concepts per segment. Even with this small amount of data, this difference is significant in the segments where SV is tutored although not in the segments where CVP is tutored (Glass et al., 1999).

We see an even more marked difference in the use of the term *primary variable* (the first variable in the Prediction Table to change in the DR stage). The experts use this term to each other and to the developers to explain what happens in the tutoring session; they do not use it to describe the underlying physiology. It is not a concept that the students need to learn. In the 22 sessions examined here, they never use it with students. The novice tutors use it with their students in 12 of the 14 novice tutoring sessions. This difference is significant at the .001 level using Fisher's Exact Test.

We have identified some clear differences in the behavior of novice and expert tutors, but we have not been able to determine what impact particular differences have on student learning. In Chapter 18, we discuss some of the problems associated with this kind of research.

10.3 WHAT ACCOUNTS FOR THE OBSERVED DIFFERENCES IN TUTOR BEHAVIOR?

There are now many descriptions of one-on-one tutoring sessions (Chi et al. 2001; Fox, 1990, 1993; Graesser, 1993a, 1993b; Graesser & Person, 1994; Graesser et al., 1995; Lepper, Woolverton, Mumme, & Gurtner, 1993; Littman, Pinto, & Soloway, 1991; McArthur, Stasz, & Zmuidzinas, 1990; Merrill et al., 1992; Ohlsson, 1987; VanLehn et al., 1998) focused on students learning subjects such as physics, programming, algebra, experimental design, or physiology. On a superficial reading of these descriptions, it is easier to see the differences in tutor behavior than it is to see the similarities. These differences are, of course, very real. We then must again ask, does the tutoring being described "work" and does it "work" better than something else? To the extent that the answer to both questions is "yes, one-on-one tutoring, regardless of how it is done, works," we need to ask what is common to all of the seemingly different tutoring being examined.

We have argued that the commonalities lie in the use of natural language dialogue to establish an environment in which the student is kept as active as possible while being guided to successful completion of a problem-solving task. If tutoring, whether conducted by novice or experts, works, it is because the process incorporates the features just described.

The sources of the differences in tutoring behavior are many and varied, but understanding them can contribute to our understanding of how tutoring works. We believe that the differences arise from several factors:

- The level of expertise of the tutors (peers vs. cross-age tutors vs. content experts).

- The domain of subject matter being tutored (reading vs. algebra vs. physics or physiology).
- The nature of the task being tutored (learning to read vs. acquiring new knowledge vs. learning to solve problems).
- The context in which tutoring is occurring (a school setting vs. an experiment).

Much more needs to learned about how to do one-on-one tutoring most effectively, whether the tutoring is done by human tutors in the classroom or by intelligent tutoring systems.

10.4 TAKE-HOME MESSAGE

One-on-one tutoring works (students do learn from their interaction with a tutor) and in many situations it works better than other more "conventional" educational treatments (students learn more). Our experiments have shown that even students as intelligent and motivated as first-year medical students learn significantly more from one-on-one tutoring than from reading. Their abilities to solve problems improve most of all. The measurable consequences of one-on-one tutoring clearly depend on a multitude of factors, however, including the characteristics of the students being tutored, the subject matter being learned, and the expertise of the tutors. Furthermore, the complexities of the usual educational environment make it difficult to do experiments to definitively demonstrate the benefits of one-on-one tutoring. Novice tutors behave differently than expert tutors (the characteristics of their interactions with the student are different). Our experiments suggest that novice tutors obtain less substantial learning gains, but more studies are needed to demonstrate this conclusively.

PART III: Building CIRCSIM-Tutor: An Intelligent Tutoring System With Natural Language Capabilities

Gordon McCalla, the keynote speaker at the Intelligent Tutoring System Conference in Montreal in 2000 (ITS 2000), set out to predict the future of ITS in the first 10 years of the new millennium. One of the predictions was that after 10 years there would still be no natural language tutoring systems.

The CIRCSIM-Tutor project has already proven him wrong. The CIRCSIM-Tutor system carries on a tutorial dialogue in natural language with the student. Although it is limited to the domain of cardiovascular physiology and although it does not always understand the student, it manages to communicate effectively and teach students to solve problems in cardiovascular physiology.

As we show, every step of the design process was based on the analysis of human tutoring sessions described in Part II. Thus, the system is designed to implement Michael and Rovick's ideas about tutoring, and it is based on their belief that students learn best when they have to put their ideas into words at every step. The system is designed to prod students into solving the problem and constructing explanations for themselves. The focus is on asking questions and providing hints, rather than on producing cogent explanations. Because decisions about what questions to ask and what hints are most helpful depend on a detailed model of the student's conceptions and misconceptions, the system postpones interventions until it has had a chance to collect predictions from the student and analyze them in a large and complex student model.

We determined to handle all the tutoring with words, not pictures, to demonstrate the value of dialogue in tutoring, although we suspect that some combination of words and pictures provides the best learning environment and we have built several tutorials based on the concept maps described in Chapter 5.

Even a simple dialogue requires a complex system to support it. Knowledge about cardiovascular physiology, knowledge about how to teach it, knowledge about parsing, knowledge about language generation, knowledge about student modeling, and knowledge about dialogue planning, all have to be harnessed and used in concert. Building the modules to understand the student input, turn it into a logic form, incorporate that form into the student model, and generate an appropriate response, turned out to be even more complicated than we expected when we started out. Existing grammars of English and text generation techniques were built to understand and produce complete and correct declarative sentences, not questions, elliptical answers, hints, and comments. This meant that we needed to build our own sublanguage grammar and come up with our own rules for generating turns and conducting a dialogue.

The chapters in Part III describe the construction of CIRCSIM-Tutor. Chapter 11 begins by describing what the system looks like to its users and then describes the architecture of the system designed to support tutoring dialogues of this kind. The following chapters discuss the major modules of the system one by one, describe what each module contributes to the tutorial dialogue, and then explain how that module does its job. Chapter 12 describes the growth of planning as it became a central issue in the system. Chapter 13 discusses the evolution of the Input Understander and the important role that spelling correction plays in making sense of the student input. Chapter 14 explains our solution to the student modeling problem. Chapter 15 follows the revolutionary changes that have taken place in the knowledge base and the problem solver over the years. Chapter 16 describes our Text Generator, the focus of the dialogue generation process. Finally, Chapter 17 describes the design of a Screen Manager capable of supporting all these other activities.

11

The Architecture of an Intelligent Tutoring System

In this chapter, we give an example of CIRCSIM-Tutor in action, explain its software architecture, and give a brief description of the main components of the system. We then discuss some architectural issues and how the architecture has changed over time in response to these issues. We have attempted to illustrate these changes in Table 11.1. The overriding necessity of performing spelling correction, parsing, modeling, planning the response, and actually generating the output within 2 sec, dominated our thinking as we built the system. Then we briefly recount how the time problem and the natural language problems affected some software engineering decisions and we give a brief history of the system development process. Finally, we close with some lessons learned.

11.0 CIRCSIM-TUTOR IN ACTION

CIRCSIM-Tutor begins a session by asking the student to choose a problem from a menu. Each problem describes a perturbation in the

TABLE 11.1
Changes in the CIRCSIM-Tutor Architecture

Version 2.1 to 2.6	*Version 2.7 to 2.9*	*Version 3.0*
Tried out by a few students	Tested with classes from 1998 to 2002	Under construction; not yet tested with students
Woo's Controller-Planner	Woo's Controller-Planner	Freedman's APE Planner + Separate Controller (written in APE)
Fixed list of four problems	Fixed list of eight problems	Curriculum Planner with 40 problems
Knowledge stores owned by separate modules	Some knowledge stores accessible to all modules	All knowledge stores accessible to all modules; New Tutoring History
Zhang-Woo Discourse Planner + Chang's Sentence Generator	Larger variety of Discourse Plans + Chang's Sentence Generator	Kim-Freedman Discourse Planner + Turn Planner + GenKit

normal operation of the cardiovascular system. The system asks the student to make predictions about how this perturbation will affect seven important parameters during the DR period. These predictions are qualitative—the student is asked whether the CO will go up, go down, or stay the same, not how many milliliters of blood are output from the heart each minute. The system makes sure that the student gets the first variable correct, but then waits to make further comments until the whole column has been filled. As soon as the student clicks on the "Done Predicting" button, the system marks any wrong predictions with a slash across the box and launches into a tutorial dialogue with the student to discuss any errors and probe for misconceptions to which those errors might point. When this dialogue is successfully concluded, the system asks the student to make predictions about the RR period, and embarks on another remedial dialogue. Finally, the student is asked to predict what will happen in the SS and a third round of dialogue begins. At the end, the system produces a summary of the physiology involved in this perturbation and then puts up the menu again so the student can choose the next problem. The algorithm for solving a CIRCSIM problem has been described in greater detail in Chapter 2.

Figure 11.1 shows how the main screen looks at the end of a dialogue about the DR errors made by the student. The dialogue window takes up the whole length of the screen on the left side, because this is where the main tutorial interaction occurs. The tutor contributions are marked with a "Tutor>" at the beginning. The student input is marked "Student>." The system keeps as much of the dialogue visible as it can fit on the screen. This window is scrollable so that the student can look back at the whole dialogue involving this perturbation. A description of the perturbation appears in the window on the upper right and the Prediction Table appears below it. Here the student makes a series of predictions and winds up with two errors. The system marks these boxes with slashes and then launches into the tutorial dialogue shown on the screen in Fig. 11.1 (also shown in Example 11.1).

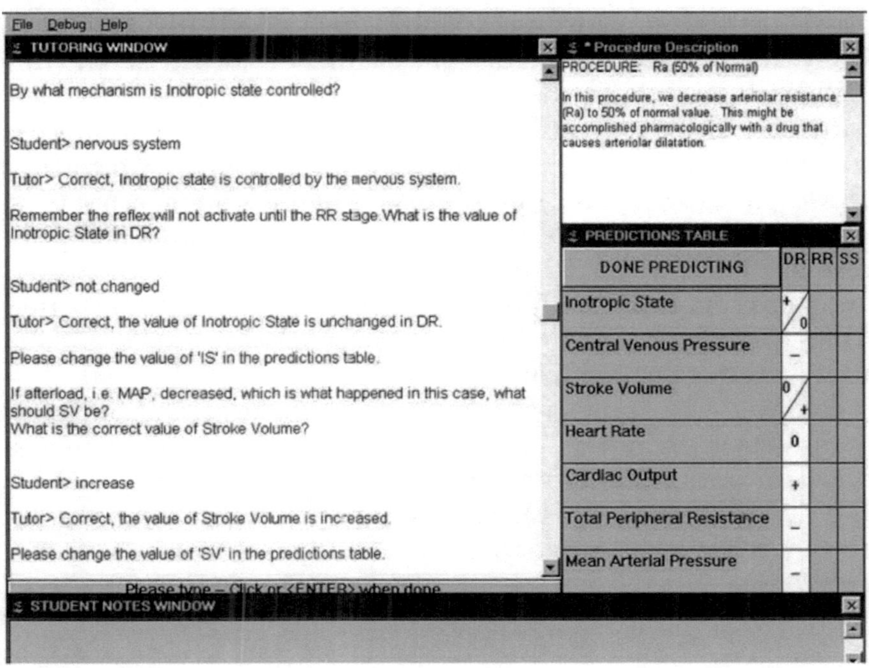

FIG. 11.1. A CIRCSIM-Tutor screen from Version 2.9 (November 2002).

Example 11.1: The Text from Figure 11.1 (From Version 2.8 in 1999)

Tutor>	By what mechanism is Inotropic State controlled?
Student>	nervous system
Tutor>	Correct, Inotropic State is controlled by the nervous system. Remember, the reflex will not activate until the RR stage. What is the value of Inotropic State in DR?
Student>	not changed
Tutor>	Correct, the value of Inotropic State is not changed in DR. Please change the value of 'IS' in the predictions table. If afterload, i.e., MAP, decreased, which is what happened in this case, what should SV be? What is the correct value of Stroke Volume?
Student>	increase
Tutor>	Right, the value of Stroke Volume is increased. Please change the value of 'SV' in the predictions table.

The dialogue fragment in Example 11.1 (and in Fig. 11.1) comes from an actual CIRCSIM-Tutor session in November 1999, when approximately 40 students used the system in a regularly scheduled first-year physiology laboratory. The Planner decides to start off the dialogue by addressing the error in the neural variable because this particular error suggests the possibility of a serious confusion about the meaning of the DR phase. The student gives two correct answers in a row and the tutor decides that this student is not confused after all. In any case, the tutor always asks the student to correct the value in the Prediction Table. Experience with earlier programs suggests that students remember the correct value better if they insert it themselves (Rovick & Michael, 1992). The tutor then addresses the second error.

Example 11.2 shows a slightly more sophisticated example of the system in operation. The system suspects that the student has a misconception about the relationship between Cardiac Output and Central Venous Pressure, probes to confirm this suspicion, and then gives an explanation, in the hopes of remedying the problem.

Example 11.2: Output from CIRCSIM-Tutor Version 2.8 in November 2002

Tutor>	Your prediction for Central Venous Pressure is right, but let's talk a little bit more about it. What is the determinant of Central Venous Pressure?
Student>	map
Tutor>	No, Mean Arterial Pressure is not a determinant. Central Venous Pressure is determined by Cardiac Output. Is the relationship from Cardiac Output to Central Venous Pressure direct or is it inverse?
Student>	direct
Tutor>	Sorry, you got the wrong answer. A change in Cardiac Output has an inverse effect on Central Venous Pressure. When CO decreased, less blood will be taken out from the central venous compartment, CVP will go up.

The generation of this short stretch of dialogue involves all the modules in the system diagram in Fig. 11.2. The central position of the Instructional Planner in this diagram reflects the fact that the planner serves as a main program, calling the other modules in turn.

During the first turn in the sample dialogue, the Planner decides it is time to ask the student for the determinants of Central Venous Pressure. It calls the Text Generator and passes it the logic form,

(ASK(affected-by CVP ??))

The Text Generator turns that logic form into the question, "What is the determinant of Central Venous Pressure?" and returns this question to the Planner, which calls the Screen Manager to display it to the student. The student, who is indeed confused about this relationship, thinks that the determinant is Mean Arterial Pressure and types in the answer, "map."

The Input Understander looks at this answer and produces the following logic form:

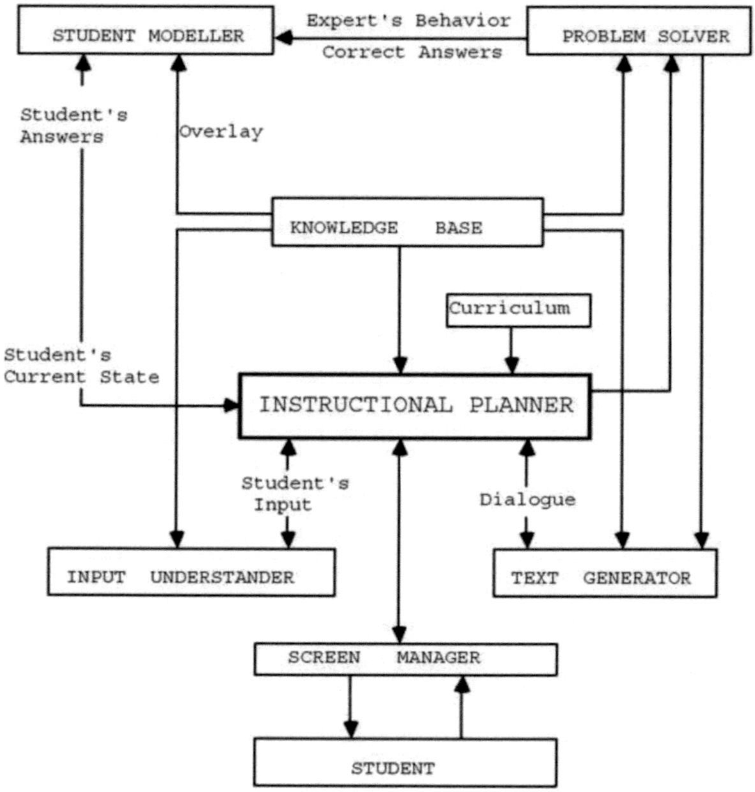

FIG. 11.2. The top-level architecture of CIRCSIM-Tutor Version 2 (adapted from Woo, 1991, p. 21).

(Answer (affected-by CVP MAP))

The Input Understander then sends this logic form to the Student Modeler. The Student Modeler consults the Problem Solver, which, in turn, consults the Domain Knowledge Base, and discovers that this answer is wrong. It updates the Student Model with the information that the student is indeed confused about the relationship between CO and CVP, and reports to the Planner, which decides that it has found a real relationship error, that a hint is useless, and that it needs to tell the student about the mistake and try to explain why CVP is determined by CO and not by MAP. It generates the following logic form:

(NEG-ACK (affected-by CVP MAP))

The Planner sends it to the Text Generator, which returns the following sentence: "No, MAP is not a determinant."

The Planner sends this sentence to the Screen Manager for display in the dialogue window. Then it realizes from its discourse plan that it has more to say and produces the following logic form describing the correct relationship:

(STATE (affected-by CVP CO))

The Planner sends this to the Text Generator and gets back the following sentence: "Central Venous Pressure is determined by Cardiac Output."

The Planner sends the sentence to the Screen Manager for display to the student. Finally, the Planner generates the following logic form:

(ASK (relation CO CVP ??))

The Planner sends this logic form to the Text Generator, and gets back the actual question: "Is the relationship from Cardiac Output to Central Venous Pressure direct or is it inverse?"

The Planner then sends the question to the Screen Manager for display as well.

This process may sound rather complex, but it can be accomplished within 2 sec (about as long as users are willing to wait for a response; Norman & Draper, 1986) and it provides us with the flexibility to execute the kind of complex plans that we see in human dialogues. The fact that these sentences are generated separately makes the output sound somewhat disjointed. One important improvement currently under development is overall turn planning (Yang, Kim, Glass, & Evens, 2000b). Figure 11.3 gives a synopsis of the tutoring process.

11.1 THE SYSTEM ARCHITECTURE

The architecture of CIRCSIM-Tutor differs from the standard intelligent tutoring system architecture only because of the extra components needed to carry on a tutorial dialogue. Like other tutoring

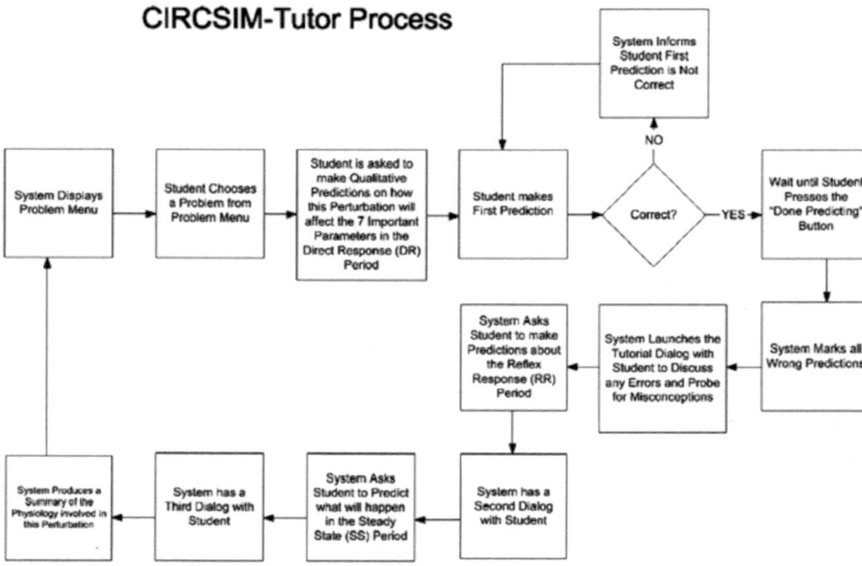

FIG. 11.3. The tutoring process in CIRCSIM-Tutor (from Yusko & Evens, 2004, p. 192).

systems (VanLehn, 1988), CIRCSIM-Tutor has an expert problem solver module, a knowledge base, a student modeler, and a pedagogical module. Due to the demands of carrying on a dialogue, we decided to split the student interface module in a typical intelligent tutoring system into three pieces: one to parse and interpret the student input (the Input Understander), another to generate the natural language output (the Text Generator), and a third to handle the various windows and make sure that the system responds promptly to the student (the Screen Manager). Also, the need for dialogue planning as well as lesson planning soon convinced us to turn the pedagogical module into a full-scale hierarchical planner. This led to the architecture of the current version of CIRCSIM-Tutor as seen in Fig. 11.2.

Our choice of a software architecture may seem very conservative. In fact, this choice has served us well, so perhaps it is justified by our success. We considered two alternative architectures (described briefly below) and decided against them because we were so worried about time problems, about whether we could parse the input, create a semantic form, update the student model, plan the next move, generate the output from the logic form, and display it on the screen in less than 2 sec on a Macintosh or an IBM PC. With the hardware available to us in 1990 it was not obvious that we would be able to meet this 2-sec limitation. Two sec was the maximum time that human interface experts stated that people were willing to wait for a program to respond (Norman, 1990, 1992; Norman & Draper, 1986).

We briefly considered using some kind of parallel programming approach to natural language processing like the one developed by Winograd (1972). In spite of the charm and theoretical attractions of this approach, we decided that it was potentially inconsistent with our determination to arrange for large numbers of medical students to try out the program. For that we needed a program that ran easily on a variety of cheap machines.

We gave much more thought to using a blackboard architecture, which we had already used in building a system for the diagnosis and management of stroke patients, another large system implemented by a number of students over time (Hill, Curt, Hier, & Evens, 1985). In a blackboard architecture, the component modules exchange information by reading and writingto a common storage medium (the blackboard). Control is passed through the blackboard as well. A blackboard approach makes it even easier to isolate modules from each other and to support alternate competing student implementations. W. R. Murray (1989) argued that the blackboard approach, which has been so successful in handling complex interacting rule sets in many expert systems, was an ideal way to build a tutoring system. He designed a blackboard style planner especially for tutoring systems. This architecture allowed him to separate the discourse management rules from the hierarchical sets of pedagogical rules. We were so concerned about the timing problems that we did not attempt it, but this approach would certainly work well on the PCs available today.

11.2 HOW THE ARCHITECTURE HAS CHANGED AND WHY

Although we have made major changes in most of the component modules and are planning for major changes in the rest, the overall architecture of CIRCSIM-Tutor has changed relatively little over the past 14 years. About a year after the system staggered into being, Ramzan Ali Khuwaja pointed out a serious problem in our original plan (Khuwaja, Rovick, Michael, & Evens, 1992). Originally, the knowledge base was accessible only through the problem solver. Khuwaja remarked that the Input Understander and the Text Generator also need direct access to the knowledge base. What is more, the Input Understander and the Text Generator had separate lexicons, the result of being developed on different machines, which produced inconsistencies that bewildered the users. He proposed that all the knowledge stores be made accessible to all the major modules. He also pointed out the importance of creating separate journal files, dialogue histories, and tutoring histories—we were trying to make the dialogue history do all three jobs with messy results. These changes were so clearly desirable that they were unanimously accepted and immediately adopted. The official list of knowledge stores became: the Curriculum, Lexicon, Grammar, Tutoring History, Dialogue History, Journal File, and Domain Knowledge Base.

A new journal file is created for each user and tagged with the user's name and date. It records all calls to major modules, the logic forms and structure trees for the sentences being parsed and generated, along with the sentences themselves. This makes it a very useful debugging tool. Glass wrote an ICON program to extract dialogues from the journal file and label the sentences, like those in Examples 11.1 and 11.2.

11.3 A VERY BRIEF HISTORY OF THE SYSTEM DEVELOPMENT

Readers can skip this section and go on to the next unless they are interested in tracking down the work of one particular student or discovering the makeup of a particular fielded version of the system.

This project has been fortunate enough to attract the interest of a large number of talented people from around the world, who made major contributions. The majority have come from South Korea, because of the national focus on computer-aided education in that country, but others have come from China, Kuwait, Pakistan, and Taiwan, as well as the United States. Nakhoon Kim wrote a Prolog prototype of CIRCSIM-Tutor in the spring semester of 1989, which he demonstrated at a conference (N. Kim, Evens, Michael, & Rovick, 1989). This system contained a student modeler, a screen manager, a problem solver, and a domain knowledge base, which gave us a chance to try out our ideas about the Prediction Table, the Domain Knowledge Base, and the Student Model. Although Michael and Rovick thoroughly tested the system, we did not try it with students because it had no natural language processing components.

At the behest of ONR, we set out to design and implement our ideas on a Xerox LISP machine, which supported Interlisp. This choice seemed especially fortunate to us because Ron Kaplan's LFG Grammar Writer's Workbench ran on this same machine and Kaplan arranged with Xerox to give us a copy. Yoon Hee Lee (1990) wrote the first Input Understander and Yuemei Zhang (1991) wrote the first Text Generator on that machine. Jun Li was working on a screen manager when disaster struck; Xerox decided to stop making Lisp machines.

We were eager to move the system to Macintoshes, because Rush Medical College has recently built a teaching laboratory full of Macintoshes, and ONR agreed on the basis that we were doing basic research, not building a system that the Navy planned to deploy. We plunged ahead; Jai Seu translated Yoon Hee Lee's Interlisp program into the new Procyon Common Lisp, which ran on both PCs and Macintoshes, and when it was compiled, ran very fast. We decided that maybe our disaster was not all bad news. Zhang developed a new version of the Domain Knowledge Base to provide knowledge to the Planner and the Problem Solver. Ru-Charn Chang (1992) wrote a new Text Generator combining Zhang's work with her own ideas about sentence planning. Chong Woo (1991) wrote an instructional planner that also doubled as a system driver and integrated all of these modules and Shim's (1991) Student Modeler into a running whole.

On December 17, 1991, Version 2.0 debuted at Rush Medical College with two student volunteers trying it out. The hints were terrible—they just told the student the right answer, but the system asked sensible questions and it often understood the answers. When it failed to understand, it apologized, "Sorry I did not understand you, please rephrase." Although they did not complain about the generated text, the Rush Medical College students got very tired of seeing this phrase over the next 2 years.

During the next year, Chang made some major improvements in the text generation process, so that the system could produce the subordinate clauses essential to causal explanations. We tried it out with several students in February 1992 (Version 2.1) and again in November 1992 (Version 2.2) and the output text was much better, but the system crashed when a student typed "abcd" in one turn and "efgh" in the next. Muhammad Elmi (1994), with a professional programming background developed at Reuters, did a lot of work to make the system more robust, and Version 2.3 underwent trials in November 1993. Elmi's special focus was spelling correction, but he also improved the coverage of the Input Understander.

At this point, Michael and Rovick decided against using the system with the whole class, because of the bad hints, the interface problems, and the many failures by the Input Understander. For this reason, Ramzan Ali Khuwaja urged us to start working on the new Version 3, instead of continuing to improve Version 2, and he also argued for a number of new experiments with human tutors.

Khuwaja (Khuwaja, Rovick, Evens, & Michael,1994) designed a whole new architecture for Version 3 based on CLOS (the Common Lisp Object System) and he and Hume (1995) built a new domain knowledge base, problem solver, and student modeler using CLOS. We finally scrapped these modules because of performance problems. We have never been sure whether these problems were due to bad programming on our part or to the new and almost untried CLOS software. At the same time, we returned to our old architecture for Version 2, except for the addition of several knowledge sources that are now accessible from all of the other modules.

It was not until Michael Glass (1999, 2000) built a whole new Input Understander based on Information Extraction techniques and Stefan Brandle (1998) built a new Screen Manager that we went back to serious tests with Version 2. We did a trial using Version 2.6 with a group of students from the Alternative (problem-based learning) Curriculum. (These students were ready to study cardiovascular physiology in April, rather than the usual November time-frame.) A bigger trial in November 1998 with Version 2.7 (described in Michael, Rovick, Glass, Zhou, & Evens, 2003) included a number of improvements to the Input Understander, and increased the number of available problems from four to eight. Version 2.8, tested in November 1999, with the whole class participating, contained Yujian Zhou's implementation of answer analysis and hinting. She went on to add her student model during the next few months. Glass added open questions to the system and improved the spelling correction before the trials of Version 2.9 in November 2002. Table 11.2

summarizes the different versions and the dates on which students tried them.

11.4 SOFTWARE ENGINEERING ISSUES

Because the computer science community is not the sole target of this book, we have decided to keep our discussion of software engineering issues to a minimum, but we could not resist the opportu-

TABLE 11.2

Development Time Line for the CIRCSIM-Tutor Project
(Version 2.0 Was the First to Be Tested by Students)

	Planner	*Input Under-stander*	*Student Modeler*	*Domain Knowledge Base*	*Text Generator*	*Screen Manager*
Prolog 1989	N. Kim		N. Kim	N. Kim		N. Kim
Version 1 1990		Y. H. Lee			Zhang	
Version 2.0 December 1991	Woo	Y. H. Lee Seu	Shim	Zhang Woo	Chang	Kim Woo
Version 2.1 February 1992	Woo	Y. H Lee Seu	Shim	Zhang Woo	Chang	Kim Woo
Version 2.2 November 1992	Woo	Y. H. Lee Seu	Shim	Zhang Woo	Chang	Rama -swami
Version 2.3 November 1993	Woo	Seu E mi	Shim	Zhang Woo	Chang	Rama -swami
Version 2.6 April 1998	Woo	Glass	Shim	Zhang Woo	Chang	Brandle
Version 2.7 November 1998	Woo	Glass	Shim	Zhang Woo	Chang	Brandle
Version 2.8 November 1999	Woo	Glass	Zhou	Zhang Woo	Chang	Brandle
Version 2.9 November 2002	Woo	Glass	Zhou 4 level	Zhang Woo	Chang	Brandle
Version 3.0 November 2005	Freedman APE	Glass	Zhou	Freedman Abbas Yusko	J..H. Kim Freedman Yang Mills Lulis	Brandle C. H. Lee H .S. Roh Y. W. Kim

nity of mentioning a few basic principles that have guided our work. Obviously, software engineering and development methodology are extremely important in a project of this size, as many different students participate in the building process over a long time span. Three early decisions have helped keep the software functional. We decided to store a working reference copy of each module in a special directory on a separate machine. We decided to define names and parameters for the main modules in advance and make sure that people used them. We also decided to label all code changes with the names of the people who made them.

We started out with the conviction that it was important to construct and maintain a working version of the system that experts and students at Rush Medical College could use as much as possible. This was one of the wisest decisions that we made. Comments and complaints from our colleagues as they used the program have been an extremely valuable part of the communication between us; these interchanges have had significant effects on the development process. Feedback from students has motivated many other changes, especially improvements in the language and the error messages produced by the system.

Because our major interest was in the natural language processing problems that we faced, we planned from the beginning to do the programming in Lisp. Lisp was originally designed for natural language interaction (McCarthy, 1960, 1962). Natural language understanding systems have been written in Lisp, beginning with the pioneering work of Winograd (1972), Woods (1970), and Schank and Riesbeck (1981). The major work in natural language generation has also been written in Lisp, beginning with McDonald (1980, 1983) and McKeown (1985). What is more, Kaplan's software for Lexical Functional Grammar, which we have used extensively, was written in Lisp. The advent of Common Lisp simplified our lives tremendously. Ever since Procyon stopped supporting its version, we have used the Allegro Common Lisp package from Franz, Inc.; the staff at Franz has provided excellent support over the years. If this project were starting now, we might well have used the Common Lisp Object System.

The architecture for Version 3.0 is much like that of Version 2.0, except that Woo's Planner has been replaced by Freedman's (2000a, 2000b, 2001) APE system and the Controller (the main program) has been separated from the Planner. In addition, Curriculum Planning and Turn Planning modules have been added. The details of the planning interaction in Version 3 are given in the next chapter. Readers interested in exploring alternative architectures for tutoring systems should look at the recent work of Johanna Moore's group at the University of Edinburgh, especially Zinn, Moore, and Core (2002). The way that they support mixed initiatives is particularly interesting (Core, Moore, & Zinn, 2003).

11.5 TAKE-HOME MESSAGE

We believe that we have indeed made the case that it is to build an intelligent tutoring system that carries on a dialogue with its users today. When we first built CIRCSIM-Tutor, it was alone in its field. It is not so lonely any more and we welcome the company. We discuss some of the outstanding new systems in Chapter 19, and we hope that this book will encourage the building of many more.

The increases in PC speed and size have made architecture issues less important and have made it possible for builders of new systems to concentrate on the language issues and the educational issues. The task still involves the construction of a large piece of software, however, and so software engineering issues are important.

If we were starting over today, we would make even more use of existing software packages and we would design the system to serve a wider variety of domains. We still believe it will not be difficult to move the present system to other domains with a focus on causal reasoning.

12

Plans and Planning in the CIRCSIM-Tutor Project

Planning has been a key issue from the very beginning of the CIRCSIM Tutor Project—we have discovered that planning is necessary at many different levels, from curriculum and protocol planning to producing instructional goals to discourse planning to turn planning to the planning of individual sentences.

Dynamic planning is essential in any system designed to tailor a tutorial dialogue to respond to the student's answers and initiatives, because we cannot predict what the student is going to say. Leinhardt and Greeno (1986) showed that experienced teachers use multiple levels of planning. At the global level, they determine instructional goals. When it is time to carry out a particular goal, they plan individual actions and make decisions about what to do next. This means that dynamic hierarchical planning is a necessity in any system that hopes to emulate human tutors.

In Chapters 6 through 9, we have described the planning carried out by our expert human tutors. As we saw, the experts plan constantly at every level from the top level, where the protocol and procedure are chosen, to the bottom level, where they pick the next hint, or decide whether this particular student is likely to be able to interpret a gentle nudge toward self-correction or needs an explicit "No."

We see them make reactive plans—"this student told me the answer to my next question when he answered the last one, so I had better skip the next question." We see them make opportunistic plans, as in "this student betrayed a possible confusion about the length-tension relationship, let's attack it right now," or in a happier example, "this student seems to understand the difference between the sympathetic and the parasympathetic system, let's check whether she knows how different parts of the heart are affected."

In this chapter, we begin with a brief mention of some of the early planning systems and the types of planning used in some early Intelligent Tutoring Systems. Then we describe Woo's hierarchical planner, which has powered the current version of CIRCSIM-Tutor since 1991. Although this planner has been very successful in supporting our original vision, we have gradually discovered the need for more facilities to support reactive planning and opportunistic planning. We then give a brief description of Freedman's Atlas Planning Environment, the core of the emerging Version 3 of our system. Figure 12.1 illustrates some of the most salient differences between these two systems. Finally, we describe planning in this new system.

12.0 SOME EARLY LANDMARKS IN PLANNING

The first planning systems like STRIPS (Fikes & Nilsson, 1971) and HACKER (Sussman, 1975) focused on robot motion or on stacking blocks in a toy world. These systems input planning rules and a description of the situation and output a list of actions. These systems are based on the "linear assumption" that one ordering of actions is as good as another. Because even in the robot world, this assumption may not be true (the robot needs to open the door before it walks through the doorway and not afterward), the planner may need to be able to backtrack (Tate, 1975) and plan again to produce a workable series of actions. Sacerdoti (1974) came up with a new planner, ABSTRIPS, which can solve the same planning problems as STRIPS, but much more rapidly, because it solves problems at a more abstract level and thus avoids much of the backtracking. ABSTRIPS separates subgoals into different priority levels with the more ab-

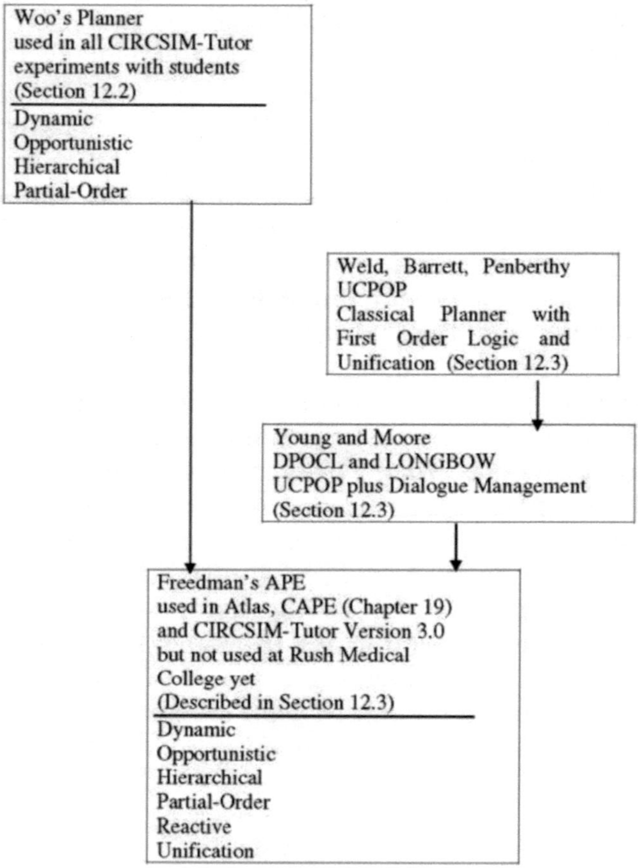

FIG. 12.1. Improvements in planning tutorial dialogues.

stract goals at a higher level and more detailed goals at a lower level. Sacerdoti (1977) went on to build NOAH, a true hierarchical planning system that uses partial ordering with a least-commitment strategy instead of linear ordering. MOLGEN (Stefik, 1981) and NONLIN (Tate, 1977) were based on NOAH's approach to planning, but use other strategies for deciding what to postpone.

The next important step was to allow the planner to monitor execution and adapt the plan to new circumstances (Hendler, Tate, & Drummond, 1990). An ITS needs this capability, because the system can never predict the student's next response with certainty. Hayes-Roth (1985) developed a methodology for opportunistic planning, a particularly apt strategy for a coaching system, which waits until the student asks for help and then seizes the chance to tutor on relevant material. Derry, Hawkes, and Ziegler (1988) made especially good use of this approach. Wilkins (1984, 1988; Wilkins, Myers, Lowrance, & Wesley, 1995) focused on a methodology for replanning. Hammond (1989; Edelson, 1996) adapted case-based strategies to do both planning and replanning.

12.1 EARLY APPROACHES TO INSTRUCTIONAL PLANNING

The builders of the earliest Socratic ITSs, SCHOLAR (J. R. Carbonell, 1970) and WHY (Stevens & Collins, 1977), made a serious effort to discover and implement both discourse strategies and pedagogical strategies, but they did not conceive of their problems as planning problems. The next round of systems, SOPHIE (J. S. Brown et al., 1982), WEST (Burton & Brown, 1982), WUMPUS (Goldstein & Carr, 1977), and WUSOR (Goldstein, 1979), deliberately represented knowledge in the form of rules (Goldstein, 1982). Clancey (1982) represented these rules as the production rules made popular by MYCIN and the other early expert systems and organized them into discourse procedures.

Beverly Woolf (1984) reorganized the discourse procedures of GUIDON into a discourse management network for Meno-Tutor to provide a style of tutoring in which the student raises a problem and the tutor helps with the solution. Many current task assistance dialogue systems use a finite-state model much like Woolf's system. This kind of planning makes sense when the goal of the system is to respond to a variety of requests from the public, and where the major goal is to figure out what users are asking and then tell them what they need to know. We decided early on that this kind of approach to planning was not powerful enough for our tutoring system, which starts out with a complex agenda of its own, diagnosing the students' ability to solve problems and providing them with practice in their areas of weakness. As Chapters 6 through 9 revealed, expert tutors make multistep plans at many different levels, responding to many different kinds of changes in the student model.

Wenger (1987, p. 400) argued that tutoring systems should combine both hierarchical and opportunistic approaches to obtain the best results. Hierarchical control helps keep the tutoring session on target and ensures that the pedagogical goals are accomplished; opportunistic control helps the tutor respond effectively to student initiatives.

Another historically important system was Dan Russell's (1988) IDE Interpreter, designed to carry out instructional units written in IDE (Russell, Moran, & Jordan, 1988). An instructional unit is a set of rules for teaching a particular topic. These rules operated at different levels in the process; some rules expanded other rules, so the IDE Interpreter was a hierarchical rule interpreter, doing a kind of hierarchical planning.

Wilensky's UNIX Consultant (UC) is an important landmark in the use of natural language in tutoring systems (Wilensky et al., 1988). UC is a coach that carries on a natural language dialogue with a UNIX user whenever the user asks for help. Before he began this project, Wilensky had already written a book on planning (Wilensky, 1983), and UC embodies his sophisticated approach. UCEgo, the system controller, calls the planners as it needs them. The functions of the original planner, PANDORA (Faletti, 1982), have now been divided between a goal analyzer (PAGAN) and a domain planner (KIP). KIP produces plans expressed in the system knowledge representation system (KODIAK), so that they can be used in reasoning just like other kinds of domain knowledge.

12.2 WOO'S HIERARCHICAL PLANNER FOR CIRCSIM-TUTOR

After considering these alternative models in the literature, Chong Woo (1991; Woo, Evens, Michael, & Rovick, 1991a, 1991b) decided to build a just-in-time hierarchical planner for CIRCSIM-Tutor. We needed a hierarchical planner because we have a hierarchy of plans. The system must choose a goal, determine a strategy to achieve that goal, and then identify the tactics needed to carry out that strategy. It is important to be able to do those things in separate steps at different times, to do just-in-time planning. We wanted a just-in-time planner that expands plans at the lower levels of the hierarchy just at the point that the system is ready to use them, because otherwise constant revision is required whenever the student gives an unexpected response. It is easier to throw out old plans and make new ones than revise old plans at multiple levels. This also seems to reflect what expert human tutors do, perhaps because of memory limitations.

When Woo started to write rules to describe the approach to tutoring used by Joel Michael and Allen Rovick, he divided these rules into two groups: lesson planning rules and discourse planning rules. The lesson planning rules analyze the Prediction Table entries, identify inconsistencies, and pick the topics to be covered in the natural language interaction. Three of these goal generation rules are shown in Table 12.1. The planner applies these rules and generates the list of goals in the Goal Stack in the order that they should be tutored (Table 12.2).

New goals can be generated during the interactive tutoring process if the student betrays further confusion. These new goals are

TABLE 12.1
Rules for Generating Lesson Goals in CIRCSIM-Tutor (Adapted From Woo, 1991, p. 73)

IF	Current Primary Variable is CC and Student Answer is not NOCHANGE for TPR
THEN	Build Lesson Goal (NEURAL-CONTROL; TPR)
IF	Current Primary Variable is RAP and Student does not know CAUSAL-RELATION (RAP, SV)
THEN	Build Lesson Goal (CAUSAL-RELATION; RAP, SV)
IF	Current Primary Variable is RAP and Student does not know CAUSAL-RELATION; SV, CO)
THEN	Build Lesson Goal (CAUSAL-RELATION; SV, CO)

Note. CC = Cardiac Contractibility; TPR = Total Peripheral Resistance; RAP = Right Atrial Pressure; SV = Stroke volume; CO = Cardiac Output.

TABLE 12.2
Snapshot of the Lesson Goal Stack (Adapted From Woo, 1991, p. 73)

Order	*Lesson Goals*
1.	NEURAL-CONTROL (TPR)
2.	CAUSAL-RELATION (RAP, SV)
3.	CAUSAL-RELATION (SV, CO)

Note. TPR = Total Peripheral Pressure; RAP = Right Atrial Pressure; SV = Stroke Volume; CO = Cardiac Output.

queued after the other goals unless they represent major misconceptions, in which case, they are stacked on the top. If the student asks a question or otherwise initiates a new topic, the associated goals will also be stacked on the top of the goal stack, so that they get an immediate response

The discourse planning rules describe how to achieve the goals set up by the lesson planner. After months spent writing and rewriting rules, Woo divided these rules into Strategy Rules like those in Table 12.3 and Tactical Rules like those in Table 12.4. The tactical rules provide recipes or schemas for carrying out the strategies.

The goal stack mechanism makes it possible to do opportunistic planning with Woo's planner. When the tutor notices a student misconception, the system can dump a stored plan for remediation on the top of the goal stack.

TABLE 12.3

Examples of Strategy Rules (Adapted From Woo, 1991, p. 15)

1.	IF	Goal = CAUSAL-RELATION and Student does not know CAUSAL-RELATION and Direction is incorrect
	THEN	Strategy = TUTOR-CAUSALITY
2.	IF	Goal = CAUSAL-RELATION and Student does not know CAUSAL-RELATION and Direction is correct
	THEN	Strategy = REMIND-RELATION
3.	IF	Goal = NEURAL-CONTROL and Procedure = first and
	THEN	Strategy = TUTOR-DEFINE-NEURAL

TABLE 12.4

Tactical Rules Translate Strategies Into Subgoals (Adapted From Woo, 1991, p. 76)

IF	Strategy = TUTOR-CAUSALITY
THEN	Tactic = DETERMINANTS, ACTUAL-DETERMINANT, RELATIONSHIP, VALUE
IF	Strategy = TUTOR-NEURAL-CONTROL
THEN	Tactic = MECHANISM, VALUE
IF	Strategy = TUTOR-SS-PHYSICAL-VARIABLE
THEN	Tactic = VALUE-DR, VALUE-RR, VALUE-SS

The result is a list of subgoals in the subgoal stack as shown in Table 12.5. Then the discourse planner pops a subgoal off the stack and turns it into a call to the text generator to produce a sentence as shown in Table 12.6.

Woo (1991) implemented a hierarchical planner-interpreter to develop lesson goals and expand them into subgoals using strategies and tactics. This planner operates depth-first and it waits to expand a plan until the system is ready to use it, to simulate just-in-time planning. It does only minimal plan monitoring, because we decided to use replanning as an alternative to plan repair. Replanning is faster

TABLE 12.5
Subgoals Stacked for Execution (Adapted From Woo, 1991, p. 77)

Order	*Subgoals*
1.	Determinants
2.	Actual-determinant
3.	Relation
4.	Value

TABLE 12.6
Example of Goals, Plans, and a Call to the Generator (Adapted From Woo, 1991, p. 78)

Goal Generation	
Student Model:	Do-not-know (SV)
Goal Stack:	CAUSAL-RELATION (RAP, SV) CAUSAL-RELATION (SV, CO)
Current Goal:	CAUSAL-RELATION (RAP, SV)
Plan Generation	
Strategy:	TUTOR-CAUSALITY
Tactics:	(determinants) (actual-determinant) (relation) (value)
Current Plan:	(ask determinants)
Subgoal Stack:	(actual-determinant) (relation) (value)
Call to Text Generator:	(Question—Determines, ??, SV) "What are the determinants of SV?"

Note. SV = Stroke Volume; RAP = Right Atrial Pressure; CO = Cardiac Output.

and we observed human experts constantly discarding old plans and making new ones.

The goal stack approach also makes it relatively easy to implement responses to student initiatives. Once the initiative is recognized, the system can stack a plan to respond on the top of the goal stack, execute that plan, and then go back to its earlier goals. At this point, the system can only handle a few simple initiatives of the form:

- What is Intropic State?
- I don't understand Inotropic State.
- Tell me about Inotropic State.

All of these lead the system to produce a definition. The difficulty here is not in the system planning but in the system's ability to recognize the student's plan. We are trying to apply Carberry's (1989, 1990, 1991) work on plan recognition, to figure out whether the student is trying to ask a question or answer one. We have undertaken a study of initiatives (Shah, Evens, Michael, & Rovick, 2002) with the hope of expanding our capabilities here.

For the last 10 years, Woo's planner has served as the backbone of the CIRCSIM-Tutor system as we implemented a new input understander (Glass, 1999), experimented with different interface designs (Brandle, 1998), implemented hints (Zhou et al., 1999a, 1999b), and built a new four-level student modeler (Zhou & Evens, 1999). But over the years, we have discovered that there are some kinds of planning that we want to do that are not well supported by Woo's planner. It is not easy to do reactive planning with Woo's planner. One of the most frequently executed plans used by the system asks the student for the name of the next variable to change, waits for the student to type the name of that variable, and then asks for the direction of the change. For example,

T1: *What variable will be affected next?*
S2: *CO*
T3: *Right, and how will it change?*
S4: *Increase*

The system has plans to respond to a variety of alternative wrong answers typed instead of S2, but suppose that, instead of typing S2, the student types the perfectly correct S2':

S2': CO increases

The system sounds really dumb if it goes ahead and asks question T3 at this point, but it is messy to write the rules to eliminate T3 in Woo's framework. This kind of problem often arises with task assistance dialogues as well. Bratt (personal communication, October 19, 2004) gave the following example from the Communicator Travel Planning system:

Communicator: What city are you departing from?
Traveler: Chicago on Tuesday the 13th.

The system needs to recognize and record the date of travel and also delete the plan to ask for the date. Julitta Vassileva (1995) defined a reactive planner as one that can recognize and react to any changes that occur in the world while the system is running. The situation just described is one of many that calls for reactive planning. One way to provide this capability is to develop a better way to express preconditions.

There were other considerations that made us believe it was time to think about a new planner. Reactive planning and opportunistic planning both provide ways to tune the tutoring process to the needs of each particular student. Reactive planning allows the system to modify existing plans when the student reveals new knowledge. Opportunistic planning allows the system to do dynamic planning, to seize the opportunity to move the session in a new direction. Both types of planning have become even more significant as we have attempted to implement the multiturn discourse structures discussed in Chapter 8. Reactive planning goes hand in hand with the opportunistic planning needed to support student initiatives. Woo's planner makes it easy to do some kinds of opportunistic planning, but it lacks some facilities for handling variables and it does not support reactive planning well.

12.3 RECENT RESEARCH IN PLANNING FOR DIALOGUE MANAGEMENT

During the last 10 years, while we have been using Woo's planner, the planning community has made significant advances in general-purpose planning engines. Weld (1994) stressed the value of "partial-order planning." This approach to planning is designed to reduce backtracking by postponing commitment until the last possible moment. A partial-order planner uses a graph to represent the necessary relationships between individual steps and it does not linearize them until just before execution. UCPOP, a partial-order planner, has been shown to be sound and complete (Penberthy & Weld, 1992). It provides universal quantifiers, first order logic, and unification for feature matching (Barrett & Weld, 1994). Ever since the appearance of UCPOP, dialogue planners have demanded these features along with support for natural language interaction.

Michael Young and Johanna Moore (1994a) wrote an article entitled "Does Discourse Planning Require a Special Purpose Planner?" that begins by telling us that the answer to this question is "No." Apparently, they soon discovered that, although it is possible to use a general-purpose planner for planning discourse, it is much more convenient to use one that it is tailored for the job. Less than a year later, they produced DPOCL, based on UCPOP (Young & Moore, 1994b). A year of work with DPOCL inspired them to write Longbow, a text planning system that met their needs even better (Young, 1994; Young, Moore, & Pollack, 1994).

Reva Freedman's (1996c) dissertation outlines a whole new approach to dialogue planning and dialogue management. As we mentioned in Chapter 3, her work led us to use dialogue markup and machine learning to explore the structure of human tutoring dialogues in new ways. She then argued for better dialogue planning facilities to generate the new tutoring schemas discovered.

Freedman worked with Longbow to generate natural language tutoring dialogue for a time at the University of Pittsburgh and then built her own text planning system, the Atlas Planning Engine or APE, to function as the core of the Atlas tutoring system (Freedman, Rosé, Ringenberg, & VanLehn, 2000). APE is a just-in-time, opportunistic, reactive hierarchical planner that supports variables and unification (Freedman, 2000a, 2000b, 2001). APE represents goals in first order logic; goals are then matched using unification. APE planning operators have preconditions; they also support plans (called recipes) with multiple steps, which make it simple to do multiturn planning. Recipes have three powerful mechanisms that can be used to change the agenda. The "Fact" mechanism evaluates a condition, and, if that condition is true, then the rest of the recipe is skipped. This gives us an easy way to skip asking a question that the student has just answered or to do other types of reactive planning. The "Retry-at" mechanism lets us back up to a choice point and make a different decision. This mechanism makes backtracking easy; it also lets us do complex reactive planning. The "Prune-Replace" mechanism removes goals from the agenda and replaces them with new ones. This makes it easy to handle unexpected responses and to do other kinds of opportunistic planning. If the student produces an initiative or betrays a misconception, the system can totally change the agenda to follow this new path.

APE (Freedman, 2000a, 2000b) has been used to build the Atlas system at the University of Pittsburgh (VanLehn et al., 2000; VanLehn, Jordan, et al., 2002; VanLehn, Lynch, et al., 2002) and the CAPE system at Northern Illinois University (Freedman, 2001). Freedman (2001, p. 201) described CAPE as "a stripped-down prototype of the next version of CIRCSIM-Tutor." Tutor functions that had not yet been rewritten as planning operators were replaced by simplified Lisp functions. Bruce Mills (2001) is now implementing Freedman's ideas about discourse planning in Version 3 of CIRCSIM-Tutor using APE. Byung-In Cho (Cho, Michael, Rovick, & Evens, 1999, 2000) has already implemented curriculum planning (see Section 12.4) and protocol switching (see Section 12.5) in APE, but we have not yet tested this version of the system with a class of medical students.

12.4 CURRICULUM PLANNING

In the world of intelligent tutoring systems, the term *curriculum planning* denotes the choice of problems to present to the students and the determination of the order of presentation (cf. Brecht, McCalla, Greer, & Jones, 1989; Lesgold, 1988). In a tutoring system like ours with a focus on problem solving, the choice of problems is a major issue (Halff, 1988). The various versions of CIRCSIM-Tutor so far tested with students at Rush Medical College have included some or all of the eight problems that Michael and Rovick designed for the CIRCSIM system in 1986. Although we have allowed the students to choose to do these problems in any order they like, all but a very few (1 out of 66 in the fall of 2002) have worked steadily down the menu on the screen. Cho (2000) read the work of Khuwaja (1994) and decided that it was time to implement the curriculum and the curriculum planning that Khuwaja had proposed. Cho implemented the new curriculum and the curriculum planning rules to support it as part of Version 3.0. The curriculum planner has been thoroughly tested in the laboratory at IIT, but it has not yet been used by students at Rush Medical College.

Over the years, Michael and Rovick have identified a number of examples of perturbations in the blood pressure that occur in important physiological states, or arise with the use of therapeutic drugs such as beta-blockers. They have written up several descriptions of ways in which these perturbations can occur for use as examination questions or in small group sessions. As we began to implement the new Version 3 of CIRCSIM-Tutor using Reva Freedman's APE, Cho realized that the curriculum planning could be implemented in this same framework (Cho et al., 1999, 2000). Cho interviewed Allen Rovick at length and the two of them devised a complete set of planning rules. They worked out all the corresponding prediction tables. Then, Rovick rewrote the problem descriptions and Cho (2000) implemented the curriculum planning rules in APE.

The goal of curriculum planning is to make sure that the student sees a wide variety of problems that cover the most important points in the curriculum, and at the same time to ensure that the student is not bored by problems that are too easy or frustrated by problems that are too hard. Every student starts with the same initial problem, which contains detailed instructions for using the system, but after that we attempt to present a choice of five different problems that the student can choose from. Every time the student finishes a problem, the curriculum planner develops a fresh assortment of problems and presents them in a menu on the screen, so that the student can choose one. A typical menu appears in Table 12.7.

We have established four levels of problem hardness. In addition, the problem descriptions can differ in difficulty as well, depending mainly on how easy it is to figure out what variable is the first one affected by the problem and which prediction table variable will be affected first. The student who gets these variables correct is much more likely to do well in making predictions. Table 12.8 shows three different descriptions for the same problem that differ only in the description difficulty level.

The curriculum planning rules make use of the problem hardness level and the description difficulty level as well as the student's performance in the problems solved so far, to decide what problems to

TABLE 12.7

Menu With Five Different Procedure Descriptions (Copied From Cho, 2000, Fig. 5.4, p. 63, by the Permission of the Author)

1. A medical student donated 1 liter of blood to a patient about to undergo surgery. Predict the effects of the blood donation on the student.
2. Predict the effects of simultaneously increasing both heart rate and cardiac contractility (cardiac inotropic state) using the maintained infusion of a drug.
3. What would be the effects of continually infusing an individual with a potent, long-acting cholinergic muscarinic antagonist (blocking agent)?
4. A group of teenagers were experimenting with drugs. One of them swallowed some pills that contained a specific arteriolar smooth muscle relaxant.
5. A mother was preparing for her 5-year-old's birthday by blowing up balloons. One very large balloon was particularly stiff. What would be the cardiovascular effect of her effort to inflate this balloon? Assume that she tried to blow it up in a very long, sustained, suspiratory effort.

TABLE 12.8

Three Different Descriptions of the Same Procedure With Increasing Description Difficulty Level (Copied From Cho, 2000, Fig. 6.1, p. 68, by the Permission of the Author)

1. Predict the effects of decreasing venous return. Assume that no change in venous capacitance or venous compliance occurs.
2. A patient was admitted to the hospital after experiencing a fainting spell. After a series of tests her problem was determined to be an abdominal tumor that was compressing her vena cava, reducing her venous return.
3. Certain agents are known to cause veno-constriction, without affecting venous compliance or capacitance. What would be the effect of administering this agent to a patient?

choose for the next round. In addition, students are asked if they want harder problems, easier problems, or problems that are about the same, the next time around. The problems are organized in groups that cover different parts of the curriculum and that are designed to attack particular misconceptions. The curriculum planning rules make sure that the student sees problems from every group. We decided to rate the description difficulty levels on a scale of four, just like the equally important problem hardness level, because we felt that these two considerations should be treated as equally important. Table 12.9 shows some of the first few curriculum planning rules.

The problem hardness and description difficulty levels used in the curriculum planner are based on Rovick's estimates (Cho, 2000). His many years of teaching physiology during which some of these problems were used in small group sessions give us confidence in these estimates, but we should try to collect some empirical observations to support them. Susan Chipman has suggested that we record the number of prediction errors that students make in predicting the primary variable as a measure of description difficulty. Then we could use the number of initial errors in the rest of the DR column before tutoring begins as a measure of problem hardness. We could even use the initial errors in the RR and SS columns as well.

12.5 SWITCHING TUTORIAL PROTOCOLS

Among the top-level decisions that the tutor must make is when to begin the tutoring after the student begins making predictions. In CIRCSIM, corrective feedback is provided only after the entire table has been filled in. Our expert tutors usually begin tutoring after all

TABLE 12.9
Some Curriculum Planning Rules
(Adapted From Cho, 2000, Table 6.3, p. 71, by the Permission of the Author)

The Core Procedures are:

1. Decrease Arterial Resistance (Ra) to 50% of Normal
2. Decrease Inotropic State to 50% of Normal
3. Increase Venous Resistance to 200% of Normal
4. Denervate the Baroreceptors
5. Reduce Ra by 50% after Denervating the Baroreceptors
6. Hemorrhage—Remove 0.5 Liters.
7. Hemorrhage—Remove 1.0 Liters

The first procedure is Core Procedure 1.

The second procedure set is set (2, 3, 4).

If the global assessment is low repeat the set (2, 3, 4 else present (5, 6, 7).

If the student selects procedure 6, then suggest procedure 7.

the predictions in a column (phase of the response) have been made, and CIRCSIM-Tutor proceeds in the same way, with the exception that the tutor ensures that the first prediction in the first (DR) column is made correctly. On occasion, however, the expert tutors tutor after each individual prediction is made. Each of these approaches to generating a tutorial interaction is what we call a "protocol." Khuwaja analyzed the different tutoring protocols used by our experts in human tutoring sessions and found at least three different approaches (Khuwaja, Rovick, Michael, & Evens, 1994b).

Byung-In Cho (2000; Cho et al., 2000) was the first to recognize that Michael and Rovick switch protocols in a systematic fashion as recounted in Section 7.1. He was fascinated by this process and felt it was important for us to provide the capability of switching protocols for the tutoring system. We encouraged him to go ahead with this implementation using APE in the hope of carrying out some long-term research goals, to compare the effectiveness of different protocols. We have not been able to test this capability with students yet, however.

Now we turn from planning at the highest level (making decisions about which tutoring policies to use and which problems to ask the student to solve) to planning at the level of individual tutor turns.

12.6 FITTING TURN PLANNING INTO THE PLANNING SEQUENCE

The current version generates sentences one at a time from the logic forms sent to the text generation component by the planner. Students have no problem in understanding the program output but they do sometimes tell us that they find it repetitious. It certainly does not sound natural. One of our goals is to generate more natural-sounding text with the hope of making the students more comfortable with working through a longer curriculum and making them more likely to take the initiative during the dialogue.

It was Reva Freedman (1996a, 1996b, 1996c) who first argued for the necessity of turn planning. She pointed to a number of turns that sounded clumsy and long-winded, because of too much repetition and a lack of anaphora. She also recommended that we analyze the use of discourse markers in human sessions and add them to the text; the results of this analysis are summarized in Chapter 4 (for more details, see J. H. Kim, Glass, Freedman, & Evens, 2000).

In 1998, Feng-Jen Yang volunteered to investigate turn planning for the new CIRCSIM-Tutor using Freedman's APE and we suddenly needed to determine how to fit turn planning into the rest of our system (Yang, Kim, Glass, & Evens, 2000a, 2000b). It was Michael Glass who came up with the best proposal. He drew a diagram that inserted the turn planner between the discourse planner, which determines the content of the turn, and the sentence generator, which outputs a sentence at a time. The result is shown in Fig. 12.2, which displays all the levels of planning to be deployed in Version 3. In this model, the planning in CIRCSIM-Tutor begins with the Curriculum Planner, which chooses a problem or an assortment of problems for the student to work through. The Protocol Planner then goes to work and initializes the protocol. Unless we have some special research plan in mind or some reason to expect that this student will have special difficulty, the system will start the session with the standard protocol and that protocol will only be changed if the student seems really confused.

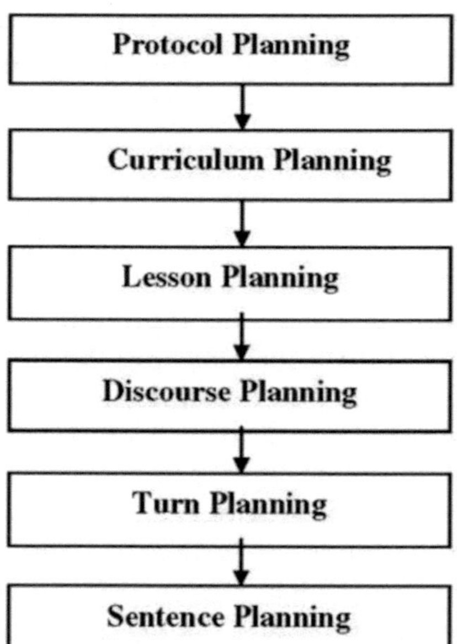

FIG. 12.2. Levels of planning in Version 3 of CIRCSIM-Tutor. (The current version, Version 2, has only three levels of planning, Lesson Planning, Discourse Planning, and Sentence Planning. The Curriculum Planning and Turn Planning have been implemented and tested but not used by students. The Protocol Planning has not been fully implemented.)

The system presents the student with the chosen problem and the student makes a first set of predictions for this new problem. Now the Lesson Planner generates a series of topics to be taught to the student to remedy any prediction errors. If the student does not make any errors, then the Lesson Planner picks a topic area where misconceptions are frequent and asks an open-ended question, searching for problems. The Discourse Planner plans some discourse to handle the first lesson goal and the Turn Planner is assigned the task of planning the first turn as a series of logic forms. The Turn Planner attaches features to the logic forms. One set of features, for example, determines whether the variable name is to be spelled out, abbreviated, or pronominalized. Finally, the Sentence Planner is called to generate the actual sentences. Note that in the new version of the system, these "planners" (except for the sentence planner) are really separate sets of rules used by Freedman's APE to produce appropriate plans at different levels of the system. Turn planning, like curriculum planning, has been tested in the laboratory but not used in an experiment with students at Rush Medical College.

Unfortunately, the situation is not quite as simple as it looks in Fig. 12.2. The highly successful plan to remedy an answer that is correct but incomplete begins with the tutor saying "And?" This plan combines discourse, turn, and sentence planning into one step. Sometimes we want protocol planning to control the whole process. If we were to carry out an experiment on the value of giving immediate feedback, for example, then protocol planning would have to dominate the whole system. But Cho's (2000) research suggests that ordinarily we want to be able to change the protocol during the session when a student gets into trouble with a part of the lesson. Much of the time the tutoring schema limits the appropriate dialogue plan. For example, a tutoring schema like "tutor-another-neural-variable" determines the dialogue plan needed to carry out the next stage in a lesson plan. Freedman (1996a, 1996b) pointed out that Joel Michael and Allen Rovick clearly make sustaining the tutoring dialogue their prime concern. For this reason, our tutoring system is designed to end every turn with a question or an instruction to update the Prediction Table. More recently, Freedman (2001) has argued that dialogue planning should subsume lesson planning. This suggests that Fig. 12.3 is a more realistic picture of the planning that we need to do than Fig. 12.2.

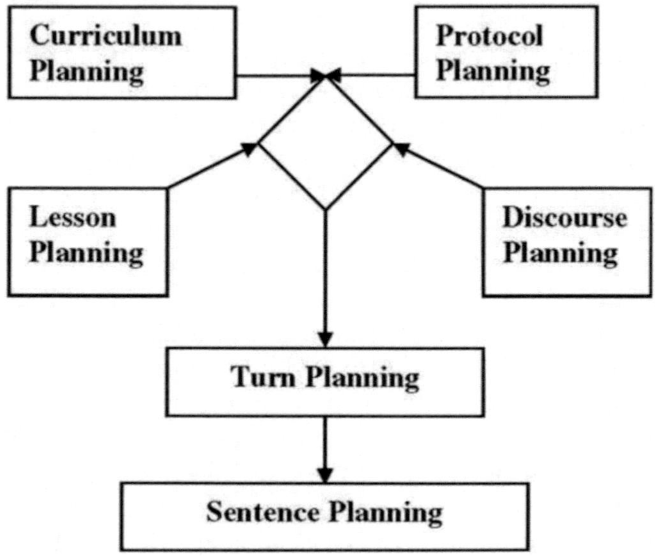

FIG. 12.3. A more realistic view of planning levels.

We have not discussed sentence planning in this chapter, because our current sentence planning is being done separately, not using the main planner, through a set of text generation algorithms (Chang, Evens, Michael, & Rovick, 1994). The emerging Version 3 of CIRCSIM-Tutor uses Genkit for sentence planning (Nyberg & Tomita, 1988), which also has its own special-purpose planning algorithm. These issues are discussed in Chapter 16, which also gives a detailed description of the turn planning process in the context of dialogue generation.

Is it reasonable to treat sentence planning as a separate issue? It has developed historically as a separate problem with separate solutions, although it has long been recognized as a planning problem (Appelt, 1985). Could we do sentence planning also using Freedman's APE system? We have not even explored this issue, because we have been so involved with using APE to do the dialogue planning, instructional planning, and turn planning that it was designed to do, but it seems like a provocative question—one that should be explored sometime soon.

12.7 TAKE-HOME MESSAGE

When we started to implement CIRCSIM-Tutor, we did not appreciate the tremendous amount of planning that human tutors do before and during tutoring sessions, and we did not realize that planning would become a central issue in the design and development of the CIRCSIM-Tutor system. Tutoring sessions that generate a natural language dialogue require a tremendous amount of planning at every level—from protocol and curriculum planning to lesson planning, discourse planning, turn planning, and sentence planning. There are good arguments for making sure that the planner that creates all these plans is capable of hierarchical, reactive, opportunistic, just-in-time planning.

Our experience provides further testimony of the value of repeated student trials with a running system. We would never have discovered the need for turn planning if we had not tried the system with a number of students and looked at the clumsy-sounding text that the system sometimes produces.

We should emphasize again that although we have implemented protocol planning, curriculum planning, and turn planning with much care and consideration, because they seem to us to be essential components of a natural language tutoring system, we have not tried them out with a large class of students. The system that the students have used is still controlled by Woo's planner, although Glass's new Input Understander is processing the student input and Zhou's Student Modeler has replaced the old package, to take advantage of the improved analysis made by the Understander and to allow for the generation of more hints and better ones. In the next chapters, we go on to explore other components of this system.

13

Understanding the Student Input

This chapter addresses the spelling correction issues, describes the lexicon, and then discusses the two very different parsers that we have used and the trade-offs between them. Readers who are uncomfortable with discussions of parsing can skip this chapter, but we hope that some of you will continue reading long enough to realize how much you can do with a very small and simple grammar and lexicon, if you tailor it to the problem at hand.

Figure 13.1 attempts to summarize some of the changes in spelling correction and parsing.

13.0 SOME BASIC PRINCIPLES

The job of the Input Understander, as we originally designed it, was to perform three major tasks: correct the spelling, parse the input, and then produce a logic form. Recently, the Input Understander has been extended to cooperate with the Student Modeler to classify the answers in terms of both correctness and appropriateness.

From the very beginning, processing speed has been a major concern. Most experts in human factors agree that computer users get

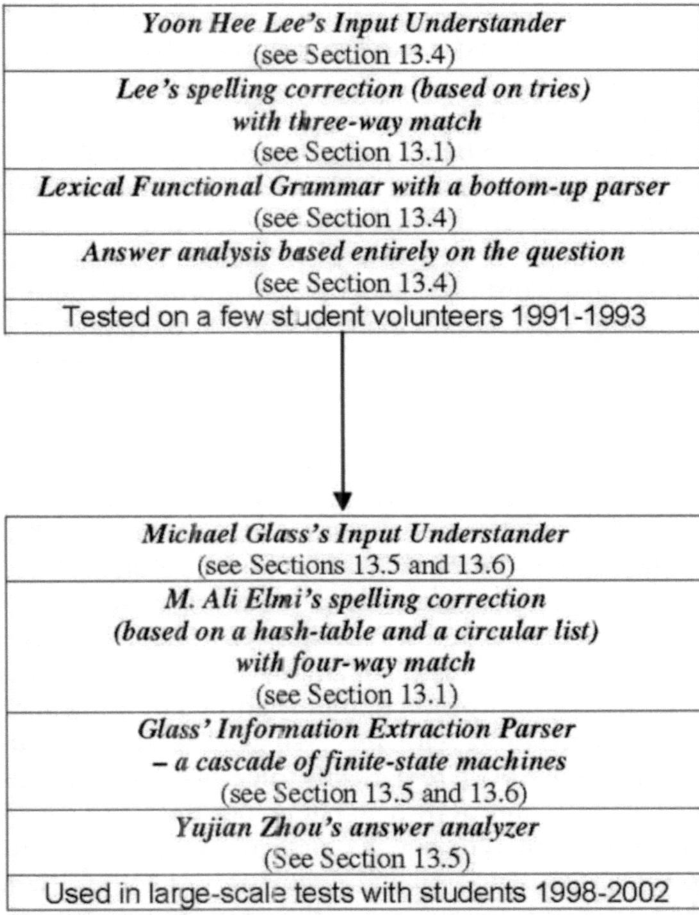

FIG. 13.1. Changes in the CIRCSIM-Tutor Input Understander.

annoyed if systems do not respond in less than 2 sec (Norman, 1990, 1992; Shneiderman, 1984). In CIRCSIM-Tutor, this implies that the Input Understander has to produce a logic form, which the Student Modeler uses to update the model. The Planner can then plan a response, which the Text Generator turns into a sentence that the Screen Manager can display on the screen. And all of this must be accomplished within 2 sec. Our concern about speed affected the design of all the component modules of the Input Understander, and our decisions about time and space trade-offs always sacrificed space for speed. As a result, we were terrified that we would run out of main memory.

Spelling correction is absolutely essential to any system like ours; it has also turned out to be a much more difficult problem than we expected and it is still giving us trouble. Even the most sophisticated parser cannot function without spelling correction if it is handling unrestricted student input. The kind of familiar spelling correction provided by most word processors is not appropriate here. We do not want to interrupt students in the middle of a deep discussion of a tricky point in physiology with a demand that they fix the spelling of a word. It is essential that the system figure out what the student means whenever possible.

The system response to communication failures is also critical to carrying on a dialogue. The earliest version of our system told the student periodically, "I am sorry. I don't understand you. Please rephrase." The students found this very annoying. Human tutors, like other people faced with a misunderstanding, ask a clarification question or try to explain what it is that they want. Replacing the "I am sorry" message with a message explaining what kind of input the system was expecting improved communication and immediately increased student comfort with the system. The students at Rush Medical College have been remarkably tolerant of much clumsy and repetitive language output by the system, but the "I am sorry" message apparently seemed to signal a total communication failure.

Our original focus was on the generation of tutorial language rather than on the understanding of ill-formed input. But a tutorial dialogue, like any other kind of dialogue, requires language understanding as well as language generation. Experiments by Aleven, Koedinger, and Cross (1999) have shown that pushing students to explain something indeed helps them to learn, but they are still reluctant to continue to produce explanations when the system is not attempting to understand them. Aleven (Aleven, Koedinger, & Popescu, 2003; Aleven, Popescu, & Koedinger, 2001) is now attempting to add language understanding to his system.

After we had worked for several years, Michael and Rovick decided that the language understanding in CIRCSIM-Tutor was still not adequate, and we replaced our original, simple, bottom-up parser with a cascade of finite-state machines. The new system, built by Michael Glass (1999, 2000, 2001), made such a pronounced improvement that Michael and Rovick decided to try the system out with the 24 students in the problem-based learning curriculum in April 1998, and then on the whole first-year class that fall (November 1998).

13.1 SPELLING CORRECTION

Although Shortliffe (1976) stressed the importance of providing spelling correction in any medical system attempting to communicate with users in natural language, and although we had some prior experience with the problem (McElwain & Evens, 1962), we still did not realize the urgency and the size of this problem. In fact, spelling correction continues to be a source of system errors today. Fortunately, we were aware of the work of Peterson (1986), which convinced us of the importance of keeping the vocabulary small to simplify the recognition of spelling errors. Kukich (1992) provides a still valuable review of the spelling correction literature.

Yoon Hee Lee (1990; Y. H. Lee & Evens, 1998) was the first in our group to recognize the crucial nature of the spelling correction problem. When Lee started his thesis research, we had not yet collected any tutoring transcripts. Joel Michael provided the implementation team with a set of examination papers with short answer questions and essay questions. Lee found many sentence fragments and relatively few correct whole sentences. He collected a lot of useful words for our new lexicon, including a large number of common abbreviations. He discovered that medical students also coin new abbreviations frequently. When they get far enough along in a word so that they think the professor can understand what they mean, they just stop and go on to the next word.

When we began to study our first set of eight keyboard-to-keyboard transcripts, we observed the same phenomena. In addition, the student responses were often very telegraphic in style, as we had expected from reading Bozena Thompson's (1980) study of naval personnel using a natural language interface to a database. Lee also discovered a number of typical typographical errors like "teh" and "hte" for "the" and "fo" for "of" in words too short for any known spelling correction algorithm to handle. He immediately decided to create lexical entries for these strings so that our system could indeed correct them, although commercial systems had not yet started to use this approach.

As Lee analyzed the transcripts, he discovered that most frequent errors were word boundary errors, which turn "heart rate" into "heartrate" or "he artrate" or "hear trate." Next most frequent were errors involving a single letter that is dropped ("heart" garbled to "hert") or added ("heart" garbled to "hesart") or replaced by another ("heart" garbled to "heast"). Reversals of two letters are also very common ("heart" garbled to "herat").

Lee analyzed the way that these different types of errors show up in matching unknown strings with strings already in the lexicon. Suppose that we are trying to match "hert" with "heart" as in Fig. 13.2. The first two letters "h" and "e" match, but then we try to match "r" against "a" and find a mismatch. So we compare the "r" in "hert" with next letter "r" in "heart" and find a match and then we compare the "a" in "heart" with the next letter "t" in "hert" and find a mismatch. This tells us that we probably have a dropped letter. We confirm that by successfully matching the "t" in "hert" with the "t" in "heart." In Fig. 13.3, we show what happens in the case of an added letter. Here we are trying to match "hesart" with "heart" and again the first two letters match, but when we compare the "s" in "hesart" with the "a" in "heart," we find a mismatch. So we compare the "s" in "hesart" with the next letter "r" in "heart" and find a mismatch, but when we compare the "a" in "heart" with the next letter "a" in

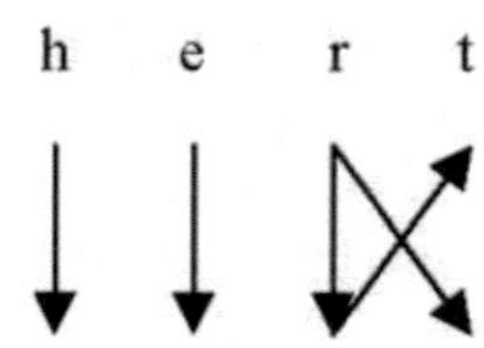

FIG. 13.2. Lee's algorithm identifies a dropped letter (here "hert" is an unknown word and "heart" is a candidate correction).

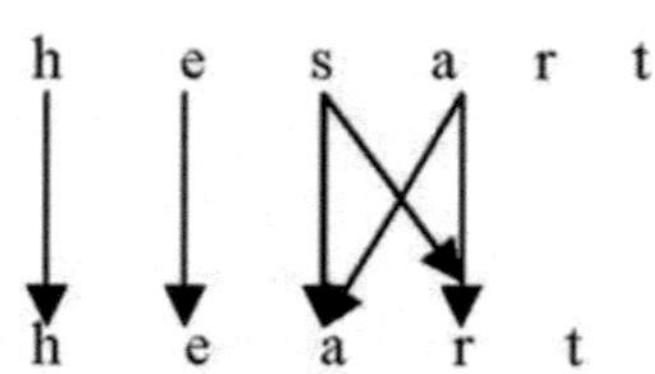

FIG. 13.3. Lee's algorithm identifies an added letter (here "hesart" is an unknown word and "heart" is a candidate correction).

"hesart," we find a match and this suggests an added letter. Again we can confirm this by matching the "r" in "hesart" with the "r" in "heart" and the "t" in "hesart" with the "t" in "heart."

In Fig. 13.4, Lee's algorithm identifies the case where two letters are reversed. Here we are matching an unknown string "herat" against the word "heart." Again the first two letters "h" and "e" match, but when we compare the "r" in "heart" with the "a" in "heart" we find a mismatch. So we compare the "r" in "herat" with the next letter "r" in "heart" and the "a" in "heart" with the next letter "a" in "heart" and we find two matches and we suspect that we have reversed letters. We go on to confirm this by finding that the "t" in "herat" matches the "t" in "heart."

It is now easy to see how the general case works. Suppose we have an unknown string with s characters m_1 m_2 … m_{k-1} m_k m_{k+1} … m_s and we are matching it against a candidate word from the lexicon with t characters n_1 n_2 n_3 … n_{k-1} n_k n_{k+1} … n_t as shown in Fig. 13.5. Suppose the first k–1 characters have been matched and are exactly the same, that is, $m_1 = n_1$, $m_2 = n_2$, … and $m_{k-1} = n_{k-1}$, but m_k and n_k are different. When Lee's program detects the mismatch between m_k and n_k, it immediately compares m_k with n_{k+1} and m_{k+1} with n_k. If $m_k = n_{k+1}$ and

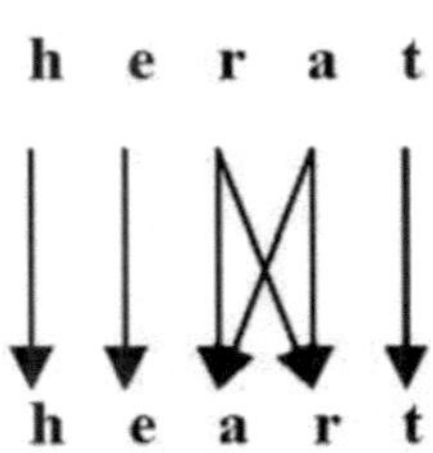

FIG. 13.4. Lee's algorithm identifies reversed letters (here "herat" is an unknown word and "heart" is a candidate correction).

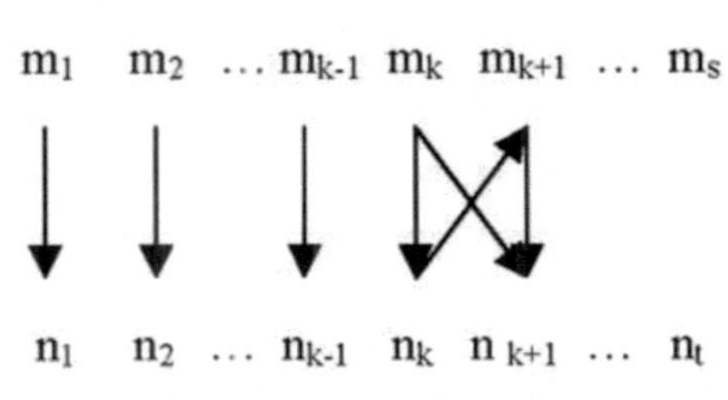

FIG. 13.5. String matching in Lee's algorithm (m_1m_2 … $m_{k-1}m_km_{k+1}$ … m_s is an unknown word and $n_1n_2n_3$ … $n_{k-1}n_kn_{k+1}$ … n_+ is a candidate correction).

$m_{k+1} = n_k$ then it attempts to confirm that two letters are reversed, as in the "herat" → "heart" example shown earlier. If $m_k = nk+1$ but $m_{k+1} \neq n_k$, then it looks for an inserted letter, as in the "hesart" → "heart" example. If $m_k \neq n_{k+1}$, but $m_{k+1} = n_k$, then it suspects a deleted letter, as in "hart" → "heart." Like most conventional spelling correction programs, Lee's program assigned a weight to each change. This approach is fast and it allows the system to handle multiple errors in a word so long as they are not adjacent. To compensate for the student propensity to invent new abbreviations by stopping part way through words, Lee gave lower weight to missing characters at the end of a word.

Another crucial decision in spelling correction is how to store the word list. Lee decided to use a trie (Knuth, 1972). The argument for this approach is the speed of search. Students almost never get the first letter of a word wrong, or if they do, they backspace and correct it, so it made sense to search only the trie of words beginning with the same first letter.

All this time, we were trying to push Lee into writing a parser. He finally did so, but he insisted on solving the spelling correction problems first. The passage of time has certainly proved him right. Spelling correction is essential to a program like ours.

After Lee returned to Korea, Jai Seu (1992) translated the Input Understander into Common Lisp, but he was much more interested in our studies of language described in Chapter 4 (Seu et al., 1991) than in the spelling correction and parsing issues, so he made no real changes in the design.

Four years later Mohammad Elmi decided to redo the spelling correction. He was convinced that he could write a smarter, faster, more space-efficient algorithm and after he had rewritten the program half a dozen times, he proved his point. He threw out the trie and replaced it with a hash table. He organized the lexicon as a circular list and started the lookup process with the first letter of the garbled word. This approach was considerably faster than the trie and required much less space in main memory.

Instead of starting off with a spelling correction pass, Elmi arranged for the parser to call the spelling correction module every time it is ready for a new word (modern compilers do this with their lexical analyzers). This makes it possible to try to correct the problems created when one word garbles into another, for example, "from" is misspelled as "form" (Elmi & Evens, 1998).

Elmi also added a fourth-way match to Lee's three-way matching algorithm. That is, the system compares m_{k+1} with n_{k+1} after it compares m_k with n_k and m_{k+1} with n_k and m_k with n_{k+1}. This allows us to recognize situations in which a single letter was substituted for another and distinguish them from interpolations and deletions. Consider an example in which "pressure" is garbled to "prewsure." The three-way match algorithm decides that the "w" is an interpolated letter, changes "prewsure" to "presure" and then matches this new string to "pressure" again. Now it decides to add an "s." So it makes two corrections instead of one. The four-way match program detects the letter substitution at once and corrects the word in one step. In a long word like "pressure," two changes are feasible, but with a shorter word, the correction process may fail completely. If the error had been "prews" for "press," then Lee's system would have decided that the second change was too expensive and given up, whereas Elmi's program can make the correction rapidly (Elmi & Evens, 1998). Elmi's algorithm also assigns different weights to letter substitutions, depending on the proximity of the keys, so that replacing a letter by an adjacent letter is a very low cost change. Elmi's spelling correction program was carefully preserved when a new parser was written and it still plays a major role in the current running version of the system. Glass has recently extended it to do a better job with multiple-word phrases; basically it looks for possible phrases first before it searches for single words.

After suffering from lack of interest for 10 or 15 years, spelling correction has recently returned to center stage, because of the current interest in information retrieval from unedited web pages, which often contain spelling errors. Jurafsky and Martin (2000) discussed spelling correction at length and outlined some probabilistic approaches that might help us too. Two kinds of machine-learning algorithms have proved useful (Golding & Roth, 1999). One is based on the Winnow Algorithm and confusion sets; the other is a Bayesian approach. Confusion sets seem to be most useful when one word garbles into another ("two," "too," and "to," or "form," "from"). Bayesian approaches seem to work well in restoring missing pieces of collocations.

13.2 DESIGN OF THE LEXICON

In this section, we describe the lexicon used by the current Input Understander. If you find this discussion too technical, then please go on to the next section; you do not need the details about the lexicon to understand the rest of the system. Our main goal here is to show how little lexical knowledge is needed to do the job, and explain briefly what knowledge is needed in the lexicon and how the system uses that knowledge.

Every aspect of this work is affected by the special nature of tutorial dialogue. Students who are using this system spend most of their time answering questions from the tutor and people answering questions do not usually answer in complete sentences; instead, they supply the necessary information in a simple phrase. When this habit is combined with the well-known tendency of computer users to be as terse as possible (documented first by Thompson, 1980), the result is that many student answers consist of a cryptic word or two. The fact that the system knows what question it just asked is often an important factor in decoding the answers. Natural language front ends to databases often run into this same laconic input and also solve the problem in very much the same way (Evens, 2002).

Our spelling correction algorithms require a list of all correct strings known to the system. Timing considerations convinced us to put every form of every word in our small vocabulary into the lexicon to avoid the time penalty required for the simplest morphological analysis. Thus, we have entries for both singular and plural forms of nouns. So the lexicon includes entries for both "artery,"

artery (pos noun cm count num sing plural arteries ISA blood_vessel)

and "arteries."

arteries (pos noun num plural reference artery)

with "arteries" listed first.

In our entries, "pos" stands for "part of speech" and "num" for "number" and "sing" for "singular." The attribute called "cm" tells us whether we are looking at a count noun or a mass noun

(Conlon & Evens, 1994a). Count nouns can occur with quantifiers like "three" or "many" and when they appear in the singular, they require a determiner of some kind. Mass nouns appear with "some" and "much" and they are always singular in our sublanguage, although McCawley (1979) has identified the plural mass nouns "guts" and "clothes." The count-mass indicator helps the system to generate "many arteries" but "much resistance." The ISA relation can be paraphrased as "is a kind of" or just "is a." This field tells us where the noun appears in the noun ontology, so the lexical entry encodes the knowledge that an artery is a kind of blood vessel.

Phrasal nouns also have entries. The entry for "Total_Peripheral_Resistance" reads as follows: (pos noun cm mass num singular ISA parameter abbrev TPR). The abbreviation TPR has an abbreviated entry of its own:

TPR (pos noun abbrev-for Total_Peripheral_Resistance)

The system looks in the entry for "Total_Peripheral_Resistance" to discover that it is dealing with a mass noun, so it will generate "TPR is ...." but "An artery is ...."

Adjective entries are marked with "pos adj." These entries also indicate whether the adjective is stative or not stative (i.e., dynamic). Stative adjectives cannot be used with progressive forms of the verb or in imperatives; dynamic adjectives can. So "Be careful!" is a well-formed sentence but "Be low!" is not, and "You are being careful" is appropriate and "Your prediction is being low" is not. (For more discussion of these issues, see Conlon, Evens, Ahlswede, & Strutz, 1993.)

Adjective entries also include positional information. That is, they indicate whether the adjective can be used attributively, as in "the low pressure," or predicatively, as in "the pressure is low." If the adjective can appear after the noun, like "enough" in "Do you have evidence enough to support this theory?" the pair "postpositive yes" is added to the entry. If the adjective can support sentential complements, as "certain" does in "Are you certain that HR will increase?" the information that it takes the complementizer "that" is also included. The entry for the adjective "low" has the following form:

low (pos adj stative yes attributive yes predicative yes comparative lower superlative lowest)

Comparative and superlative forms have brief entries of their own:

lower (pos comparative reference low)

lowest (pos superlative reference low)

Adverb entries (Conlon & Evens, 1994b) contain the part of speech information, some positional information, and the semantic class (time, duration, location, cause, etc.). Words that some authorities call conjunctive adverbs like "when" and "because" are classified as subordinate conjunctions (pos conjunction type subordinate), whereas "and," "but," and "for" are classified as coordinate conjunctions.

Interjections like "OK," "wrong," and "Great!" have very simple entries with just a part of speech tag (pos interjection) and an indication of whether they are positive or negative.

The most interesting entries belong to verbs. These entries contain a complete set of verb forms, an indicator of whether the verb is stative or dynamic (not stative), that is, whether it can appear in progressive forms and in imperatives), and an indication of whether it can appear in the passive. So the entry for "fall" reads as follows:

fall (pos verb stative no passive no present fall v3s falls ving falling ved fell ven fallen)

There are also entries for the other forms of the verb:

fallen (pos ven reference fall)

falling (pos ving reference fall)

falls (pos v3s reference fall)

fell (pos ved reference fall)

In addition, every verb has one or more entries in the case table. The verb "fall" has only one, but "decrease" has two, one for the intransitive sense and one for the transitive one. We use these entries to recognize that when a student says:

"The decrease in CO increased CVP"

she means that Central Venous Pressure went up, but when she says just:

"CO increased."

she means that Cardiac Output went up.

The case table has a row for each argument of the verb and five columns: the first identifies the verb sense, the second gives the grammatical role of the argument, the third gives its semantic role or case (using the inventory of cases in Allen, 1987, expanded from Fillmore, 1968), the fourth gives its occurrence information, and the fifth gives its selection restrictions in our sublanguage. The occurrence alternatives are obligatory (this argument must be present), optional (this slot may be empty), or elliptical (this slot may be empty if the filler is clear from the context, as in "We gave at the office."). The case table also includes an example for each sense for the convenience of human readers (Conlon et al., 1994; Dardaine, 1992). The entries for the verb "increase" appear in Table 13.1. This lexicon was largely built by hand, but Chung Hee Lee (Lee, Seu, & Evens, 2002a, 2002b; Lee & Evens, 2004a) is now building tools for lexicon construction that we can use in the next tutoring system (which is discussed further in Chapter 20).

13.3 WHAT THE PARSER NEEDS TO DO

The job of the parser is to turn the student's answer into a logic form for use by the student modeler and the planner. The analysis must

TABLE 13.1
Case Table Entries for the Verb "Increase"

Verb	***Syntactic Role***	***Semantic Role***	***Occurrence***	***Selection Restrictions***
increase1	subject	theme	obligatory	parameter
	Example—Central venous pressure increased.			
increase2	subject	agent	obligatory	event
increase2	direct object	theme	obligatory	parameter
	Example—The fall in cardiac output increased central venous pressure.			

depend, of course, on the question that the student is assumed to be trying to answer. If the question is, "What is the change in CVP?" then all the answers that could possibly signal an increase in CVP would be mapped into the logic form

(ANSWER (INCREASE CVP))

including all of the following:

CVP increases

It increases

up

I (often an abbreviation for "increase," not a pronoun, in our tutoring context)

+

It went up

CVP rose

Of course, the student may not know the answer, so the parser needs to consider the possibility that the student is trying to tell us that the CVP decreased or stayed the same. The student may also reasonably respond with "I don't know." If the student input cannot be interpreted as describing a change in CVP, or as a statement of inability to answer, then the Input Understander must try to interpret it as one of the few student initiatives it can handle:

I am confused about Central Venous Pressure

Tell me about Central Venous Pressure

What is Central Venous Pressure, anyway?

These initiatives all get translated into the logic form

(QUESTION (DEFINE CVP))

which indicates that the Input Understander believes that the student is asking a question rather than answering one and then gives its best guess at the substance of the request. The logic form is then sent back to the Planner, which sends it off to the Student Modeler.

Our informal logic forms are based on the work of Graeme Hirst (1987), Martha Palmer (1990), and David Kieras (Bovair & Kieras, 1985). Kieras's work is itself largely based on the work of Walter Kintsch (1974). (For a more complete discussion, see J. H. Kim, 1997.)

13.4 LEE'S BOTTOM-UP CHART PARSER

It seems as if any attempt to use classical parsing techniques to parse input that consists of short phrases with a few complete sentences sprinkled here and there, should start bottom up. That is, it should start by combining words into phrases, and those phrases into bigger phrases, and the bigger phrases into sentences. Almost all practical parsers use a chart or a table to store intermediate results so that they do not have to be recomputed.

The decision to use a bottom-up chart parser was reinforced by some of the early work on ill-formed input (Granger, 1983; Hayes & Mouradian, 1981; Jensen, Heidorn, Miller, & Ravin, 1983; Kwasny, 1981; Miller, Heidorn, & Jensen, 1981; Weischedel & Sondheimer, 1983).

When this project began, our intention was to use Bresnan's (1982) Lexical Functional Grammar approach in both parsing and generating language. At that time existing grammars of English were designed for parsing expository text full of complete and correct declarative sentences, not for parsing one- or two-word answers to questions. We had to build a grammar of our own for the fragments that medical students type in response to questions from a tutor, mostly noun phrases such as variable names and names of stages, sometimes verbs or verb phrases, occasionally an adverb or an adjective. When the students type a complete sentence, it is often a very simple one. We used Kaplan's Grammar-Writer's Workbench to develop our grammar and we strongly recommend it (Kaplan, 1999; Kaplan & Bresnan, 1982). Yoon Hee Lee (Y. H. Lee, 1990; Y. H. Lee & Evens, 1998) wrote a simple bottom-up chart parser (Winograd, 1983) to produce a parse tree or constituent structure (c-structure), and then implemented Wescoat's (1987) algorithm to build a semantic representation or functional structure (called the f-structure) from the c-structure.

Given the sentence "The Central Venous Pressure increased," the tokenization process looks up words in the lexicon, recognizes that the three words "Central Venous Pressure" name one single concept abbreviated "CVP," and produces the string "(the cvp increased)." The parser starts by looking up the part-of-speech information in the lexicon and creates a new list (DET N V) to record that it has found a determiner ("the"), a noun ("cvp"), and a main verb ("increased"). It scans the string (DET N V), recognizes that the DET and N form a legal noun phrase (NP) and that the V by itself can form a verb phrase (VP), and records the structure (NP VP), which forms a legal sentence. The corresponding tree, displayed in Fig. 13.6, is called a constituent structure or c-structure in Lexical Functional Grammar terminology.

The corresponding semantic representation or functional structure (shown in Table 13.2) is a list that records grammatical relationships and other semantic information. The functional structure tells us that the main verb is "increase," that its subject is "CVP" and that "CVP" is singular and modified by a definite determiner, "the." Then it is matched with the case frame table, which gives us the correct sense of increase—so we can tell that this sentence means that CVP itself went up, not that CVP made something else go up. As it turned out, Michael and Rovick were not satisfied with the performance of the Input Understander and thus were unwilling to try out the system with large groups of students.

13.5 GLASS'S CASCADE OF FINITE-STATE MACHINES

Michael Glass (1999, 2001) took on the challenge of building a new parser and chose an information extraction approach that capital-

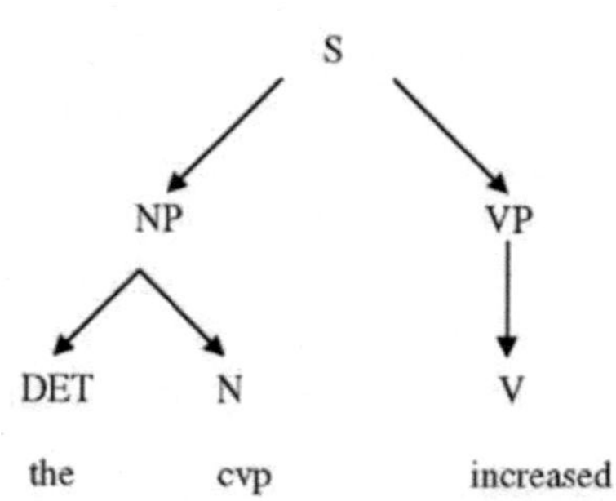

FIG. 13.6. Parse tree or LFG constituent-structure for a simple sentence.

TABLE 13.2
Semantic Representation or Functional Structure for "The CVP Increased"

```
((PRED @ increase (SUBJ)
         (TENSE PAST)
         (VOICE ACTIVE))
  (SUBJ (PRED @ cvp)
         (NUM sing)
         (SPEC the)
         (DEF+))
```

izes on the fact that the system knows what to expect from the student most of the time. The information extraction approach combines Schank's work on semantic grammars (Schank & Riesbeck, 1981) with approaches that adapt more conventional parsing techniques to handle ill-formed input (J. G. Carbonell & Hayes, 1983; Granger, 1983; Hayes & Mouradian, 1981; Kwasny, 1981). Lehnert (1997) contains an excellent review of the evolution of information extraction through the Message Understanding Conferences (MUCs) over the last 10 years and described its great strides in the processing of ill-formed input. Glass has replaced Yoon Hee Lee's parser with a parser that uses the information extraction approach, based on the emerging technology of cascaded finite automata (Roche & Schabes, 1997).

Glass created a separate finite state machine for each of the more perplexing parsing problems in our domain. He created a finite state machine to look for forms of negation (*no, not, never,* etc.). He built another one to detect forms of the verb "to be" (and distinguish the abbreviation "IS" for Inotropic State from the verb form "is"). He built still another to look for changes in parameters like "increase," "decrease," "go up," and "go down."

Most important, the new parser can build logic forms for a larger fraction of the input than the old parser and it runs very rapidly. When it cannot make sense of the input, it tells the student what kind of input it is expecting. Another change was made in the overall organization of the system, when the new parser was inserted into the system. The Input Understander now calls the student modeler directly and together the two modules determine how to classify the student's answer (Zhou et al., 1999a, 1999b). The categories recognized are "near miss" (unexpected but correct), partially correct but missing some essential information, partially correct and partially wrong, "grain of truth" (first recognized by Woolf, 1984, the wrong answers in this category contain a correct concept that the tutor can use as the basis for a productive tutoring interaction), "I don't know" answers, and totally wrong answers. This categorization enables a much wider range of responses. Also, the earlier versions of the system told the student that he or she was wrong whenever the student typed an unexpected answer, even when that answer was correct; adding the ability to make good replies to these near misses is a big step forward.

One elegant feature of Glass's (2001) Input Understander is the ability to handle "algebraic sentences" with a mixture of English and equations. There are two equations involving parameters that the system needs to discuss with the student (see Table 2.3). The students express these equations in a number of different ways:

K7-st-100-1: But isn't CO × TPR =MAP ?

K40-st-109-1: CO =SV×HR.

K13-st-52-1: Sv times hr =co

Understanding student input involving equations and making appropriate responses is well known to be a tricky problem (Gertner, 1998; Gertner, Conati, & VanLehn, 1998; Mark, Koedinger, & Hadley, 1998). Glass extended our grammar to support these expressions. Then, to make sure that the students know that the system can handle this kind of input, he and Zhou (Zhou et al., 1999b) added hints like the following:

T: MAP = TPR × what?

13.6 TESTING GLASS'S NEW INPUT UNDERSTANDER

In November 1999, we conducted a test of CIRCSIM-Tutor with the first-year class in Physiology at Rush Medical College, using the new Screen Manager (Chapter 17) and the Glass Input Understander

(1999), which had also been used in April and November 1998. We have 42 pretests and posttests but only 35 transcripts, because 14 students used the system in pairs. All 35 copies of the system were robust enough to survive an hour or more of use. Here is an example (13.1, from Session 8) of the system coping with a student near miss—"preload" is a correct answer to the question, but it is not the name of a Prediction Table parameter, so the tutor asks for another name and gets "vp," which the spelling correction program maps into "CVP" or "Central Venous Pressure," the answer that the tutor expects.

Example 13.1 Fragment of Session 8 With CIRCSIM-Tutor in November 1999

T:	What are the determinants of Stroke Volume?
S:	is, afterload, preload
T:	Right, Inotropic State is one. MAP, or afterload, does affect SV, but the effect is not quantitatively important in this case. Think about what parameter in the prediction table represents preload? What is the other determinant of Stroke Volume?
S:	vp
T:	Right, Central Venous Pressure ....

There were 1,642 student inputs in total from the 35 sessions with the system, only 6 of which (0.4%), were misinterpreted by the system. Five of these errors involved failures by the spelling correction component. The sixth involved a missing vocabulary item. In this case (shown in Example 13.2), and in two of the others, the student figured out what to do in spite of the system failure and the session continued without a hitch.

Example 13.2 Missing Vocabulary From Session 23 ("Initial Stage" Has Now Been Added as a Synonym of DR)

T:	What stage must the value of Stroke Volume follow in SS?
S:	initial
T	(as an error response): Didn't recognize a stage: DR, RR or SS.
S:	DR

T:	Correct, the value of Stroke Volume follows the value of Stroke Volume in DR.

In the other three cases, shown in Examples 13.3, 13.4, and 13.5, the student input was totally misunderstood by the system, but the students managed to recover and continue the dialogue. Two of the three cases of major confusion involved the same student (from Session 35). In Example 13.3, the student typed "storke voulme" for "stroke volume" and the spelling correction module corrected "storke" to "stores" and "voulme" to "volume." Fortunately, the student was able to figure out the answer in spite of the system's mistakes.

Example 13.3 An Embarrassing Fragment From Session 35 in November 1999

T:	Blood Volume determines CVP. However, no change in blood volume occurs in this situation. Think about another determinant.
S:	storke volume
T:	(an error response): Please respond with prediction table parameters
S:	stroke volume

The second recognition failure in Session 35, shown in Example 13.4, is even more embarrassing. The system changed "Venour" to "Veins" and totally lost track of the parameter name "Central Venous Pressure." Then it decided that "pressure" unmodified must refer to MAP.

Example 13.4 An Even More Embarrassing Fragment From Session 35

T:	Stroke Volume is determined by Central Venous Pressure and Inotropic State. Which determinant is dominant in this case?
S:	central venour pressure
T:	Nope, the important determinant of Stroke Volume in this case is not Mean Arterial Pressure. The important determinant of Stroke Volume in this case is Central Venous Pressure.

In the third example of total misunderstanding (shown in Example 13.5), the student gives a wrong answer that the system cannot interpret and gets a very unhelpful error response from the system. She finally gives a wrong answer "heart rate" that the system does understand and receives appropriate feedback.

Example 13.5 Version 2 Is Clueless in November 1999

T:	What is the other determinant of Mean Arterial Pressure?
S:	reflex
T	(error response): Please respond with prediction table parameters
S:	-
T:	(error response): Please respond with prediction table parameters
S:	clueless
T	(error response): Please respond with prediction table parameters
S:	heart rate

The first change made to the spelling correction program after this experiment was to make it look for phrases before it searches for single words. We also made some additions to the vocabulary. From the very beginning, the system has recognized "I" and "IN" as synonyms of "increase." We decided that we needed to recognize them as synonyms of "inverse" in the right context after finding multiple examples where the students tried to use them this way. We also decided to add "initial stage" as a synonym of "DR" after looking at Example 13.4 from Session 23.

There were 86 inputs out of the 1,642 (5.3%) where the system decided it could not interpret the student input correctly and issued an error message explaining what kind of input it was looking for. We scored all of these as appropriate uses of this strategy, but in a number of these situations, an expert human tutor could have made productive use of the student answer. There are several instances where the student is trying to correct the value of a variable rather than answer the tutor's current question, as in Example 13.6. We are now trying to figure out how to detect this kind of situation.

Example 13.6 Student Is Determined to Correct the Value of CO in SS

T:	What stage must the value of Cardiac Output follow in SS?
S:	no change
T	(error response): Didn't recognize a stage: DR, RR or SS.
S:	decrease
T	(error response): Didn't recognize a stage: DR, RR or SS.
S:	0
T	(error response): Didn't recognize a stage: DR, RR or SS.
S:	no change in ss
T:	Nope, the value of Cardiac Output doesn't follow the value of Cardiac Output in SS.

A problem for any system that handles typed input is how to cope with expressions of student frustration. We received several unprintable comments during the student trials in November 1998. We expect to see more when the system is more widely used, especially if the system is being used in the middle of the night on a home computer. We certainly expected to see more of the same in November 1999. But all we saw is the "clueless" in Example 13.5 and two answers "jj" and "kl" from another student who got stuck. To avoid this kind of student frustration, if the student does not get the point after two error messages, the system now gives the answer. This solution avoids, or at least mitigates, the unfortunate system behavior shown in Examples 13.5 and 13.6.

We would like to think that our improvements have made the system less frustrating to use, but it seems more likely that the student restraint was due to the presence of several Computer Science graduate students, who were there to handle system crashes (fortunately there were none) and to make sure that no medical student left without taking the posttest and filling out the survey form. At this point, we just treat this kind of input like any other input that the system does not understand. This approach lets us change the subject in a dignified way but it may not seem very responsive to an angry student. Should we add a list of curse words to the lexicon and an apology to the list of discourse strategies? We are not sure.

Several problems turned up during this experiment that we had failed to discover in earlier ones. There are several places where the system generates ungrammatical sentences. The students did not comment on these at all, but there was one place where the system announced that it was going to ask the student questions, but did not do so if the student predictions were all correct. This resulted in annoyed comments from the students, who otherwise liked the system and asked if they could use it again when reviewing for examinations.

Before we carried out another large-scale experiment in November 2002, Glass fixed the grammar and altered the spelling correction module so that it considers phrases as candidate corrections before it handles individual inputs. The resulting Input Understander performed extremely well (described in more detail in Chapter 18). There were no embarrassing failures like those seen in 1999. There were about the same number of student inputs per session (a total of 2,980 student inputs in 66 sessions for an average of 45.15 per session). There were 130 inputs (an average of 1.97 per session or 4.3% of the whole) where the system did not understand the student input and produced an error message (see Table 13.3) telling the student what kind of input it was expecting. There were 12 occasions where the student still did not answer appropriately after receiving two of these messages. The system then gave the student the answer and continued on to the next topic. In all of these cases, the session continued with no problems.

The changes to the spelling correction module were a definite success. The system corrected 104 spelling errors but made no recognizable miscorrections. It did, however, fail to correct "lood volume" to "blood volume" and "soconstriction" to "vasoconstriction."

Glass added a number of open questions to the system in November 2002. The system delivers an open question when the student

TABLE 13.3

System Messages When the Input Is Not Understood (The Column on the Right Indicates the Number of Times this Message Was Displayed in 66 Sessions in November 2002)

Please indicate increased, decreased, or unchanged.	19
Is the mechanism of control neural or physical?	24
Please respond with prediction table parameters.	61
Please indicate a stage: DR, RR or SS.	17
Please indicate directly or inversely related.	9

makes a complete set of correct predictions. Our goals were to collect data about how students would answer these questions and also to provide a richer experience for good students, who were shortchanged by the system before. Because we assumed that the system would not be able to understand the results, we rolled out a "canned" answer using example explanations from human tutoring sessions, no matter what input the student provided.

Most of the answers to open questions that students provided in November 2002 were longer and more substantive than those we see in response to ordinary system questions and we definitely want to continue in this direction (Lee, Evens, & Glass, 2004b). But most were relatively simple in sentence structure and the current Input Understander could have handled many of them. Parsing the answers to open questions is our next goal.

We hope that when the students discover that the system can understand their answers, they will begin to produce the kinds of student initiatives that we see in human tutoring sessions (Shah et al., 2002). As Freedman (1997a) has pointed out, we can only hope to respond to those initiatives that are relevant to the current tutoring goals of the system. But, in fact, the majority of the initiatives identified by Shah are attempts by the student to state a minitheory that explains a current issue. Of course, we may need to implement some understanding of the students' plan (Carberry, 1991) to recognize whether the student is trying to ask a question, confirm a theory, or just provide a long-winded answer to the last question from the tutor.

13.7 TAKE-HOME MESSAGE

The performance of the new Input Understander is much better than the old one, but we sacrificed generality to obtain this better performance. The original concept behind Lee's approach to student answers was to expand the words and phrases into complete sentences. In moving to Glass's parser, we abandoned this approach in favor of analyzing the answers as utterances in their own right, not as elliptical forms of sentence-long responses. This approach is both more manageable and more scientific. Glass's parser does a much better job of handling the main task, parsing short answers. On the other hand, it is less general, and also less able to handle long student inputs, like student initiatives.

We also lost something important in abandoning the LFG paradigm for the Input Understander. There are times when a human tutor repeats what the student said, or some part of what the student said. This behavior was easier to synthesize when both the Text Generator and the Input Understander used the same logic form, c-structure, and f-structure, and deposited these structures in the Dialogue History. Now the Dialogue History contains only strings and logic forms, because the two modules do not use the same kind of intermediate forms.

We have been asked if logic forms are really necessary. Some kind of semantic representation of the student input is absolutely essential. There are dozens of ways to say that a parameter increased and a semantic representation gives us a canonical form, which can also be used to update the representation of what the student knows in the student model. Students constantly provide partially correct answers; the system needs to be able to tell the student what was right and what was wrong in this answer. Human tutors paraphrase student answers all the time. CIRCSIM-Tutor does not paraphrase well, but it could not do so at all without a system of semantic representation.

14

Student Modeling

In this chapter, we describe various student models that we have envisioned and built as well as some of our ideas about possible future work on student modeling. Figure 14.1 attempts to summarize the variety of approaches to modeling.

14.0 ARGUMENTS FOR STUDENT MODELING

When we started the CIRCSIM-Tutor project 15 years ago, some experts in the field argued that student modeling was too difficult to be worth the trouble; some even classified the problem as totally intractable (Self, 1990). Anyone who observes human tutors in action, on the other hand, must recognize that they base decisions at all levels, from the choice of the next problem to present to the student to what kind of hint to provide, on their model of the student (Hume, 1995; Hume, Michael, Rovick, & Evens, 1996b; Katz, Lesgold, Eggan, & Gordin, 1993; Khuwaja, 1994; Khuwaja & Patel, 1996). Joel Michael and Allen Rovick were so convinced of the crucial importance of modeling that they picked the CIRCSIM domain for our tutor largely because they felt that it would be easy to construct a good student model in this subject area and that collecting predictions in the Prediction Table would give us a good basis for developing a sound model. As is clear from our discussion of tutoring protocols in Chap-

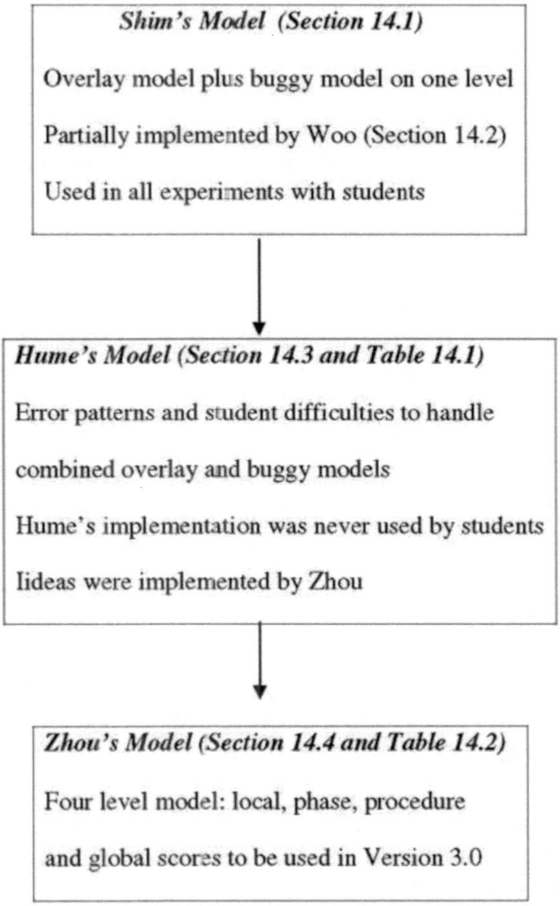

FIG. 14.1. Changes in the student model.

ter 7, they are also convinced that it is important to build a comprehensive model before starting to tutor, to ensure that the tutor can begin by attacking the most important of the student's conceptual difficulties.

Of course, when we talk about a student model, we are not really modeling what the student thinks, we are modeling the tutor's view of the student's knowledge of the task at hand. Kurt VanLehn (1988) was one of the first to make this distinction and to argue for the importance of trying to understand the student's view of the tutoring process, as well.

14.1 SHIM'S MODEL

Joel Michael and Allen Rovick found it more difficult to talk about their own internal models of the student than about any other parts of the human tutoring process. When attempts to discuss these issues failed, Leem Shim pored over our first set of eight tutoring transcripts and read the existing literature on modeling. He came up with a plan to make use of the two principal approaches to student modeling employed at the time: overlay models and buggy models.

An overlay model essentially records that part of the domain knowledge that the system believes that the student knows (VanLehn, 1988). It is called an overlay model because it can be viewed as a kind of tracing of part of the expert's model. A buggy model, on the other hand, is a record of the misconceptions or bugs in the domain that students are likely to have, along with an indication of which of these affects the thinking of the student in question (J. S. Brown & Burton, 1978; J. S. Brown & VanLehn, 1980; VanLehn, 1982).

An overlay is typically implemented either by tagging those elements in the knowledge base that are known by the student or by making a copy of those features of the knowledge base that the student knows. Shim chose the second approach because it made it simpler to leave room for a history of the student's use of that knowledge. This approach also makes it easier to store the model when the student has finished, for use in later debriefing and in evaluations of the system. It also makes it faster to start a new model when a new student starts to use the system.

For each student prediction or answer to a question involving a particular item of domain knowledge, Shim (Shim, Evens, Rovick, & Michael, 1990; Shim, Evens, Michael, & Rovick, 1991) proposed to add a "c" or a "w" to the model string for that item, depending on whether that use was correct or wrong. Thus, the string "wcc" records one error followed by two correct uses. Michael and Rovick agreed that this approach seemed reasonable, but they argued that when they are tutoring, they only remember recent answers, usually at most three for any given relationship. Also, they said, the most recent answer was certainly given more weight than older ones. So, in fact, we needed to weigh the answers so that

www < cww < wcw < wwc = ccw < cwc < wcc < ccc

Shim and James Kenevan, at that time a faculty member in the Computer Science Department at IIT, came up with the following simple convolution (see Knuth, 1972, pp. 290–294) to perform this task

$$v = \frac{1 * a_{n-m+1} + 2 * a_{n-m+2} + \ldots + (m-1) * a_{n-1} + m * a_n}{1 + 2 + \ldots + (m-1) + m}$$

where we have n recorded answers, $a_i = 1$ if the ith answer is c and $a_i = 0$ if the ith answer is w, and we are interested in the m most recent values. Obviously, the convolution ranges in value from 0 to 1. Its value is 0 if all the student's answers on this topic are wrong and 1 if all are correct, so the "value" v of a particular item can be viewed as a kind of probability estimate that the student knows this item. This formula is easy to calculate and it automatically gives more weight to recent values. If we want to consider only the three most recent answers, then we just set m to 3. In this case we get

v(www) = (1*0 + 2*0 + 3*0)/(1 + 2 + 3) = 0

v(cww) = (1*1 + 2*0 + 3*0)/(1 + 2 + 3) = 1/6

v(wcw) = (1*0 + 2*1 + 3*0)/(1 + 2 + 3) = 2/6 = 1/3

v(wwc) = (1*0 + 2*0 + 3*1)/(1 + 2 + 3) = 3/6 = ½

v(ccw) = (1*1 + 2*1 + 3*0)/(1 + 2 + 3) = 3/6 = ½

v(cwc) = (1*1 + 2*0 + 3*1)/(1 + 2 + 3) = 4/6 = 2/3

v(wcc) = (1*0 + 2*1 + 3*1)/(1 + 2 + 3) = 5/6

v(ccc) = (1*1 + 2*1 + 3*1)/(1 + 2 + 3) = 6/6 = 1

We considered just storing the three most recent values, but we rejected this alternative on the grounds that it would mean losing the historical record (Shim et al., 1990, 1991). Also, there are times when Michael and Rovick have displayed an extraordinary memory for past interactions, especially student initiatives and misconceptions. Moore's group has found evidence in their corpus analysis (Rosé, Moore, VanLehn, & Allbritton, 2001) for the same kind of tutor recollection of exchanges that the expert tutor considered especially salient.

The buggy model was simply a list of misconceptions plus a tally for each time that this particular student responded in a way that suggested the presence of this misconception, where a misconception is defined as an incorrect mental model, containing something that the individual considers to be true, although it is actually false. Misconceptions are typically much harder to dislodge than an ordinary gap in the student's knowledge, such as a missing relationship (Chi & Roscoe, 2002). Students are typically ready, even happy, to fill these gaps and can do so easily. Misconceptions, on the other hand, often give rise to a whole structure of false beliefs, which are difficult and costly for the student to relinquish (Chi & Roscoe, 2002; Ohlsson, 1987, 1992; Smith, diSessa, & Roschelle, 1993; Wandersee, Mintzes, & Novak, 1994). Feltovich, Spiro, and Coulson (1989) have shown that practicing physicians retain some of the misconceptions and faulty mental models that Michael and Rovick see in first-year medical students. Caramaza, McCloskey, and Green (1981) have studied common misconceptions in physics and Minstrell and Kraus (2001) have made an exhaustive catalog of such misconceptions. Further discussion of the ways in which Michael and Rovick treat misconceptions can be found in Chapters 6, 7, and 8.

The accumulated experience with students of our expert tutors that led them to compile the list of misconceptions can be called a *generic student model.* We argued about whether to initialize the student model using a generic model based on the accumulated experience of our expert tutors, but they decided that they did not feel comfortable starting with a "loaded model" that assumed that the student had certain common gaps and misconceptions. When tutoring themselves, they try to start tutoring a new student with an open mind about how that student will perform, although they have a list of possible misconceptions that may underlie the students' responses. They wanted CIRCSIM-Tutor to start the same way, so we initialize the student model so that it is empty of information. That is, unknown values are set to 0.5, which is halfway between belief that the student does not know about this item ($v = 0$) and belief that the student does know it ($v = 1$).

14.2 STUDENT MODEL BUILT BY WOO AND ZHANG

Chong Woo (1991) carried out the actual implementation of the modeler in the process of constructing Version 2.0 of CIRCSIM-Tutor. Yuemei Zhang (1991) and Woo added a number of frames to the knowledge base to simplify the overlay. The knowledge base already contained frames for each Prediction Table parameter, including HR and CO, but they added frames for each relationship (like that between HR and CO) to make it easier to record a correct use of that relationship or a prediction or an answer that violates that relationship. They also created frames for several more general concepts such as "neural variable" and "hemodynamic (non-neural) variable." (See Chapter 2 for an explanation of these terms.) Although the relational information was already stored in the associated parameter frames, it was faster and easier to store and query information in the model with these new frames. These new frames also made it easier to generate appropriate dialogue about these concepts and relationships. But because no current tutoring rules made use of any information in the model except the most recent answer, no answer history was stored and the convolution was never used. This discovery really brought home to us an important principle of student modeling: it is not useful to store a particular piece of information in the model unless some rule somewhere in the system makes use of that knowledge, that is, unless it is part of the precondition of some rule.

14.3 INFERRING MISCONCEPTIONS

The next major contribution to the student model was the work of Gregory Hume (1995). In the process of analyzing the transcripts to determine the hinting behavior of the expert tutors (see Chapter 8), he refined the bug list in the original model (shown in Table 6.1) into a table containing the underlying misconceptions in cardiovascular physiology and the error patterns that the expert tutors used to detect them. This list of misconceptions and associated error patterns can be seen in Table 14.1.

Hume's (1995) approach gave us a way to combine the overlay model and the buggy model into one. Hume associated a (potential) student difficulty with each item of the domain knowledge base, as well as with each misconception. Then he set up pointers from each error pattern to one or more student difficulty. This makes it possible to store both kinds of difficulties in the same way with just a flag to mark the misconceptions. The first error pattern in Table 14.1 is triggered when a student predicts that a neural variable will change in DR.

TABLE 14.1
Misconceptions and the Error Patterns That Reveal Them

Misconception	*Error or Error Pattern*
Confusion about DR	Predicted change to neural variable in DR
Confusion about difference between preload and inotropic state (both determinants of stroke volume)	IS prediction error with answer referring to preload, filling, or Frank-Starling
Preload confusion	CVP to SV relationship error
Input–output balance across the heart	CO to CVP relationship error
Afterload confusion	MAP to SV relationship error
Regulated variable confusion	MAP in RR is NOT opposite to MAP in DR
Reflex fully compensates for disturbance	MAP in SS is predicted to be 0
Neural reflex confusion	Neural variables in RR are not predicted to change in the opposite direction from MAP in DR
DR determines SS confusion	SS predictions differ from RR predictions
"Clamped" variable confusion	Neural variable that is "clamped" (held constant in DR) is predicted to change in RR
Causality/algebra confusion	Student solves equation of form A = B*C for B or C and infers causality from new equation

Note. DR = Direct Response; IS = Inotropic State; CVP = Central Venous Pressure; SV = Stroke Volume; CO = Cardiac Output; MAP = Mean Arterial Pressure; RR = Reflex Response; SS = Steady State.

Faced with this error pattern, the expert tutors typically investigate the possibility that the error was due to a slip (the student knows the correct answer but makes a careless error) or that the student is confused about whether a parameter is a neural variable. They rule out these simple possibilities before they go to work on the hypothesis that the student does not understand the definition of the DR period. This difficulty is common enough so that we have a special schema to handle it, called the *neural DLR*. They have developed complex schemas for other remediation processes, which they have discovered to be effective by repeated trial and error. (See Chapter 7 for further discussion of these schemas.)

Given the first error pattern (a prediction that an unclamped neural variable, say TPR, has changed in DR), the tutor will first probe to find out whether the student knows that TPR is indeed a neural variable, asking the following: "By what mechanism is TPR controlled?" If the student answers this question correctly, the tutor goes on to ask whether the student knows the definition of DR. If the student can answer this question correctly, and can then infer that TPR has not changed after all, the tutor assumes that the student is not in the grip of the underlying misconception and goes on to another topic. Otherwise, the tutor explains what DR means and asks the student to make the correct inference. If the student is still stuck, the tutor will deliver a brief explanation. We have tried to implement these schemas using tutoring plans.

The difficulty of detecting a misconception is increased by the fact that the list of error patterns contains some overlaps. An incorrect prediction for the neural variable once called *Cardiac Contractility* (CC) and now more often labeled *Inotropic State* (IS) can point to several different misconceptions. The tutors usually look for the DR confusion, if the session is still in the DR phase. But if the session is now in the RR phase, the problem may be the regulated variable confusion. If the student actually mentions filling or the Frank-Starling Law or the length-tension curve, then the tutors suspect that the student has IS confused with the Frank-Starling curve. The schema for the remediation of this last misconception is described in Chapter 7. As we saw there, the expert tutors usually try to complete this task in an interactive fashion, asking the student a series of questions. Because we were worried about the system's ability to sustain this approach, Zhou (2000, p. 98) produced a single-turn "canned" version for use in Versions 2.8 and 2.9:

T: By what mechanism is Inotropic State controlled?

S: It is filling.

T: Well, you are confusing the Frank-Starling effect (increased filling gives greater output) and contractility. Inotropic State (contractility) is the force of contraction at any given filling or at an end diastolic volume. An increase in sympathetic stimulation of the myocardium increases the Inotropic State of the muscle. So it is neurally controlled. (p. 98)

Hume (1995) also uncovered the depths of the experts' pessimism about misconceptions. They believe that if the student has come up with three correct answers in a row for an item in the overlay model (which corresponds to a value v of 1), then the student almost certainly knows that item. The experts are not nearly so sanguine about misconceptions, however. First of all, they expect that it will be much harder to correct a misconception than an ordinary error, because students often develop further false theories based on an underlying misconception. They have developed several special-purpose schemas for dealing with the most common misconceptions, like the plan for remediation of the confusion between IS and Frank-Starling described in Chapter 7. These plans are based on many past attempts to teach this material in class and in small-group tutoring sessions. They tend to be rather pessimistic about the success of these plans. They do not expect that two or three repetitions will succeed in demolishing a misconception. We have tentatively set a threshold of five as the number of correct repetitions that will allow the system to believe that a misconception has been cured, following evidence that a student suffers from a given misconception.

14.4 ZHOU'S FOUR-LEVEL MODEL

Some of Hume's ideas about hints and misconceptions were implemented by Zhou (Zhou & Evens, 1999) in time for the system trials in November 1999, but the majority were not implemented until after that experiment and were not tried with students until November 2002. The core of her version of the system is a new four-level student model; each level of the model (shown in Table 14.2) provides the input for a different set of planning rules. The lowest level of the model, the local assessment, contains a score for the student performance on each concept tutored. The rest of the scores are computed from the scores at the next lower level and from the Prediction Table score (Zhou, 2000).

Two scores are computed at this lowest level: the performance in tutoring this concept (What proportion of the questions received correct answers?) and the performance in responding to hints (What proportion of the hints succeeded?). The next level, the phase assessment, is based on three scores: the Prediction Table performance

TABLE 14.2
The Four Assessments in Zhou's Model

Assessment Type
Global Assessment
Calculated from the procedures completed so far.
Procedure Assessment
Calculated from the three phases.
Phase Assessment
What proportion of the initial Prediction Table entries were correct (plus the results of the local assessments)?
Local (Concept) Assessment
What proportion of the questions received correct answers?
What proportion of the hints succeeded?

in this phase (What proportion of the seven Prediction Table variables were correctly predicted in this phase?), the performance in tutoring in this phase (based on the scores computed for each separate concept in computing the local assessment), and the performance in hinting in this phase (based on the scores computed for each separate concept in computing the local assessment).

The procedure assessment also combines the Prediction Table performance in this procedure, the performance in tutoring in this procedure, and the performance in hinting in this procedure. Each of these performance values is calculated from the performance values already computed for the three phases. The global assessment is computed from the procedure assessments in the same way.

The local assessment is recomputed after each student answer. It can be thought of as an estimate of the probability that the student knows this concept at time t. If any part of the student answer contains some correct information about this concept, then the system recalculates the probability that the student knows it using the equation

$$pKnown_t = pKnown_{t-1}(1 + wCategory)(1\text{-}pGuess)$$

where *pGuess* is the probability that the student will give a correct answer even though the skill has not been mastered and *wCategory* is the weight assigned to this answer category. If the student answer seems to contain no correct information about this concept, then *pKnown* is updated using another equation

$$pKnown_t = pKnown_{t-1}(1 - wCategory)(1 + pSlip)$$

where *pSlip* is the probability that the student will make an error even though the concept has been mastered.

Each type of assessment is used as input to a separate set of rules. The local assessment is used as input to the rules that decide whether to hint or to tell the student the correct answer during the tutoring of the current concept. This assessment is also used in deciding whether to ask a follow-up question about this concept. The phase assessment is used to decide what tutoring schemas to use next (see J. H. Kim, Freedman, Glass, & Evens, 2002). The procedure assessment is used to determine the lesson plan for the next procedure and also when to probe for misconceptions. The overall strategy is to wait until the student has mastered much of the fundamental material in the procedures before raising other issues. The global assessment is used to pick the next procedure. Zhou's student model is used to trigger the analysis of student answers and the production of hints in Version 2.9, which was tried out extensively with students in November 2002, but that version still allowed the students to pick their procedures for themselves and so did not make use of the global assessment and the curriculum planner.

14.5 RESEARCH USING THE STUDENT MODEL

At roughly the same time that Zhou was figuring out how to categorize answers, Cho (2000) designed a new function for calculating the local and global assessments for use in curriculum planning and in switching protocols, as described in Chapter 12. Cho began by calculating a Prediction Table Score (PTS), based on the number of correct predictions in the prediction table. He defined

$$\mathrm{PTS} = \sum_{i=1}^{3} \sum_{j=1}^{7} (\mathrm{PT}_{ij}) / 21$$

where $PT_{ij} = 1$ if the ith prediction score in the jth column is correct and $PT_{ij} = -1$ otherwise. Then the Local Assessment (LA) is defined in terms of the sum of the Prediction Table score and a certainty factor score based on responses made by the student during the dialogue. The score for an individual response R_n is given by the formula

$$R_n = \frac{C^2}{N * D} * 2 - 1$$

where C is the number of correct items in an answer, N is the number of items in the answer, and D is the number of items in the desired answer. For example, suppose the tutor asks for the determinants of MAP. As we have seen in Chapter 2, MAP is the product of CO and TPR, so the correct answer is CO and TPR and D = 2. Suppose the student answers that HR and TPR are the determinants. Then N = 2 and C = 1, so

$$R_n = \frac{1^2}{2.2} * 2 - 1 = -\frac{1}{2}$$

So the Certainty Factor is then computed for a given response using Shim's convolution:

$$CF = (R_{n-2} + 2 * R_{n-1} + 3 * R_n) / 6$$

Then the LA is given by summing up the CF values for all the error types:

$$LA = PTS + \sum_{i=1}^{e} (CF_i) / 2e$$

The Global Assessment (GA) is then computed from the known LA values. Let n be the number of procedures already solved. Then we add up the LA values, giving most weight to the one just completed:

$$GA = LA_n / 2 + (\sum_{p=1}^{n-1} LA_p) / 2(n-1)$$

In Chapter 17, we describe how Cho's work with the GA score has changed our interface design in some unexpected ways. We suspect that there are many other ways in which we could use changes in the student model to discover improvements in the system that by themselves may not make enough difference in the overall learning gains to be visible in a large-scale experiment, but which aggregated could make the system more comfortable to use, and in time, get the student users to express themselves more, and in the process, learn more.

When Version 3.0 of the system is finally implemented, we want to try out both Zhou's and Cho's algorithms for computing global assessments and discover whether there are any differences in performance.

If we were starting this project now, we might well build Bayesian models, like those used in tutoring by Koedinger, Corbett, Ritter, and Shapiro (2000). We have used a Bayesian inference engine in medical diagnosis with great success (Trace, Evens, Naeymi-Rad, & Carmony, 1990). This approach seems particularly appropriate in the diagnosis of misconceptions where we are reasoning from uncertainty on the basis of symptoms of that misconception. We should also explore some of the new work in cognitive assessment by Corbett and others at Carnegie Mellon University (Corbett & Trask, 2000).

Can we expand on this basic concept and discover ways to use the student model as a research tool? At this point, if we want to demonstrate that one strategy or one approach is more effective than another, we need to do an experiment with a large number of students and compare learning gains between two populations. If we had a truly reliable standard approach to student modeling, thoroughly evaluated in a variety of systems, would it be possible that system builders could compare changes in the model rather than long-term learning gains? Such a technique might be much more sensitive to differences; a detectable difference in learning gains requires a really large-scale difference between the approaches being compared. It might even be possible to compare strategies in several areas in one experiment. We hope to explore this idea further.

14.6 TAKE-HOME MESSAGE

We are even more convinced than we were when we started this project 15 years ago that good student modeling is essential to good tutoring, and the numbers of papers on modeling in the ITS conferences in the last few years make it clear that this opinion is now widely shared.

Cho's (2000) work, as described in this chapter and in Chapter 17, suggests that the student model could be a potent resource in our research and that we should look for more ways to make use of it.

It has become increasingly clear to us that planning and modeling must go hand in hand. Information in the model representing what the tutor thinks that the student knows is crucial to good planning. On the other hand, there is no point in storing information in the model unless the planner can use it. In Chapter 21, we discuss some emerging questions about whether the system should try to model the student's affect as well as the student's knowledge and how the system should respond to evidence of student distress.

15

The Domain Knowledge Base and the Problem Solver

The history of our domain knowledge base is a stormy one. The whole knowledge base has been torn apart and completely rebuilt six times and Jay Yusko (Yusko & Evens, 2002, 2004) is now building a completely new seventh version. The Domain Knowledge Base contains the knowledge about the cardiovascular system that the system is attempting to help students understand and use in solving problems, so it is vital to our system. All the major modules of the system potentially make use of the Domain Knowledge Base. Its most immediate customer, however, is the Problem Solver, which generates predictions for all of the procedures presented to the students and the answers to questions. The Problem Solver and the Domain Knowledge Base are so closely linked that it has been necessary to rebuild it every time that the knowledge base was rebuilt.

As our understanding of the complexity of the planning required for tutoring and for dialogue generation increased, we built new knowledge bases to support the tutor; each new knowledge base has required us to build a new domain problem solver. To be exact, it might be more correct to say that we built four different problem solvers, and then whenever we built a problem solver, we needed a new knowledge base to support it.

The CIRCSIM-Tutor system has several knowledge stores in addition to the Domain Knowledge Base: the Curriculum, the Lexicon, the Grammar, the Student Model, the Discourse History, and the Journal or Log File. Our goal was to put all the knowledge of the cardiovascular system in the Domain Knowledge Base, to make it easier to port the system to other domains, but some of the domain knowledge is necessarily stored in other files. The Curriculum, of course, is heavily dependent on the domain. The Lexicon contains some domain-specific terminology, of course, but this seems to be a relatively small proportion of the total word count (roughly 250 words out of 5,000). The rest of the vocabulary can be reused in any tutoring system that targets causal reasoning about changes in parameters. The Student Model also contains a partial copy of the main items in the Domain Knowledge Base and a list of a dozen domain-specific misconceptions that our expert tutors have discovered in first-year medical students. This knowledge is also specific to the teaching of this particular domain. Our tutoring strategies are, in some cases, specific to tutoring students that are solving problems using qualitative causal reasoning. However, these strategies are not necessarily specific to the circulatory system except for the schemas used to attack domain misconceptions. With these exceptions, we believe that we have succeeded in capturing the domain knowledge in the Domain Knowledge Base.

In Section 15.0, we discuss Nakhoon Kim's Prolog Prototype for CIRCSIM-Tutor and the four different versions of the knowledge base that he built to support it. Next, in Section 15.1, we discuss the construction process that resulted in the collection of frames that make up the Domain Knowledge Base of the version of the system currently in use. Section 15.2 describes how different modules in the system use that knowledge base and the other knowledge stores in the system. The remaining sections of this chapter discuss three different approaches to building the ideal knowledge base for the future. All of them have contributed ideas to the knowledge base in the emerging Version 3. Section 15.3 recounts Glenn Mayer's attempt to derive a knowledge base from text. Section 15.4 explains Khuwaja's vision of the knowledge base as a series of models. Section 15.5 describes Reva Freedman's argument that the knowledge base should consist of rules. Section 15.6 discusses the Knowledge Base for the emerging Version 3. Jay Yusko's Knowledge Collective owes much to Khuwaja's vision and to Freedman's, but its knowledge architecture is very new. Table 15.1 tries to present some of these changes in a more visual way. We close in Section 15.7 with a discussion of some of the lessons learned along the way.

15.0 THE PROLOG PROTOTYPE FOR CIRCSIM-TUTOR

Nakhoon Kim (1989), the first student to work on this project, was very interested in interactive tutoring and in problem solving, but not at all interested in natural language processing. When the CIRCSIM-Tutor project began (and long before it had funding), he fell in love with our ideas for a computer tutor and jettisoned his earlier thesis topic. Although we had always planned to build the system in Lisp, like most natural language systems, he waved away our objections and wrote a prototype in Prolog to explore issues of problem solving, session planning, and student modeling. His prototype had a graphical user interface, with no natural language anywhere except in some canned instructions, but it attacked these other problems head on. His ideas survive in the way our current system describes the problem, analyzes the Prediction Table, builds the log file, and constructs the overlay part of the student model.

The first Problem-Solver calculated the correct predictions for the first four problems in the CIRCSIM-Tutor System correctly, but it did not solve those problems in the "logical order" that Joel Michael and

TABLE 15.1
Changes in the Domain Knowledge Base

Prototype	***Version 2 (Used in All Student Experiments)***	***Version 3 (Under Construction)***
Nakhoon Kim	Chong Woo and Yuemei Zhang	Jay Yusko
Prolog	Lisp	SQL and DBMS
Rules and Prolog Facts	Frames (sometimes containing rules)	Frames, Rules, Tables

Note. DBMS = Database Management System.

Allen Rovick wanted their students to learn and use. The associated Domain Knowledge Base was a collection of Prolog Rules.

It took Nakhoon Kim only a week to write the second Problem-Solver and change the rules to produce all the answers in the logical order because many of the rules were unchanged. But there was still nothing in the Domain Knowledge Base that the system could use in guiding the student to the solution of the process.

When we explained to Kim that we needed to provide this kind of guidance, he produced the third version of the Problem Solver. This version contained a solution tree for each of the four procedures implemented; each tree represented an ideal solution path for the procedure in question. Kim described how the trees could be used in guiding the student through the solution process. Yuemei Zhang, who was building the Text Generator, agreed that the solution trees were a big step forward, but she argued that the Text Generator needed to be able not only to follow the solution trace, but to generate explanations, to state the problem-solving algorithm, and discuss it with the student.

Kim was inspired to build the fourth version of the Problem Solver, along with the fourth version of the Domain Knowledge Base, based on a hierarchical set of Prolog rules that described the problem-solving algorithms and used them to solve problems. At this point, he declared victory and integrated the pieces of the prototype system so that it could request predictions, analyze the predictions entered by the student, build an overlay model of the student's knowledge of the baroreceptor reflex, determine a set of topics to be taught, and plan how to teach them. Kim's Prolog Prototype (N. Kim, Evens, Michael, & Rovick, 1989) did not attempt to carry out a natural language dialogue with the student, but it performed all the other steps in the tutoring process and we learned a great deal from building it—especially about knowledge representation (N. Kim, 1989).

15.1 BUILDING THE CURRENT DOMAIN KNOWLEDGE BASE

The Domain Knowledge Base in the current version of CIRCSIM-Tutor (the only one to be tested with large groups of students) is the fifth one built to support the CIRCSIM-Tutor system. In 1990, Chong Woo started to work on the first complete version of the system—a Lisp program designed to carry on a conversation with the student.

Yuemei Zhang seized on the opportunity to build a Domain Knowledge Base to better support her ideas about Text Generation (Zhang, Evens, Michael, & Rovick, 1987, 1990). She and Chong Woo agreed to work together to build a collection of frames in Lisp. They began by building a frame for each parameter, with the standard abbreviation, the full name, and information about each arc in the concept map connecting it with another parameter frame. If the parameter is used in an important equation, that equation is included in the frame as well. The official definition of each parameter is also stored in its frame. Table 15.2 shows the first version of the frame for SV constructed by Zhang in 1990.

As we describe in Section 15.2.5, the Text Generator uses the official definition stored in this frame if a student asks about SV. If the student makes an error in predicting the change in SV, then the system will frequently decide to tutor the student via determinants. As we saw in Chapter 7, this schema starts out by asking the student "What are the determinants of SV?" How does the system find out what the answer should be? It looks at the slot labeled "causal-relation-in" in the SV frame and discovers that the determinants are RAP and CC (now called IS). Once the student has corrected SV, the system looks to see if

TABLE 15.2
First Frame for Stroke Volume

(frame SV	
(frame-type	variable
var-type	physically-affected
frame-name	SV
class	instance
instance-of	variable
name	"Stroke Volume"
definition	"volume of blood ejected each beat"
part-of	heart
anatomy	left ventricle
equation	CO=HR*SV
causal-relation-in	causal-RAP-SV causal-CC-SV
causal-relation-out	causal-SV-CO))

Note. Var = Variable; SV = Stroke Volume; CO = Cardiac Output; HR = Heart Rate; RAP = Right Atrial Pressure; CC = Cardiac Contractibility.

there is an error in the next variable affected, the variable determined by SV. It figures out what this variable is by looking at the slot called "Causal-relation-out" and finds out that CO comes next. If there is an error in CO, then the system may choose the move-forward strategy to tutor CO and ask what the change in SV implies for CO.

One advantage of a frame-based system is that it is easy to add more frames and easy to update existing frames. In the process of building the Domain Knowledge Base, Zhang and Woo realized that the Instructional Planner and the Text Generator, like the Problem Solver, needed frames for some more general concepts like "neural variable" or "pressure," because the Instructional Planner needed to make plans about tutoring the neural variables as a group, and the Text Generator needed to explain that "neural variables do not change in DR." These frames can be found on the CD-ROM.

Why do we have code in our frames and require the text generator to synthesize sentences from the code instead of just storing it? Zhang (1991) argued that it was essential to store the problem-solving knowledge in the Domain Knowledge Base and make the Problem Solver actually execute the algorithmic knowledge in the knowledge base, so we could be sure that the system was actually solving problems in the way the Text Generator described. Her concern was that the procedural knowledge explained by the system be the actual procedure that the system carries out. Otherwise, the system may diverge from the explanation of the reasoning process that it describes to the user. This concern was originally emphasized by Elaine Rich (1982) in the context of expert systems. Zhang insisted that the Problem Solver should use the Lisp code in the frames to solve problems. This was made easier by the fact that Lisp code has the same form as Lisp data.

Zhang (1991) was determined to make it possible for the Text Generator to explain to the student what to do next at every step, so she added to this frame the information that the neural variables in RR will change in the opposite direction from MAP in DR. She included code for other portions of the problem-solving algorithm in other frames throughout the system.

Zhang and Woo also added frames to support the Student Modeler. An important part of the student model is an overlay of the Domain Knowledge Base. It is essential to record whether the student understands the relationship between SV and CO as well as the equation relating them. The frames for SV and CO both contain the relationship information, but it turned out to be much more convenient to overlay the information about a particular relationship when the relationship has a frame of its own, so Zhang created frames for each relationship.

The last group of frames that Zhang added, the anatomy frames, caused a certain amount of controversy between the expert tutors and the implementers of the CIRCSIM-Tutor system. The experts felt that including information about anatomy in a system designed to teach physiology was totally unnecessary. Zhang looked at the session transcripts, however, and saw students asking questions about anatomy (and receiving answers from the tutors) and argued that CIRCSIM-Tutor should be able to respond to questions of this type. There are even a few spots where the tutors raise anatomy issues themselves, especially when dealing with students who are thoroughly confused, because these students often have a better grasp of the anatomy than the physiology. Finally, the two sides agreed on a compromise. The anatomy frames were added to the system with a tag labeling their special status and Woo agreed not to use them in instructional plans unless the student raised an anatomy issue first.

Michael Glass changed "CC" to "IS" when Michael and Rovick decided to follow the usage in physiology textbooks and substitute "Inotropic State" for "Cardiac Contractility," although "Cardiac Contractility" remains in the IS frame as a useful synonym. At the same time, Michael and Rovick decided to replace Right Atrial Pressure (RAP) with Central Venous Pressure (CVP) because the students kept confusing RAP with MAP (Mean Arterial Pressure). Here we are not talking about a synonym but a closely related parameter that behaves in the same way (see Figure 5.2), so that a new frame was added.

More recently, Yujian Zhou (2000) has added the frames for the parameters on all three levels of the knowledge base, and she added the slot-value pair "(level top)" to the frames for the concepts in the Prediction Table.

Zhou wrote some elegant rules to implement the new student modeler for Version 3, but she implemented the new modeler and the new hints in Version 2 by making extensions to the old Domain Knowledge Base, adding some new frames and adding more information to others. The "nearmiss" slot is used when a student answers "EDV" but the system is expecting "SV." The code to support hinting then starts a series of questions to resolve this particular near miss. A slot called "refer-to-SM" tells the system where to find the relevant information in the Student Model.

This frame knowledge base has now provided the domain knowledge for all of the versions of the system used by students. The frame knowledge base has lasted for over 10 years because it was easy to build, easy to extend, and easy to use in problem solving, student modeling, and text generation.

15.2 HOW THE DOMAIN KNOWLEDGE IS USED

We include a brief explanation of how the Domain Knowledge Base is used, because most of the changes made in it were motivated by a desire to add new functions or improve existing ones.

15.2.1 How the Problem Solver Uses the Domain Knowledge Base

The Problem Solver makes more extensive use of the Domain Knowledge Base than any other module. The Problem Solver typically starts with a procedure name and a phase in the response (DR, RR, or SS) with the goal of producing the correct predictions for that phase. The problem-solving algorithms for each phase are stored in the Domain Knowledge Base along with the frames for each parameter, so that they are available to both the Problem Solver and to the Text Generator.

The main problem-solving process starts with the primary variable (the first variable affected by the procedure). The primary variable for each procedure is stored in the Knowledge Base along with its DR value (increased, decreased, or unchanged). The current protocol (see Chapter 7) requires that the student pick the correct primary variable and enter its value correctly before proceeding down the rest of the DR column. There is an ordered list of parameters to be predicted for each phase. The problem solver goes down this list making predictions using the relationship information in each parameter frame, to decide what the value of the next variable should be. Predictions for the RR column start with MAP, then the neural variables, then the rest of the parameters in the list. Predictions for the SS column can be computed "algebraically." If the DR and RR changes are the same, then the SS change will be in the same direction. If the change in one column is 0 (no change), use the change in the other column. If the two values conflict, use the DR value.

There is also an Assistant Problem Solver that can determine the change in one parameter given another. It was also designed and implemented by Zhang (1991) with the goal of supporting the tutor in asking "what-if" questions about relationships, such as the following: "Suppose CO goes up, what will happen to CVP?" Further analysis of human tutoring sessions showed us that our expert colleagues only do this occasionally, so Version 2 of our system does not use this facility, but we have left the assistant in place with the plan of using it in Version 3.

15.2.2 How the Instructional Planner Uses the Domain Knowledge Base

At the start of each procedure, the Planner uses the Domain Knowledge Base directly to retrieve procedure descriptions and to identify the proper place to start in the process of tutoring each procedure. But once a procedure is launched, it mostly calls the other major modules to find out what it needs to know. The Instructional Planner calls the Problem Solver to obtain a correct solution for the current phase and it calls the Student Modeler to discover whether the student's latest input was relevant and correct. It calls the text generator to deliver responses and explanations to the student. The rules used in developing lesson plans and discourse plans are not currently stored in the Domain Knowledge Base, but in the Planner itself.

15.2.3 How the Input Understander Uses the Domain Knowledge Base

The Input Understander makes very little direct use of the Domain Knowledge Base. This situation seems rather anti-intuitive, for certainly expert human tutors use their domain knowledge constantly in interpreting what the student says or types. This situation seems to be largely an accident of development history. The ontology and case frames, which combine domain knowledge and information about words, were built for use in the Input Understander so they are located in the Input Understander lexicon. Similarly, the identification and classification of errors and misconceptions was assigned to the Student Modeler, because it was already identifying correct answers. One of the goals for our new knowledge base is to locate as much knowledge as possible in stable structures that all the modules can easily access.

15.2.4 How the Student Modeler Uses the Domain Knowledge Base

In the first version of the system, the Student Modeler did not access the Domain Knowledge Base directly. Instead, it called the Problem Solver to decide whether a student answer (or rather a logic form derived from a student answer by the Input Understander) was right or wrong. This changed when we realized that we needed to classify answers in a more fine-grained fashion as near misses or grain of truth answers, and so forth. (See Chapter 13 for more details of this classification.) To carry out this classification process more precisely, the Student Modeler needs to associate possible near misses with certain parameters and relationships. This information is now stored in the frames in the Domain Knowledge Base and accessed there by the Student Modeler.

15.2.5 How the Text Generator Uses the Domain Knowledge Base

There are several places where the text generator just reels out canned text stored in the Domain Knowledge Base. This does not take much intelligence but it is certainly convenient. For example, the Domain Knowledge Base contains an official definition for each parameter in the Prediction Table. When the student types "What is Inotropic State?" or "Tell me about Inotropic State" or "I'm confused about Inotropic State," the Input Understander codes the input as follows:

(Request (Define IS))

The Planner passes on this request to the Text Generator and it retrieves the verbatim version of the definition from the Domain Knowledge Base and displays it in the dialogue window.

The Text Generator also uses the list of procedures in this way. Associated with each procedure, such as the blood donation procedures, we store a procedure description and a problem summary. The problem statement is displayed in a special window as soon as the student picks that procedure off the menu. The problem summary is displayed as part of the dialogue when the student finishes correcting any errors in the last (SS) phase of the problem-solving process.

The Text Generator also uses the Domain Knowledge Base to construct simple explanations, such as the following: "Central blood volume is inversely related to cardiac output" or "The increase in cardiac output will cause central blood volume to go down." The information necessary to generate these sentences can be found in the frames for central blood volume (CBV) and CO.

15.3 BUILDING A KNOWLEDGE BASE FROM TEXT

Over the same period of time (1990–1991) that Zhang and Woo were building the Knowledge Base in Version 2 (Section 15.1), Glenn Mayer engaged in a parallel but separate effort to build a knowledge base for cardiovascular physiology by parsing a chapter about the cardiovascular system written by Joel Michael.

Mayer used Naomi Sager's (1981) Linguistic String Parser, developed at New York University. This parser had a magnificent medical lexicon, even then. At that point, it had been used to parse more running text than any other parser in existence. The parser produces elegant output in tree form as well as in a fully parenthesized Lisp expression. Mayer (1992) also found Sager's approach to logical representation, her information formats, very intellectually attractive, and developed his own system of information formats for the cardiovascular domain. He then wrote a program to turn the information formats produced by the parser into frames, much like those that Zhang and Woo were building by hand.

Although Mayer's Knowledge Base was not directly used by the system, it became another source of frames for the Domain Knowledge Base built by Zhang and Woo. They read Mayer's output with care and adopted several frames that they had somehow missed. Mayer's ontology for cardiovascular terms was also the basis of later work on ontology by Freedman (1996c) and by Chung Hee Lee (Lee,

Seu, & Evens, 2002a, 2000b). Chiye Yamamoto, a master's student in Computer Science, spent many hours reading Sager's work (1981, 1986) and then creating the additional lexical entries that we needed for Mayer's parsing project (Mayer, Yamamoto, Evens, & Michael, 1989). Those entries became the nucleus of Zhang's lexicon for the Text Generator.

15.4 KHUWAJA'S VISION OF MULTIPLE MODELS

When Ramzan Ali Khuwaja joined the project, he was disturbed by our unscientific approach to knowledge representation. He argued for approaching our system as a modeling problem, on the basis that the core of our task is modeling the performance of expert tutors (1994). He also proposed a much more scientific approach to trying our systems out with students and in 1993 he persuaded Michael and Rovick to carry out a baseline experiment to demonstrate the value of human tutoring of medical students (see Chapter 10). Other demonstrations of the value of tutoring had been carried out with school children, mostly on unmotivated poor performers. There was a genuine question about whether tutoring was efficacious with adults who are highly motivated and generally excellent academic performers. As we saw in Chapter 10, although only nine students were involved, this experiment produced significant improvements from pretest to posttest, as compared with a control group of students who read material on the topic from a textbook.

Khuwaja searched through the artificial intelligence literature for ideas for a new architecture and chose the Knowledge Analysis and Design Structure (KADS) approach of Wielinga and Breuker (1990; Breuker, 1990), which has been used extensively in the European Union for a variety of knowledge-based systems including tutoring systems (Winkels & Breuker, 1990). KADS is based on the view that the development of a knowledge base is essentially a modeling activity that yields a series of models at different levels of abstraction. This modeling process starts at the level of language, where the raw data is identified, such as textbooks, interviews, and think-aloud protocols. As this knowledge is abstracted, models are constructed at the epistemological level. These models are intermediate between the linguistic level and the implementation level; they are intended to be free both of the particular form of the raw data and the details of the implementation.

Within the KADS methodology, the knowledge of the expert is itself organized into four or more levels. The first level contains the static knowledge of the domain. The second level is the inference level. The third level is the task level. The final level is the strategic level.

Khuwaja (Khuwaja, Evens, Rovick, & Michael, 1994a) adapted this approach to the modeling of the tutoring processes in the CIRCSIM-Tutor system. In his design, the Domain Knowledge Base itself has three levels, with the Problem Solver functioning as an inference level above them. The pedagogy expert, the Tutorial Planner, then uses a curriculum planning model, a tutoring strategy model, and a tutoring tactics model built on top of these lower layers. This resembles the approach used in an ITS for Lisp programming by Merrill, Reiser, Ranney, and Trafton (1992).

The three layers of the Domain Knowledge Base are nested. The top layer contains the parameters in the Prediction Table along with the Central Nervous System and the Baroreceptor Reflex—these nodes and the relationship between them are the primary knowledge that we want students to internalize while using the system. The middle layer contains all the nodes in the top layer and then additional nodes linking them at a more detailed level of discussion. The nodes in the middle layer are those that the system uses in hinting and explanations. The deep layer contains all the nodes in the middle layer and then more, including the anatomy nodes. It contains all the concepts (physiological parameters) that we expect that a student might mention in a dialogue with the system. The system needs to understand and be able to respond to questions about this set of concepts. It will not refer to those that appear only at the deep level in conversation unless the student mentions them first. These issues are discussed from the point of view of the human tutor in Chapter 5 and the Top Level Concept Map is shown in Fig. 5.1, the Middle Level is shown in Fig. 5.3, and the Deep Level is shown in Fig. 5.4.

We are motivated to support this complex structure by the experiments of Stevens and Collins (1980). They showed that if students are given more detailed explanations for relationships between parameters, then they will remember those relationships longer and be more likely to be able to apply them in reasoning. Khuwaja (1994) described our expert colleagues starting an explanation at the Top Level, and if the students do not understand, then switching to the Middle Layer or even the Deep Layer, as illustrated in Fig. 15.1. Although Khuwaja's implementation of his models using the Common Lisp Object System was discarded, many of his ideas have already been implemented in Version 2, including the three levels of the knowledge base. Others, like the protocol analysis and the curriculum planning, are central to Version 3.

It is clear that anyone starting a project like this today should make use of some of the sophisticated new modeling tools. One very attractive package of modeling tools for knowledge-based systems comes from the Institute for Scientific Information (J. Kim & Gil, 2002). Kim and Gil became specifically interested in tutoring dialogue because they want to use natural language dialogue in the knowledge acquisition process. Kim and Gil are also targeting dialogue systems as a kind of knowledge-based system that they wish their system to support. Several commercial expert systems packages come with modeling tools, but these can be expensive. The

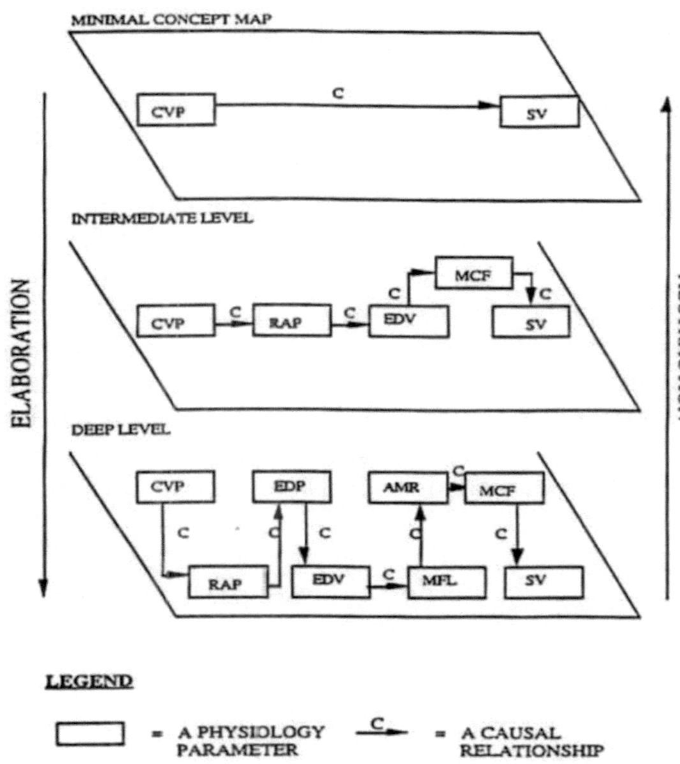

FIG. 15.1. A tutor moves from one layer to another in Khuwaja's model (adapted from Khuwaja, 1994, p. 188).

CLIPS System C Language Integrated Production System; Giarratano & Riley, 1998), supported by the Department of Energy, is an excellent system that we have used in other projects.

15.5 FREEDMAN'S VIEW OF THE KNOWLEDGE BASE

From the very beginning of the project, the Instructional Planner and the Text Generation components of Version 2 were written as sets of rules. We hoped that these components would be constantly monitored by Michael and Rovick, and they had already made their preference for this kind of knowledge representation very clear. Freedman's (1996c) thesis argued that the rest of the knowledge base should be expressed in the form of rules as well and she spent a great deal of time rewriting information from the frames as rules or tables. Thus, the top level rule for tutoring the DR phase says that if any neural variables are mispredicted, CIRCSIM-Tutor should tutor them first. Then the system should tutor other errors in the "main line" of physical variables followed by the secondary list (any variables not yet discussed). In a similar rule for tutoring the RR phase, the system starts with any neural variables that have been incorrectly predicted and how they affect MAP and then goes on to tutor any errors in the other variables. In the interests of generality, Freedman does not give a rule for what to do next from every variable. Instead, she provides a table telling what "main line" means for every procedure, because she believes that this will be easier for other people to read and understand, expert or not. Hasan Abbas (Abbas & Evens, 2000) systematically collected and retyped much of this information from Freedman's dissertation and placed it in a Microsoft® database. Some of it has become out of date owing to the development of Freedman's APE Planner and the decision to use her planning operators throughout the system, but the rest has been updated and corrected and stored in a kind of domain knowledge base called the Knowledge Collective. Freedman (Freedman et al., 2004) has also used these rules in her CAPE Tutor.

15.6 YUSKO'S KNOWLEDGE COLLECTIVE

Yusko (Yusko & Evens, 2002, 2004) has undertaken the redesign and reconstruction of the Domain Knowledge Base using a rule-based and not a frame-based approach. He began by interviewing Joel Michael about the domain and the underlying knowledge and trying to understand how he views the system. He was also interested in what kinds of tools Michael and other expert tutors could comfortably use themselves to update the system or to construct new knowledge for CIRCSIM-Tutor or the projected GASP-Tutor. Yusko has now designed a family of rulebases or databases accessed by a family of agents, each designed to optimize the handling of a different kind of data. He calls this system *The Knowledge Collective* (see Fig. 15.2).

Yusko's goal is to provide a framework, an information infrastructure, for the system, consisting of an integrated collection of databases with agents designed to collect and store data, other agents designed to make sure that related data items are consistent, and yet others to retrieve data. This approach requires explicit and accessible metadata. In other words, the definition and the semantics of the data must also be stored in the database and be made accessible to the user. This means, in turn, that the knowledge is usable in other systems or by our system for different purposes. It is a multiplayer, multiagent system that allows the agents (MicroDroids) to work together to supply information to multiple processes. All MicroDroids have access to all of the information in the knowledge base either directly or indirectly through other MicroDroids. In this way, all MicroDroids are cognizant of their environment. The Application Layer coordinates the activities of the Collective, but most of the actual knowledge resides in the Solution Layer. This layer is divided into two parts. The MicroDroids to the left of the vertical line deal with the actual domain specific knowledge. The MicroDroids to the right of the line are mapped to specific processes in an application. They supply the information for the processes to do their jobs.

The Knowledge Collective is as much a model as it is an intelligent knowledge base. It models the information needed to generate any required outputs. This can only be done if the information is stored in a form that allows a computer system to understand the structure about which it is reasoning (Yusko, 1994).

The list of knowledge stores for the emerging Version 3 of CIRCSIM-Tutor appears in Table 15.3. The new Domain Knowledge Base under construction by Yusko is a collection of rules and tables (Yusko & Evens, 2002, 2004), rather than frames. It is much easier for the expert tutors to update.

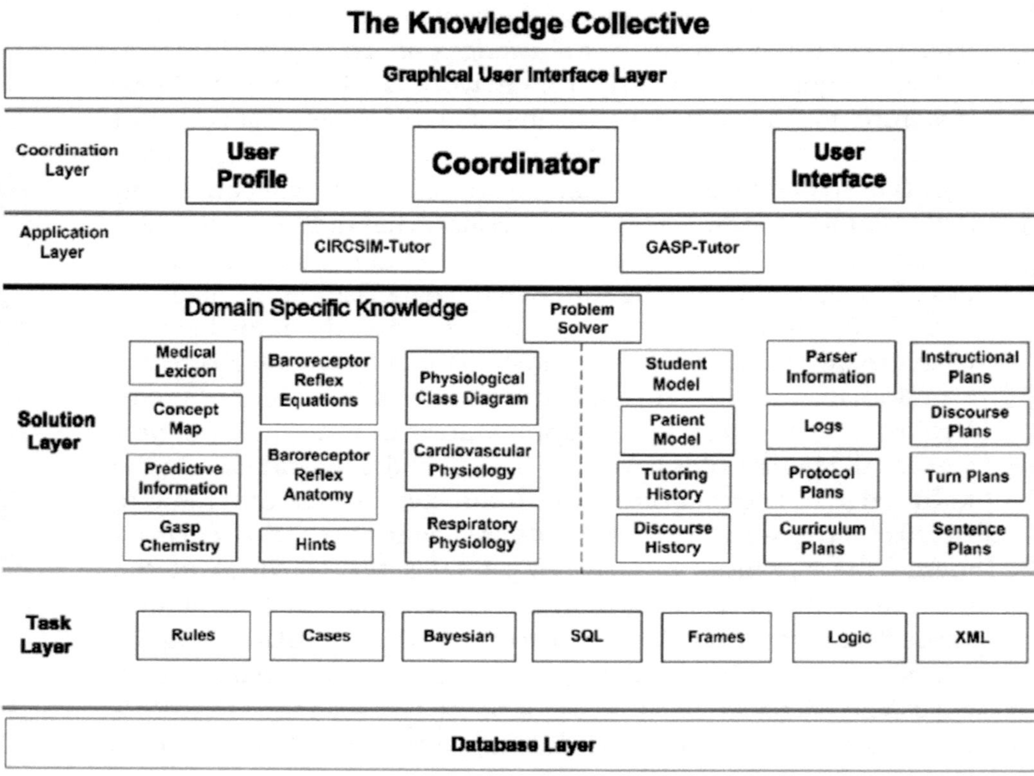

FIG. 15.2. Yusko's (2004) Knowledge Collective.

TABLE 15.3
Knowledge Stores in Version 3

The Domain Knowledge Base Tables
The Curriculum
The APE Planning Rules—for the curriculum, instructional planning, discourse generation, and turn planning
The Lexicon
The Student Model
The Discourse History
The Journal or Log File
The Tutoring History

At the center of the Knowledge Base in Yusko's version is a large collection of APE Planning Rules, for Curriculum Planning, Instructional Planning, Discourse Generation, Problem Solving, and Turn Planning. The new curriculum designed by Cho (2000) is a collection of APE Planning Rules plus a much larger file of procedure descriptions (up to 4 for each of almost 80 procedures) along with the procedure variable and the primary variable for each.

The Discourse History, as before, is a trace of the dialogue and the logic forms that the Input Understander builds and the Discourse Generation process expands.

The new Domain Knowledge Base, as we have explained, is a collection of rules, and the new Problem Solver applies those rules to the current situation.

The new Lexicon is used by both the Input Understander and the Discourse Generation process. It contains both the ontology and the case frame information. We still have two different grammars, however.

The new Log File, like the old one, is a trace of everything that happens in the session. Glass's program will still operate on it to produce a session transcript of the language exchanged between tutor and student.

The new Student Model is largely implemented in the current system but the code is necessarily spread around in pockets. The new module is much better integrated.

The Tutoring History is a list of the names of the plans executed along with an indication of whether each succeeded or failed. It is the tutoring history that makes it possible for Version 3 to choose a new and different strategy the next time around and not reuse the one that failed.

15.7 TAKE-HOME MESSAGE

When we began this project, we were overwhelmed by the problems we faced in natural language understanding and generation and the need for solutions that allow the system to respond to the student in 2 sec or less on the personal computers of the late 1980s. We were convinced that these constraints dictated a small knowledge base lodged in main memory. Advances in hardware and in database technology render many of our painful space economies unnecessary. Today we can store substantially all knowledge in a database management system, whether it consists of rules or frames or semantic networks or ontologies from a conceptual point of view. Using some kind of database management system (DBMS) provides backups and audit trails and makes it easy to build different interfaces for different users. It is also easy to store different models for different students and maintain different knowledge bases for different experts, so any system designer should seriously consider this alternative.

It seems as though anyone contemplating a project like this today should start with the most advanced knowledge modeling and construction tools available and aim for an approach that allows the expert tutor to decide directly what that knowledge should be and then update that knowledge easily and often. The real moral of this story is "think first," so you do not wind up building seven different versions of your Domain Knowledge Base, as we have done.

16

Generating Tutorial Dialogue

Now that we have described most of the other major components of the system, we have laid the necessary foundations for this chapter on the dialogue generation that is the core of our work. From the very beginning, the focus of our funding from the Office of Naval Research was on the generation of tutoring language. We contemplated trying to base this project on an intelligent tutoring system to which we could add language generation without building a whole system from scratch. We seriously considered trying to develop our research on top of the hypothetico-deductive problem-solving tutor under development at Rush Medical College and at IIT (Chen, 1999; Luksa, 1994; Michael, Haque, Rovick, & Evens, 1989). We finally decided, instead, to add dynamic planning, student modeling, a domain knowledge base, and natural language understanding and generation to CIRCSIM, so that we could build on the experience of Joel Michael and Allen Rovick. This was also the domain in which they felt most comfortable carrying out the extensive series of human tutoring sessions that we planned to use as a basis of our study of sublanguage and of tutoring strategies. In the event, we built a totally new system. As Moser and Moore (1995) pointed out, if a tutoring system is going to benefit from a natural language interface, it must be provided with the properties that make human tutoring language so effective and much more research is needed to establish just what these properties are.

Because a tutoring dialogue, like any other dialogue, is based on communication between two people, we could not make progress without understanding student input. That is, we could not generate dialogue without building an input understander. Because tutoring requires domain knowledge and problem solving, we had to build modules to carry out those tasks as well. We realized also that dialogue generation would require planning, although we did not by any means understand the scope and the sophistication of the planning carried out by human tutors at that time.

We describe how we constructed the Text Generation module in Version 2, which has been used in all of our major classroom experiments, and also, how and why we decided to move from this approach to the Dialogue Generation process in the emerging Version 3, which is still under construction, although the new components (curriculum and turn planning) have been tested separately. Figure 16.1 summarizes the differences between the two versions.

We begin our discussion of dialogue generation with a brief review of the literature in Section 16.0. We discuss discourse planning in Section 16.1 and sentence planning in Section 16.2. Questions of lexical choice have arisen at many points in our research; they are discussed in Section 16.3. Finally, in Section 16.4, we argue the need for turn planning in any dialogue system and describe how it can handle some problems unresolved by our current discourse planning processes and how it can implement the kind of lexical choice that we want. Then we wind up this chapter with a summary of what we have learned in Section 16.5.

16.0 SOME MILESTONES IN GENERATION

Although research in understanding natural language started in the late 1950s with the BASEBALL project (Wolf, Chomsky, & Green 1963), research on natural language generation did not start until 20 years later. This was partly because the basic research in linguistics on which computational linguistics depends provided much more support for analysis than for generation. In the meantime, interactive systems survived by using "canned" (prewritten) output

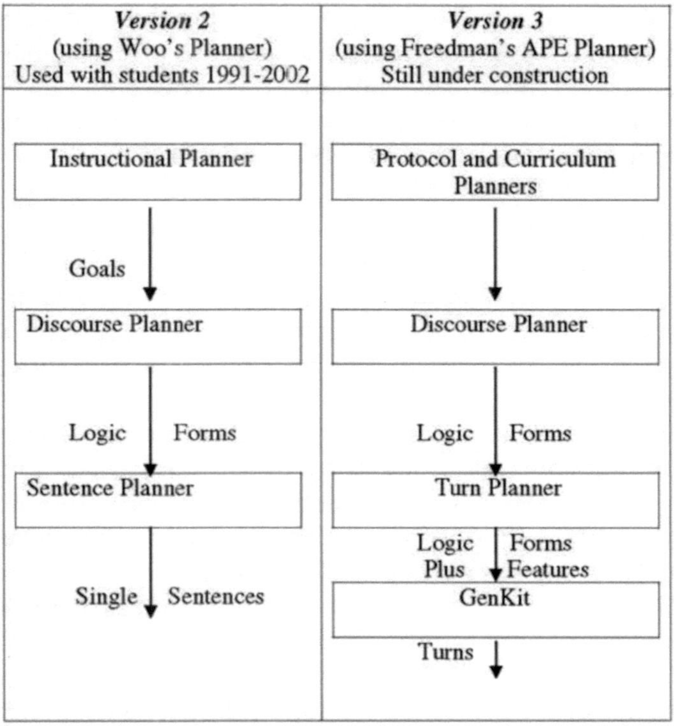

FIG. 16.1. Discourse Generation in Versions 2 and 3.

or fill-in-the-blank templates (Evens, 2002; Reiter, 1994; Reiter & Dale, 1999).

David McDonald (1980, 1983) produced the Mumble system, which embodied important pioneering work on sentence level generation and lexical choice. During the next few years, with his students at the University of Massachusetts, he produced an adaptable version of Mumble suitable for use in a wide variety of sublanguages, which was freely available and widely used in other experiments.

During the same period, Kathleen McKeown at the University of Pennsylvania developed schemas for generating definitions from a database of information about Navy ships and also for generating paragraphs that compare and contrast these same ships. Descriptions of language generation systems still begin with an explanation of how they differ from McKeown's (1985) Text system. Both McDonald and McKeown divided the generation problem into two tasks: deciding what to say and figuring out how to say it. Douglas Appelt (1985) described the role of planning in sentence generation as well as in determining the schemas to be used. Hovy discussed the problems of planning longer texts (1998a, 1998b, 1991).

McKeown's student, Cécile Paris (1985, 1988), began a research program on tailoring text to fit the needs of the individual user and how to build a model of the user to represent those needs. Today, she and her student, Vibhu Mittal (1999), are generating user-appropriate manuals. Another of Paris's students, Johanna Moore, did pioneering work on the generation of tutoring language (Moore, 1993, 1995; Moore, Lemaire, & Rosenblum, 1996).

This progress could not have happened without fundamental research on text and text structure by anthropologists and linguists. Vladimir Propp (1928/1958), George Lakoff (1972), and Perry Thorndyke (1977) set out to describe how people tell stories; they wound up devising story grammars for folk tales. Ethnographers like Oswald Werner (1974) studied cultural plans and sublanguage dialogues and developed ontologies for them. Joseph Grimes (1975) organized a group at Cornell University to study narrative structures. His student, Bonnie Meyer (1975, 1985), developed a theory of discourse relations for expository text and used these relations to carry out detailed analyses of the internal structure of that text. Eduard Hovy (1993) added to Meyer's list of relations and started to use them in generating text for machine translation. In the meantime, William Mann and Sandra Thompson's Rhetorical Structure Theory (1986, 1987) provided a badly needed theoretical basis for representing and generating text structure.

Computer scientists looked at this developing theoretical structure and began to adapt it to describe dialogues. Jane Robinson (1982) developed a dialogue grammar called DIAGRAM. Barbara Grosz and Candace Sidner (1986, 1990) studied task assistance dialogues, came up with a theory of discourse contexts, and described how they interact to determine anaphora and other elements of dialogue structure. Bonnie Webber (1982) analyzed the use of conjunctions in dialogue. Moore and Paris (1989, 1993; Moore & Pollack, 1992) produced some valuable extensions to Rhetorical Structure Theory to support dialogues and higher level planning. Barbara di Eugenio applied her study of centering and anaphora to tutoring language (Di Eugenio, Thomason, Moore, & Trolio, 1998, 2000).

This led to research by Di Eugenio (Di Eugenio, 2001; Di Eugenio & Trolio, 2000) which demonstrated that improving the generation of the output text significantly improves user learning.

16.1 PLANNING TUTORIAL DISCOURSE

Yuemei Zhang was the first to tackle the problem of planning discourse for CIRCSIM-Tutor. She started before we had transcripts to analyze, so she began by learning as much as she could about the physiology of the baroreceptor reflex, helped by her experience as a "barefoot physician" in China. She was very closely involved in the construction of the first few versions of the knowledge base. As described in Chapter 15, she argued for the inclusion of both problem-solving knowledge and domain knowledge that the discourse planner would need to construct explanations for students (Zhang, Evens, Michael, & Rovick, 1987). Deciding what to assume and what to explain is a perennial problem (Reiter, Cawsey, Osman, & Roff, 1997).

Zhang read Kathleen McKeown's (1985) book, *Text Generation,* and decided to develop schemas for a variety of generation tasks, beginning with the problem of defining the parameters. As the frames took shape, Zhang and Chong Woo developed several tutoring scenarios. Based on these scenarios, Zhang worked out several discourse schemas. One of these is the schema for tutoring neural variables in the DR period that we are still using today. In this schema, the tutor begins by asking for the mechanism. If the student gets that right, then the tutor asks for the meaning of the DR period; otherwise, the tutor explains its meaning. In any case, the tutor then asks the student to give an amended prediction for this variable. The dialogue in Example 16.1 between a student and CIRCSIM-Tutor on November 11, 2002 (Transcript T77), shows this scenario in operation.

Zhang (1991) also developed patterns or schemas for "forward tutoring," starting with the variable just tutored and figuring out how it will affect the next variable and "backward tutoring," or asking for the determinants of the current variable to figure out how it will change. These schemas are displayed in diagram form in Fig. 16.2.

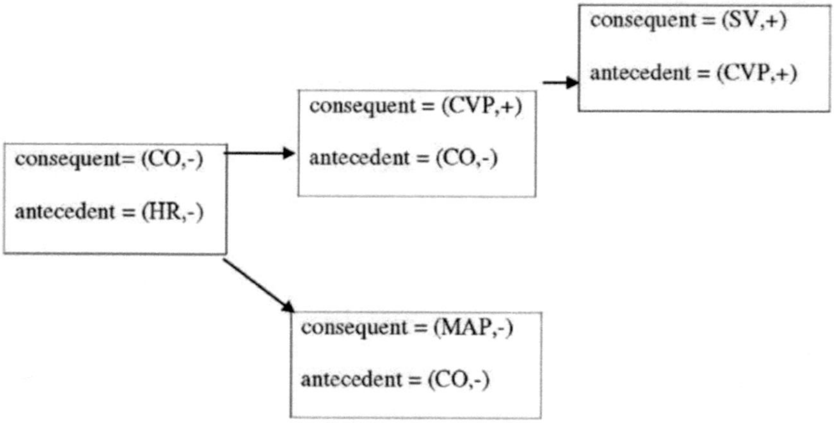

FIG. 16.2a. A forward tutoring pattern (adapted from Zhang, 1991).

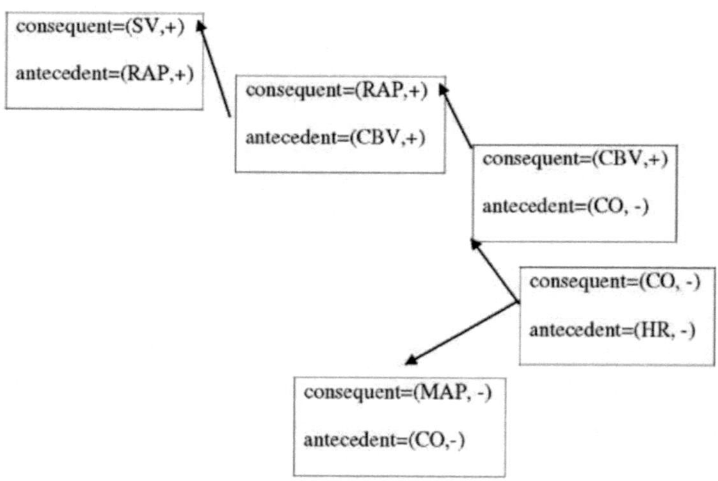

FIG. 16.2b. A backward tutoring pattern (adapted from Zhang, 1991).

Example 16.1 Neural Variable Schema Used by CIRCSIM-Tutor in 2002

T: By what mechanism is Total Peripheral Resistance controlled?
S: arteriole resistance
T: Is the mechanism of control neural or physical?
S: neural

T:	Correct, Total Peripheral Resistance is controlled by the nervous system.
T:	Remember the reflex will not activate until the RR stage. What is the value of Total Peripheral Resistance in DR?
S:	unchanged

In the forward tutoring pattern in Fig. 16.2a (cf. Section 7.2.2), the tutor has just succeeded in getting the student to establish that if HR goes down then CO will also go down. In the next step, the tutor gets the student to affirm that the decrease in CO will cause an increase in Central Blood Volume (CBV), which in turn will cause an increase in RAP, which will cause SV to go up as well. The decrease in CO also causes a decrease in MAP. In the backward tutoring pattern in Fig. 16.2b (cf. Section 7.2.1), the tutor is trying to get the student to correct the value of SV by using the fact that SV is determined by RAP. To find RAP we need to look at its determinant CBV. But CBV is determined by CO, which also determines MAP.

Because Zhang did her programming on a Xerox Lisp machine, we are not using her actual code but her discourse generation ideas were implemented by Chong Woo and she implemented much of the Version 2 knowledge base herself.

In the mid-1990s, Reva Freedman took over the main responsibility for discourse generation and she has had a strong influence over everything we have done since. She began by comparing the human tutoring transcripts and the CIRCSIM-Tutor transcripts of that day, and asking how some of the richness of the human transcripts could be implemented in CIRCSIM-Tutor. Human tutors use many different strategies and they express those strategies in many different ways.

Freedman rewrote Zhang's forward and backward teaching strategies in terms of formal "if-then" schemas and then added a number of more sophisticated strategies that she found in the human transcripts, like "show-contradiction" (see Example 16.2 and Section 7.2.3).

Example 16.2 A Human Tutor Uses the Show-Contradiction Strategy

K32-tu-226-2: What are the determinants of MAP?
K32-st-227-1: CO and TPR.
K32-tu-228-1: Correct.

K32-tu-228-2: And you have predicted CPO increases and TPR increases.
K32-tu-228-3: So how can you say MAP decreases?

Freedman (1996c) went on to build a catalogue of high and intermediate level discourse moves that defined a number of different scenarios for teaching whole phases, for teaching single neural variables, for remedying particular misconceptions, for trying again when a student failed to get the point the first time. These moves were presented as scenarios of alternative move choices, on the way to a more formal description as higher level schemas organized into hierarchical plans. An example is shown in Fig. 16.3.

Our experts were delighted with Freedman's schemas because they felt comfortable with reading them themselves. In spite of our efforts to make frames and discourse rules readable, Michael and Rovick never felt at home with them. Freedman argued that we should rewrite the whole knowledge base in rule form and table form. She did a great deal of work on this problem herself.

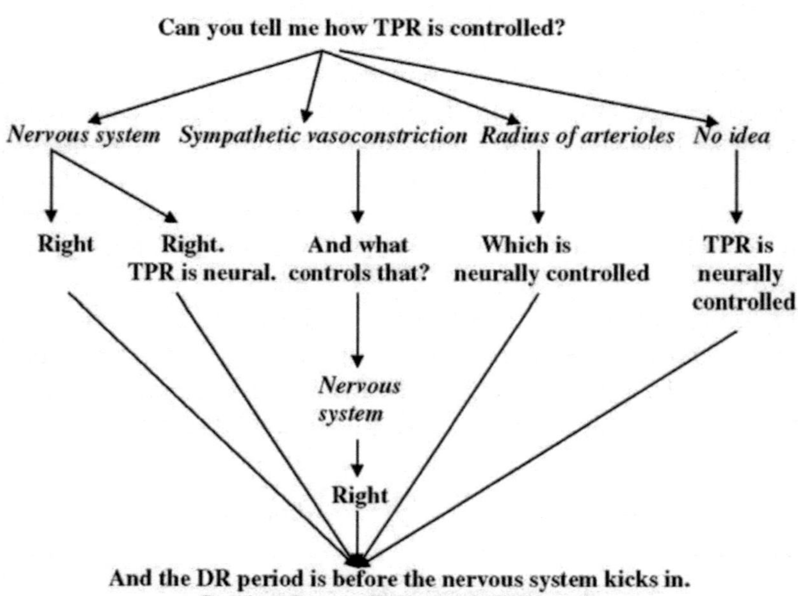

FIG. 16.3. A CIRCSIM-Tutor dialogue scenario copied with permission from Freedman, 1996c, p. 203, tutor contributions in boldface, student contributions in italics.

Freedman not only provided us with a number of ways of deciding what to say, she also attacked the question of how to say it. She collected several alternative realizations for every schema, like these four different ways to realize the "introduce-phase" schema:

T: Now let's review some of your predictions. (K32-tu-46-1)
T: Let's take a look at some of your predictions. (K10-tu-29-2)
T: Let's talk about your predictions. (K27-tu-50-1)
T: There are some errors here. Let's start with this issue. (K14-tu-31-2,3)

She pointed out that these could be delivered verbatim, if followed by an appropriate question. Most realizations need parameters, however, like these examples illustrating the first step in the "move-forward" schema:

T: And what happened to RAP? (K28-tu-8-2)
T: What effect would this have on RAP? (K32-tu-62-1)
T: ... what must happen to SV? (K28-tu-10-1)
T: How will that affect SV? (K30-tu-74-1)

Freedman also searched for more scientific methods of studying text analysis. She introduced us to the methods of conversational analysis, beginning with the work of Sinclair and Coulthard (1975). She insisted that we investigate some formal methods of SGML markup. At that point, it had been used in task assistance dialogues but not in tutoring dialogues. Electronic markup not only gave us a way of storing text annotations electronically and analyzing them by electronic means, it provided us with data for machine learning experiments (as described in Chapter 3). Freedman's work was fundamental to Zhou's analysis of different student error patterns and to her implementation of tutor hints and other responses to errors in the current Version 2 (Zhou 2000; Zhou et al., 1999a, 1999b). It was also the basis for many of the studies of tutoring strategies described in Part II of this book.

16.2 SENTENCE GENERATION

The sentence-level planner in the current version of CIRCSIM-Tutor was written by Ru-Charn Chang (1992) within the framework of Joan

Bresnan's (1982) Lexical-Functional Grammar (LFG). We found LFG very attractive because of its emphasis on the psychology of language and because it combines semantic analysis (using functional structures or f-structures) and syntactic analysis (using constituent structures or c-structures) into a unified whole. We needed to add a number of grammar rules, because the literature, which was full of analyses of complex declarative sentences, did not provide much help in generating the questions and hints and requests that make up most of our system's output. We also added to the variety of adverbial clauses available to discuss causal reasoning effectively. It is these clauses, which begin with words like "because," "since," "so that," "before," and "after," that allow us to talk about causes and changes over time. In all of our work with LFG, we made heavy use of Kaplan's Grammar-Writer's Workbench from Xerox PARC.

Let's begin with a very simple example of generation with LFG, starting with the instruction from the discourse generator to ask for the determinants of CO:

(QUESTION (determine (?? CO))).

This logic form is turned into the functional structure shown in Table 16.1. Using an algorithm of Michael Wescoat (1987), the functional structure is then mapped into the constituent structure shown in Fig. 16.4.

Applying a couple of simple punctuation rules gives us the finished sentence ready for output: "What determines CO?"

Chang (1992) did a detailed study of sentence structure in the dialogues and discovered that although the students often input just a word or two or short and simple sentences, the tutors often produce sentences with multiple clauses, especially sentential complements and adverbial clauses. If the discourse generator decides that it is

TABLE 16.1
Functional Structure for "What Determines CO?"
(Adapted From Chang, 1992, p. 337)

PRED 'DETERMINE<WHQ, [CO]>'	
SUBJ	PRED 'WHAT'
	Q-FOCUS '+'
OBJ	PRED 'CO'
	NUM SG

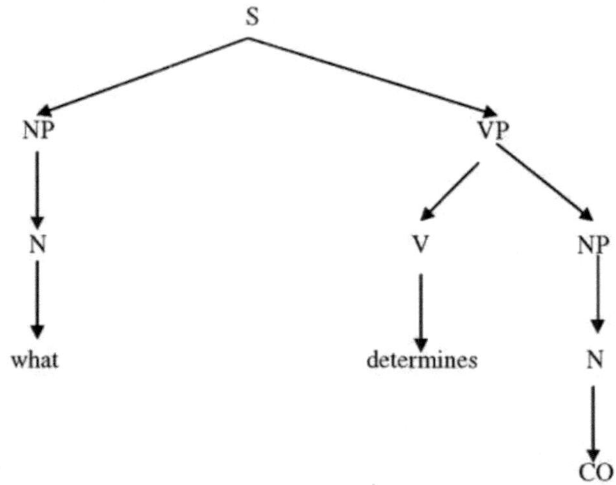

FIG. 16.4. Constituent structure for "What determines CO?" (Adapted from Change, 1992, p. 37.)

time to ask the question, "What causes RAP to rise?" it generates the following logic form:

(QUESTION (CAUSE(??, (+ RAP))))

The sentence generator turns this logic form into the f-structure in Table 16.2 (from Chang, 1992, p. 36). This f-structure is then transformed into the c-structure tree in Fig. 16.5. Again, a simple punctuation rule puts the capital "W" on "what" and adds the question mark at the end. The sentence generator returns the complete sentence to the instructional planner, which outputs it to the screen.

We give one last example of an f-structure and c-structure for a sentence with an adverbial clause, because they are so frequent in our tutoring dialogues. Suppose we want to generate the sentence "Tell me what happens to CVP when CO rises." Imperatives are treated as having the understood subject "you." The direct object of the verb is the sentential complement "what happens to CVP when CO rises," whereas "me" is an indirect object. The clause "when CO rises" is classified as an adjunct in LFG. "When" is the subordinating conjunction to choose when you are trying to describe two coordinated simultaneous activities. This gives us the functional structure shown in Table 16.3. The constituent structure (tree) generated

TABLE 16.2
Functional Structure for "What Causes RAP to Rise?" (Adapted from Chang, 1992, p. 36)

PRED 'CAUSE <WHQ> <RISE, [RAP]>'	
SUBJ	PRED 'WHAT' Q-FOCUS '+'
OBJ	PRED 'RAP'
VCOMP	PRED <RISE, 'RAP'> CTYPE '+' INF c+ SUBJ [RAP]

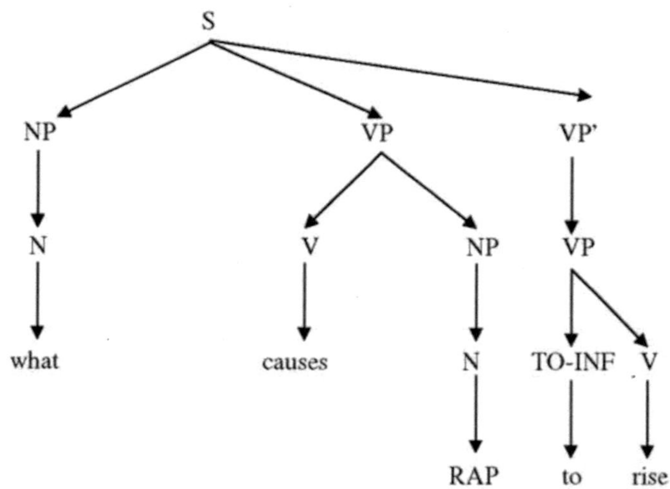

FIG. 16.5. Constituent structure for "What causes RAP to rise?"

from this diagram has the form shown in Fig. 16.6. The algorithms for building the structures and walking the trees to produce the actual sentence output are given in detail in Chang, Evens, Michael, and Rovick (1994).

We are experimenting with the use of Nyberg and Tomita's (1988) GenKit for sentence generation in Version 3.0. This will enable us to generate all text output from the same source. In Version 2, we use Chang's sentence generator to generate the remedial component of

TABLE 16.3

Functional Structure for "Tell Me What happens to CVP When CO Rises?"

PRED TELL 'YOU>' <S-COMP >		
SUBJ	PRED 'YOU'	
	PERS 2	
	CASE NOM	
	NUM SG	
INDOBJ	PRED 'ME'	
	PERS 1	
	CASE DAT	
	NUM SG	
S-COMP	PRED HAPPENS <WHQ> <P-COMP>	
	SUBJ	PRED 'WHAT'
		Q-FOCUS '+'
	P-COMP	PREP 'TO'
	HEAD	<CVP>
ADJUNCT	PRED	'RISE' <CO>
	CASE	AT-TIME
	TENSE	PRESENT
	SUBJ	PRED 'CO'
		NUM SG

the dialogues dynamically, but the introductory screens, the procedure descriptions, the instructions to the student, and the long explanations rolled out at the end of each procedure, are "canned," that is, written in advance and then stored.

This decision is a really painful one. From a practical point of view, it is desirable to produce all the different kinds of text from the same generator. From a principled point of view, we are still enthusiastic about the LFG approach. VanLehn, Jordan et al. (2002) are using Lavoie and Rambow's (1997) RealPro from CoGenTech to generate sentences in Why/Atlas with impressive results. Their system, however, generates comparatively long swatches of text as comments on long explanations from the student, as opposed to the highly interactive text that we are trying to generate. Our approach allows us to alternate between principled generation and "prewritten" text segments in a seamless fashion.

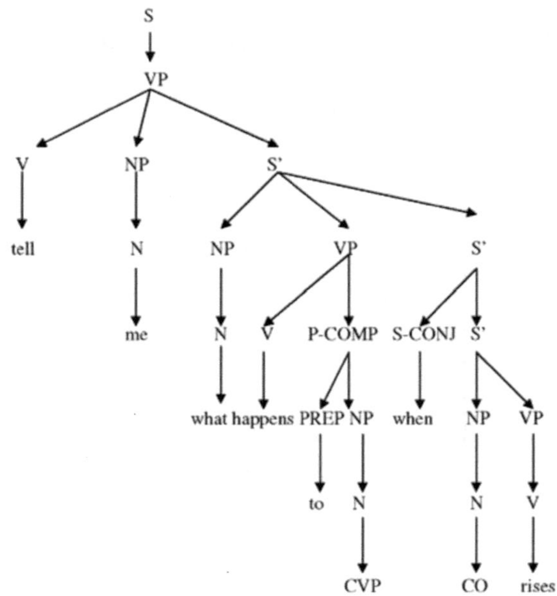

FIG. 16.6. Constituent structure for "Tell me what happens to CVP when CO rises?"

16.3 LEXICAL CHOICE

The problem of lexical choice is the problem of picking out the right word to generate at the right time. This problem is so important that it has been a central issue in language generation from the very beginning and almost all the best researchers have said something useful about it (Elhadad,1992; Elhadad & McKeown, 1990; Matthiessen, 1991; McDonald, 1991; Reiter, 1991).

Yuemei Zhang (1991) pointed out some problems of lexical choice in the CIRCSIM tutoring transcripts at the very beginning of this project. She was particularly concerned about the choice of words in discourse about causal reasoning. She noticed the relationship between the use of words like "cause" and "result" and the choice of topic and focus. She tried to ensure that the lexical choice here would fit into the discourse plan. (See Section 7.8 for a discussion of lexical choice in human tutoring.)

Zhang collected a large number of collocations and pointed out to us that generation of explanations in physiology requires the graceful manipulation of many long phrases. This problem was addressed by Hovy (1988c) for machine translation contexts and by Paul Jacobs (1988) for Wilensky's UC; we found their ideas very useful.

Zhang also commented on the large number of synonyms for "increase" and "decrease" and the importance of making consistent choices among them. This problem is complicated by the fact that increase and decrease both have causal meanings when used transitively but not intransitively. As synonyms of "increase," we find "go up," "raise," and "rise." Synonyms of decrease include "go down," "depress," "fall," and "drop." But it is important for the generator to understand that "go up" and "rise" are synonyms of the intransitive sense of "increase," whereas "raise" is a synonym of the transitive sense. In the same way, "fall" and "drop" are synonyms of the intransitive sense of "decrease," whereas "depress" is a synonym of the transitive sense.

Zhang pointed out that these verbs cannot be chosen randomly by the generator, even when the sense alignments are understood, because they form pairs of preferred antonyms like the adjectives investigated by Justeson and Katz (1991). They discovered, in investigating actual language usage, that "big" and "little" co-occur, and so do "large" and "small," but "little" and "large" do not. Zhang discovered the same phenomenon in verbs of change in our tutoring sessions: "increase" and "decrease" are paired, so are "go up" and "go down," and "rise" and "fall." Thus, the generator cannot make random choices of verbs of change to express these concepts.

Ramachandran (1994) investigated these phenomena further and gave this kind of lexical choice the name *cohesive choice*. He showed that cohesive choice of this type appears not only in the 16 transcripts examined by Zhang, but in all 50 transcripts available when he began work. It appears in the first set of novice tutoring transcripts as well. It may, in fact, be an aspect of language use in general and not a special property of tutoring language.

Ramachandran (Ramachandran & Evens, 1995) also noticed another kind of lexical choice, which he named *user-driven lexical choice*. The tutors make use of the verb that the student has chosen to describe a change, unless they find it inappropriate. So, if the student uses "increase," the tutor will use "increase" or "decrease" in the next turn to describe a change, whereas, if the student picks "go up," the tutor will use "go up" or "go down." When we asked the tutors whether this behavior was a result of conscious choice, they assured us that it was indeed planned, as a matter of validating the student's use of language. For more examples and discussion, see Chapter 7.

Ramachandran (1994) was a passionate believer in the importance of lexical choice. One advantage of effective lexical choice, he argued, was that we could make sure that students were exposed to both the full names and the abbreviations for all the parameters discussed by the system. He insisted that it is important for students to learn to recognize Cardiac Contractility, CC, Inotropic State, and IS as names for the same parameter, and he wrote a lexical choice program that cycled through the alternatives for this parameter and for others.

This proved to be a mistake. Random choice and cyclic alternation are not good ways of handling lexical choice, where the crucial point is to choose the right word for each context. When it comes to parameter names, human tutors typically use the full name when they introduce a variable and then abbreviate them all the time to speed up the typing process. Medical students trying out the system with Ramachandran's lexical choice program running assumed that a full-length variable name appearing after an abbreviation must be a hint of some kind and became confused. Because character output is no longer a problem for us with today's screen speeds, it seems appropriate for our program to choose the full name of a parameter when it is introduced in any phase and then abbreviate further occurrences within that phase. We still need to find some principled way to alternate between Inotropic State, the term preferred in the most current textbooks, and Cardiac Contractility, which seems to be more descriptive for most students.

Reva Freedman (1996a, 1996b, 1996c) looked at some of the text generated in this way and reasoned that we needed to plan the output a turn at a time, not just a sentence at a time. We believe that she should be credited with the invention of the concept of "turn planning," so we feel that this experiment indeed had a beneficial outcome. She was so distressed by the problems she saw that she insisted we turn off Ramachandran's lexical choice programs entirely. We are now reimplementing cohesive choice and user-driven choice in Version 3 as part of turn planning.

Another important issue for the generation of cohesive text is the choice of discourse markers. Goldman and Durán (1988) found that otherwise competent second language learners sometimes had difficulty in comprehending scientific texts, because they failed to understand the function of the discourse markers. More recently, T. J. M. Sanders and Noordman (2000) have demonstrated that adding appropriate discourse markers to text significantly improves reading comprehension scores of native speakers. In addition, cue words of all kinds significantly improve coherence (T. J. M. Sanders, 1997). Earlier work by T. J. M. Sanders (T. J. M. Sanders, Spooren, & Noordman, 1992) provided a taxonomy of discourse markers. Louwerse and Mitchell (2003) examined a wide range of discourse markers and produced a larger taxonomy. The work of Moser and Moore (1995), who investigated cues of various kinds, proved to be a useful guide to the methodology of studying these phenomena in our tutoring dialogues.

Jung Hee Kim became convinced that a wise choice of discourse markers would improve the coherence of the dialogue generated by CIRCSIM-Tutor. As we described in Chapter 4, she used the machine learning program C4.5 (Quinlan, 1993) to identify the discourse markers used by our expert tutors during each phase of a number of different tutoring strategies. She discovered that our expert tutors mostly stick to the discourse markers "But," "So," "And," "Well," and "Then," and they use these words especially frequently to mark the beginning of a new tutoring strategy or to ask the student to make a new inference (J. H. Kim, Glass, Freedman, & Evens, 2000).

16.4 TURN PLANNING—THE NEED AND THE PROCESS

We agreed that turn planning was the best solution for the daunting problem of implementing our ideas about lexical choice and cohesion, including the insertion of discourse markers. We were delighted when Feng-Jen Yang volunteered to carry out this task. Freedman had just completed a new planner for the ANDES/ATLAS Project at the University of Pittsburgh (2000a, 2000b) named APE (Atlas Planning Environment). We decided to use this new planner throughout Version 3. Freedman generously gave us an advanced version and Yang started to work.

Yang (Yang, 2001; Yang, Kim, Glass, & Evens, 2000a, 2000b) decided to explore a number of components of cohesive tutoring language, including anaphora. He began by marking up the RR phase of many of the same transcripts so as to have a larger database for his machine-learning experiments. (Kim's (2000) markup covered only the DR phase.) Then he needed to combine his new rules with the mass of rules that had already been collected, add more rules to insure turn cohesion, figure out how to organize the rules, and express them in terms of APE planning operators. The rules included Zhang's (1991) and Ramachandran's (1994) rules on lexical choice, Freedman's (1996a, 1996b, 1996c, 1997) rules for surface generation, and J. H. Kim et al.'s (2000) rules for discourse markers.

Yang's Turn Planner (Yang, 2001; Yang et al., 2000a, 2000b) also included the results of Zhou's machine learning experiments on hinting and other tutor responses to student errors and his own rules for softeners, pronominalization, abbreviation of parameter names, and acknowledgments. As we saw in Chapter 12, the Turn Planner gets input from the Discourse Generator and turns it into a complete tutor turn. It divides the logic forms into individual sentences and annotates them with features that determine the use of discourse markers, anaphora, and particular lexical items. (The Turn Planner has been tested separately, but because it is designed to run as part of Version 3, it has not been tested with students.)

What changes does the Turn Planner actually make in the text to make it sound more natural? Let's look at a simple example of text (Example 16.3) produced by Version 2.8 (see Table 11.2) in fall of 1999 and see how turn planning can improve it. So far we have developed rules for improvements in five different areas of surface generation: softeners, abbreviation of variable names, pronouns, discourse markers, and acknowledgments.

Example 16.3. An Example Dialogue Before Turn Planning

T1: What are the determinants of Mean Arterial Pressure?
S2: co
T3: Right, Cardiac Output is one determinant of Mean Arterial Pressure. The other determinant is neurally controlled. What is the other determinant of Mean Arterial Pressure?
S4: tpr
T5: Right. The other determinant of Mean Arterial Pressure is Total Peripheral Resistance. MAP is determined by CO and TPR. Which determinant is dominant in this case?
S6: co
T7: Correct. CO is the dominant determinant in this case. Is the relationship from CO to MAP direct or is it inverse?

S8: direct
T9: Good, you got the correct answer. What is the correct value of Mean Arterial Pressure?
S10: -
T11: Correct. The value of Mean Arterial Pressure is decreased. Please change the value of 'MAP' in the predictions table.

16.4.1 Softeners

Yang noticed that, although the machine tutor always asks questions directly, our expert tutors often phrase questions more politely, by prefixing the phrase "Can you tell me" or "Do you know." He discovered several of these phrases, which he calls *softeners,* in our tutoring sessions. He also carried out a machine learning experiment from which he derived rules for how and when to generate softeners.

These phrases turn the question into an indirect question and require a change in word order, which is one of many reasons why turn planning needs to be done before sentence generation. In Example 16.3, it seems appropriate to insert "Can you tell me" at the beginning of turn T1, to obtain the following: "T1: Can you tell me what the determinants of Mean Arterial Pressure are?"

16.4.2 Abbreviation of Variable Names

It is important for students to learn both the full name and the standard abbreviation for the important parameters of the cardiovascular system. Our current rule is to use the long form first and then abbreviate it. If we apply this rule to T3 in Example 16.3, we get the following: "T3: Right, Cardiac Output is one determinant of MAP. The other determinant is neurally controlled. What is the other determinant of MAP?"

16.4.3 Pronominalization

Another machine learning experiment on pronoun use confirmed Judy Walters's work on anaphora (Fox, 1987; Walters, 1993). The defining context for pronouns follows the plan boundaries for tutoring plans. Guindon (1988) showed that the defining context for pronouns follows the ACT-R structure. Based on the work of Dale (1992), we had expected to see a lot of referring expressions. The tutors do use such definite expressions, like "the resistance" for TPR or "the pressure" for MAP, but only on the relatively infrequent occasions when they give extended explanations; they use pronouns much more frequently. We suspect that this is because referring expressions of this kind are typical of the kind of expository text that appears in a monologue. The tutoring dialogues use relatively informal language. The availability of two or three letter abbreviations for the parameters in this domain may also affect the expert behavior.

On this basis, we have chosen to implement rules for pronominalization first.

Substituting "it" for "the other determinant of MAP" in T3 gives us the following: "T3: Right, Cardiac Output is one determinant of MAP. The other determinant is neurally controlled. What is it?"

16.4.4 Discourse Markers

Yang implemented the rules for discourse markers developed by J. H. Kim (J. H. Kim, Glass, Freedman, & Evens, 2000). Kim found that human tutors often use "now" when they ask a question for the second time, whereas "so" is used to indicate that the student should now be able to draw a correct conclusion from the information just given. These rules tell us to insert "Now" in front of the third sentence in T3, to give the following: "T3: Right, Cardiac Output is one determinant of MAP. The other determinant is neurally controlled. Now, what is it?"

Because the discussion in T5 through T9 gives the student enough information to correctly predict the change in MAP, our rules mark T9 with "So," to give the following: "T9: So, what is the correct value of MAP?"

16.4.5 Acknowledgments

Another area where the system needs improvement is in the choice of acknowledgments, which often seem obtrusive and overly emphatic. Yang wrote rules to carry out the policy that Li and Rovick implemented in ABASE (Li, Rovick, & Michael, 1992), to generate low key positive acknowledgments like "Yes" and "Right" most of the time, but to express warm enthusiasm in situations when the student has finally produced a correct answer after a struggle. (See Section 7.3 for a brief description of the work of Li and Rovick on ABASE.)

In the next section, Section 16.5, we describe how Brandle (1998) developed new rules for acknowledgements based on H. Clark's (1996) theory of joint actions. These rules are actually executed by the Turn Planner. In particular, human tutors often repeat wrong answers (giving the student a chance to correct them), but seldom repeat correct ones. These rules allow us to shorten T3, as compared to the form in the aforementioned example, so that it becomes the following: "T3: Right. The other determinant is neurally controlled. What is it?"

The transformed version of T5 sounds much more natural, and T7 and T11 are also shortened to half of the original size: "T5: Right, MAP is determined by CO and TPR. Which determinant is dominant in this case?"

Example 16.4 shows what this passage looks like before (above the line) and after (below the line) turn planning:

Example 16.4. The Passage in Example 16.3 Before Turn Planning (above the line) and After Turning Planning (below the line)

T1: What are the determinants of Mean Arterial Pressure?

S2: co

T3: Right, Cardiac Output is one determinant of Mean Arterial Pressure. The other determinant is neurally controlled. What is the other determinant of Mean Arterial Pressure?

S4: tpr

T5: Right. The other determinant of Mean Arterial Pressure is Total Peripheral Resistance. MAP is determined by CO and TPR. Which determinant is dominant in this case?

S6: co

T7: Correct. CO is the dominant determinant in this case. Is the relationship from CO to MAP direct or is it inverse?

S8: direct

T9: Good, you got the correct answer. What is the correct value of Mean Arterial Pressure?

S10: -
T11: Correct. The value of Mean Arterial Pressure is decreased. Please change the value of MAP in the prediction table.

T1′: Can you tell me what the determinants of Mean Arterial Pressure are?
S2: co
T3′′′′: Right. The other determinant is neurally controlled. Now, what is it?
S4: tpr
T5′: Right. MAP is determined by CO and TPR. Which determinant is dominant in this case?
S6: co
T7′: Correct. Is the relationship from CO to MAP direct or is it inverse?
S8: direct
T9′: Good. So, what is the correct value of MAP?
S10: -
T11′: Correct. Please change the value of MAP in the prediction table.

16.4.6 How Turn Planning Works

Feng-Jen Yang drew the diagram in Fig. 16.7 to explain how the turn planning process works. As we saw in our discussion of planning in Chapter 12, the Turn Planner operates on the output of the Discourse Planner and produces input to the Sentence Generator. The Discourse Planner deposits its discourse plans and their contents (expressed as logic forms) in a buffer until it decides that it is time for the tutor to ask a question. At this point, the system must output a turn. The turn planner reads the discourse plans for that turn from the buffer, adds features, and decides how to divide the annotated logic forms into sentences. The sentence generator picks up the annotated logic forms and generates a sentence at a time, but now these sentences fit into the turn plan that includes softeners, discourse markers, anaphora, and principled lexical choice.

Thus, the turn planner can be viewed as a collection of rules that operate after dialogue planning and before sentence generation. Until Bruce Mills (2001; Mills, Evens, & Freedman, 2004) completes the task of writing the top levels of Version 3.0 as APE planning opera-

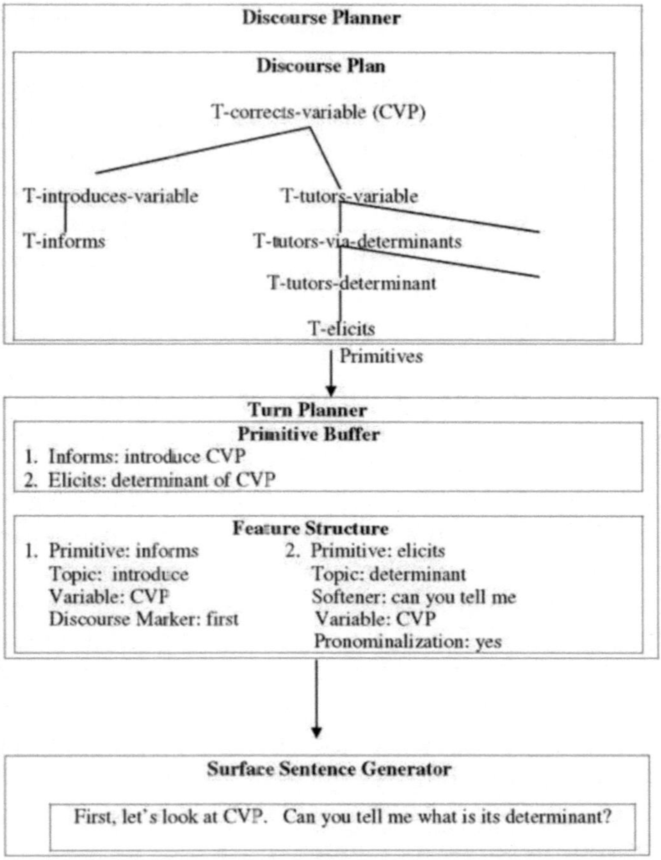

FIG. 16.7. Discourse generation with turn planning in CIRCSIM-Tutor Version 3.

tors, it will be hard to tell how well the Turn Planner meets its goals to add features to the content descriptors so that the turn comes out sounding like a coherent whole, rather than disjointed pieces.

16.5 GENERATING ACKNOWLEDGMENTS

In the original design of CIRCSIM-Tutor, the tutor responds with "Right" to every correct answer and "Wrong" to every wrong one. Then Susan Chipman came on a site visit just before the 1991 Cognitive Science Conference at the University of Chicago. She tried out the system, and pointed out that real tutors avoid telling students that they are wrong.

Chipman's comments were based on the work of Barbara Fox (1993b) and reflect the findings of Fox's Human Tutoring Project at the University of Colorado. Michael and Rovick seem to be much less reluctant to give an explicit negative response than Fox's tutors, but they only do this about a quarter of the time. They certainly do not say "Wrong" every time. In Chapter 7, we describe our study of negative acknowledgments and our gradual realization that students can often infer that their answers are wrong if the tutor does not proceed to the next topic. The students can often then make the correction themselves. Because the goal of our tutor is to get students to figure out the right answers for themselves, we really want to take advantage of this kind of opportunity.

It became clear in our study of negative acknowledgments that generating "Right" after every right answer was just as unnatural sounding as generating "Wrong" after every wrong answer. Because this practice did not seem likely to have such a bad effect on student morale, however, we left it in place. Because we did not understand when and why human tutors decide to generate or omit positive acknowledgments, we did not know what else to do. Then, in 1996, Stefan Brandle heard Herbert Clark talk about his theory of joint actions at the summer meeting of the Society for Text and Discourse and realized that Clark's (1996) work provided an ideal basis for studying acknowledgments in human tutoring.

Brandle (1998) noticed that Clark's discussion of closure (the termination of a topic) could explain an important question involving positive acknowledgments, the fact that apparently the tutor can leave many positive acknowledgments implicit without confusing the student. In fact, the student can infer that, if the tutor is ready to go on to a new topic, then he or she must be satisfied with the student's last contribution to the old topic. Thus, the tutor's decision to move on has indeed communicated an implicit positive acknowledgment. In the same vein, the student may conclude that if the tutor does not move on but continues to discuss the same topic, then there is a tacit negative acknowledgment attached. Brandle persuaded two fellow students to analyze 153 dialogue sequences and classify the acknowledgments in terms of several criteria: polarity (positive, negative, or neutral), the marking (explicit and marked, or implicit), the closure (closure expressed, closure deferred, and closure not relevant), whether the segment initiates discourse repair, and whether a judgment of the answer is expressed. He was able to obtain good interrater reliability scores (kappa values; Di Eugenio, 2000) for polarity, closure, and judgment.

The marked transcripts for these 153 segments were then used in a machine learning experiment, along with assessments of the student hand-calculated at the point when the acknowledgment was issued. Using Quinlan's C4.5 (1993), Brandle obtained the following model, which we hope to implement in Version 3.0 (1998, p. 81):

1. If the student assessment is good
   and the student's statement is correct
      then issue an implicit positive acknowledgment
   and the student's statement is incorrect
      then issue an implicit negative acknowledgment.
2. If the student assessment is fair
   and the student's statement is correct
      then issue an implicit positive acknowledgment
   and the student's statement is incorrect
      then issue an explicit marked negative acknowledgment.
3. If the student assessment is poor
   and the student's statement is correct
      then issue an explicit marked positive acknowledgment
   and the student's statement is incorrect
      then issue an explicit marked negative acknowledgment.

You might conclude from this model that the expert tutors pour a torrent of negative comments on students who are doing poorly. In fact, they do not do this at all. Instead, when a student becomes truly confused, they completely restructure the tutoring protocol as we described in Chapter 7, to provide much more guidance and more immediate feedback. They change the level of questions so that the student can succeed. The motivation for this, they say, is to provide a better learning environment for these weaker students. One of the major goals of the new version is to enable CIRCSIM-Tutor to make the same kind of protocol switches.

As Zhou (Zhou et al., 1999b) added to the hinting capabilities of the system, she inserted hints after near misses and removed the explicit negative acknowledgments. She also eliminated negative acknowledgments before some other relatively mild hints, so that the negative face of the system has been somewhat softened. As a result of Zhou's work, the current version of the system (Version 2.9) has eliminated some of the negative acknowledgments, but it is still producing redundant positive acknowledgments.

16.6 TAKE-HOME MESSAGE

A tutoring dialogue is, first and foremost, a conversation, and the first priority of the tutor (whether human or machine) is to keep that conversation going. This means that the system must end each turn with a question or a request to the student to ensure that the student knows what to do next. If the system cannot make sense of the student input, it must explain to the student what it expects or else change the topic to an area where it can understand.

We are very enthusiastic about our new Turn Planner. It is not until the system is capable of generating a tutoring dialogue that the need for turn planning becomes apparent, so it is not surprising that ours is the first in the field. Some kinds of dialogue management systems may be able to solve these problems in other ways, but our approach is both simple and effective.

The generation of tutoring dialogues requires knowledge of several different kinds—of the domain, of the problem-solving algorithms that we want the student to learn, of ways of engaging the student, of ways of remedying misconceptions.

17

The Screen Manager

The Screen Manager is responsible for enabling communication between the user and the system. It paints windows and menus on the screen, it collects the student's menu choices and Prediction Table entries, and it locates the text that is input by the student and transmits it to the Planner.

Much of the literature on screen design for intelligent tutoring systems is directed at important problems of GUI manipulation and is not particularly relevant to our research, so our review of the literature is brief. We outline some of the principles of user-centered design that guided our work in Section 17.0 and then go on to describe that work.

Most of the screens that CIRCSIM-Tutor uses, like the login screen and the introductory instruction screens, are quite simple. But the Main Screen, where most of the user work is done, has been redesigned and re-implemented several times. We describe the opening screens briefly in Section 17.1 and then discuss the major design problems of the Main Screen in Section 17.2. Finally, we summarize this chapter in Section 17.3. Table 17.1 illustrates some of the major changes described in this chapter.

TABLE 17.1
Changes in the CIRCSIM-Tutor Screen Manager

Version 2.1 to 2.5	*Version 2.6 to 2.9*	*Version 3.0*
Tried out by a few students and colleagues	Tested with classes from 1998 to 2002	Under construction; not yet tested with students
Woo's Screen Manager based on work of Nakhoon Kim and Jun Li fonts improved by Ramaswami (1993)	Brandle's Screen Manager	Brandle's Screen Manager + Screens added by Y. W. Kim and H. S. Roh to support curriculum planning
Separate windows for student input and tutor output	Dialogue screen with interwoven input and output	Dialogue screen with interwoven input and output
Menu of procedure names	Menu of procedure names	Menu of procedure descriptions (Cho)
No window for student notes	Window for student notes	No window for student notes

17.0 SOME DESIGN ISSUES AND DESIGN LITERATURE

One of the ideas that all of us who worked on this project agree on is the value of user-centered design (Hix & Hartson, 1993; Norman & Draper, 1986). The central philosophy here is that users should be involved in every stage of the design process. This philosophy implies that observation of users in action is a fundamental step, and that it is essential to fit computer tools into the user's existing work environment. What is more, the design should make the user feel in control. We have used this philosophy in building several successful tools. Shanthi Robert built a medical record input system and then Natasha Ma constructed a progress note system on top of it using user-centered design (Ma, Evens, Trace, & Naeymi-Rad, 1992; Robert, 1991; Robert, Prakash, Naeymi-Rad, Trace, Carmony, & Evens, 1991). They followed an expert around and watched what he did. Then they built a prototype and observed the expert as he worked with it and asked him for suggestions. They rebuilt the prototype and again watched the expert use it. After many cycles, we had a usable system that was later developed into a commercial product.

Translating these ideas into the domain of tutoring systems, we began by observing human tutoring sessions. We designed a system to function as a regularly scheduled computer laboratory exercise for a particular course. Then we built a working prototype and observed both experts and students using it. This led to repeated cycles of redesign and experiments with students. None of this would have been possible without the expertise of Joel Michael and Allen Rovick and the perceptive and creative suggestions of many different students at Rush Medical College.

In observing users, it may be especially beneficial to take note of errors that they make in using the system. The work of Fraser and Smith (1992) contains valuable ideas about how to study cognitive errors made by users. We found it worthwhile to write software to trap user clicks and backspaces and other key strokes. In Chapter 13, we noted how studying user errors in spelling and grammar contributed to the development of the Input Understander. Studying user clicks and backspaces made it clear to us that early versions of the system were difficult to navigate because they asked users to click on too many different buttons. (This kind of analysis is now called clickstream analysis; Barfield, 1993.) We also realized that the system often failed to make clear to users which window they should be working with at any given time.

In discussing his screen design for CIRCSIM-Tutor, Stefan Brandle (1998) pointed out that the major problem, communicating through a restricted bandwidth, has much in common with the central issue of the tutor itself, the problem of carrying on a natural language dialogue in a keyboard-to-keyboard manner without the body language, intonation, and timing information that are important components of face-to-face tutoring sessions.

Brandle was particularly influenced by the work of Donald Norman (1990, 1992) as he attacked the problem of making the system as consistent and as self-explanatory as possible. Norman's (1992) book, *Turn Signals Are the Facial Expressions of Automobiles,* pointed out that the invention of the turn signal light on the dashboard was a real step forward in communication between the car and the driver. Brandle (1998, p. 96) extended this metaphor to our screen problems: "We activate turn signals to notify other drivers of our intentions, but there is also the problem of letting the driver know whether the turn signals are on." To help our users figure out what the system was doing, Brandle designed the Screen Manager to highlight the window where we want the user to enter information at the current moment. Similarly, when the student is making predictions, we highlight the column in the Prediction Table where those predictions should go. As soon as the user finishes entering a full column of predictions, the system colors the boxes with errors red and draws diagonal lines across those boxes so the user can see immediately where the errors occur.

To help the user feel in control of the system, Brandle made it possible for users to exit or restart the system from any point. He also made it possible for users to indicate that they have finished using a screen by either pressing the <ENTER> key or clicking on the "Continue" button that he placed at the bottom of every screen.

17.1 THE OPENING SCREENS

The first screen seen by the user introduces the system; it displays the name "CIRCSIM-Tutor" and tells the user that the system comes from Rush Medical College and Illinois Institute of Technology. Then it asks the user for a name. This name is used to create a log file for this user session. If the system already has a file using this name, the old file is located and extended with this new material. During experiments with students at Rush Medical College, we assign code names for them to use in logging in as well as on the pretest, the posttest, the questionnaire, and this file, so we can collect the data that we need without any risk of invasion of privacy.

As soon as the user has logged in, the system displays three instructional screens that explain how the system works. It would be possible to fit all this material on one screen with a small font, but since it falls naturally into three different paragraphs, so we turned it into three screens, each with its own heading and a large comfortable font, in hopes that the users would actually read these instructions. Some users do, but many do not, so we have endeavored to make the other screens self-explanatory.

The design of the log file is an important issue in practical system design, an issue that raises more user interface questions. There are trade-offs between gathering the maximum amount of useful material and making the output too complicated to read. Our log file contains a great deal of information, including the names of the major modules called during the processing of each student input and the generation of the output, as well as the logic forms passed from module to module and any changes made to the student model.

This information is invaluable in debugging the system, but it is rather overwhelming to read, so Michael Glass wrote a utility program to extract just the material needed in our surface language studies, the text generated by the system and the material typed in by the student.

17.2 THE MAIN SCREEN

The original version of the Main Screen can be seen in Fig. 17.1. The current version appears in Fig. 17.2. There have been three major changes in screen design over the years. The first, and probably the most important, was the switch from separate dialogue screens for student input and tutor output to one dialogue screen with interleaved input and output. The second was the switch from using procedure names on the screen to the use of procedure descriptions. The third was the addition, and then the removal, of a window across the bottom of the screen intended for student note-taking.

17.2.1 Changes in the Window Structure

Originally, the system had separate windows for student input and tutor output and also a separate window for instructions, as shown in Fig. 17.1. This screen was constructed by Chong Woo (1991) and Jai Seu (1992), but it was based on Nakhoon Kim's (1989) work on the Prolog prototype version and on Jun Li's screen for Version 1 on the Xerox Lisp machines. We decided on this design for several reasons. It made it easy to manage the input and output separately. We had initially planned to reflect spelling changes back to the user, because we thought the user would want to see those changes. There was an even bigger motive after we implemented the first try at spelling correction. We were afraid that the time required for spelling correction would prevent us from getting back to the user in 2 sec with an appropriate response, so we divided the problem into two steps. First, we got back to the user with the results of the spelling correction. Then, as soon as the user approved those results, we began the actual dialogue processing.

When we read Barbara Fox's reports on her Human Tutoring Dialogue Project (1988a, 1988b; 1989) we acquired a more principled

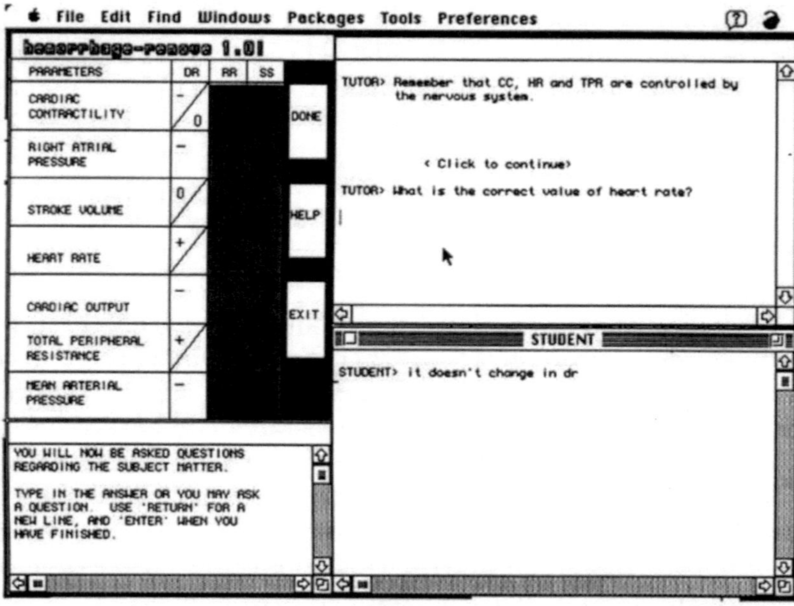

FIG. 17.1. The original Main Screen for Version 2.

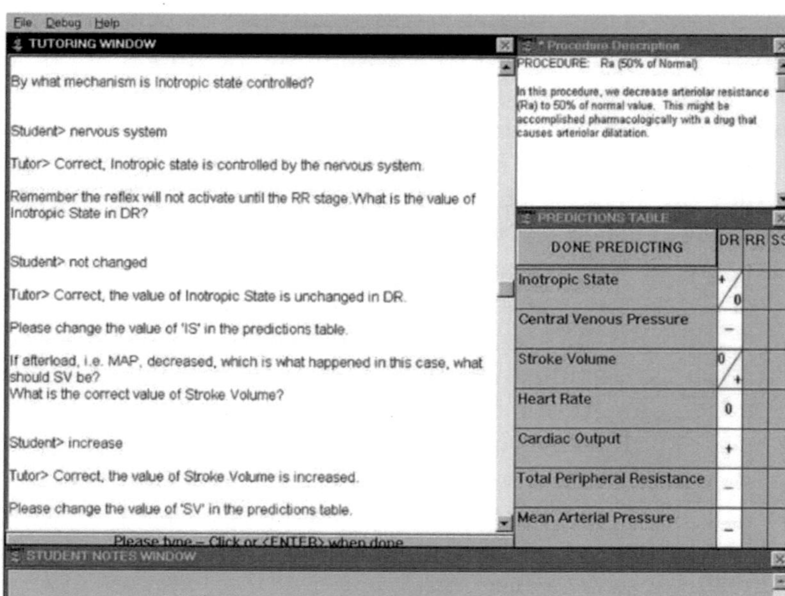

FIG. 17.2. The current main screen for Version 2 of CIRCSIM-Tutor.

motive for using two screens. She describes the student and the tutor talking at the same time. In particular, she talks about the important role of back-channel communication (when the tutor produces a string of "OK" and "Yes" responses and other encouraging noises while the student is working). Maintaining an input screen and an output screen at the same time would allow us to support this kind of back-channel communication, we thought, and we tried issuing encouraging responses while the student was typing.

It took only a few trials with students to convince us that they did not want to see spelling changes reflected back to them. They found the spelling correction feedback to be a nuisance and a waste of time. Instead, they wanted to get on with the dialogue and solve the problem. Fortunately, the speed of the new (circa 1992) Macintosh computers and the excellent Procyon implementation of Common Lisp, combined with some good programming on our part, solved the worst of our time problems. Shripriya Ramaswami (1993) improved the fonts and made the screen much more readable. Although we still believed in the back-channel argument for two screens, as more students used the system and found the two-window format confusing, we started to wonder about whether we should combine the input and output windows into a single dialogue window. The fact that system instructions came from one window and system dialogue output from another was also confusing. One student asked if there were two different systems, one issuing instructions and one taking part in the dialogue.

Brandle's change to a single window with interleaved dialogue was an immediate success. Users felt that the system had made a great leap forward. Several colleagues who were familiar with the system refused to believe that we had only changed the Screen Manager, and nothing else. The interleaved dialogue was easier to understand and it felt more natural to users, although the content was unchanged. The interleaved dialogue was easy to scroll, so students could look back to earlier stages if they lost their place in the dialogue or wanted to check an earlier point. (Scrolling is limited to the current procedure because of implementation problems.)

Because we did not do a controlled study when we made the changeover, we do not know exactly why the interleaved dialogue was such a hit with the users. We conjecture that the interleaved dialogue is not only easier to read, but emphasizes that the student is actively constructing the solution to the problem with the tutor. Fox

(1993b) described students and tutors building the answer to the problem together. The interleaved dialogue provides a record of this cooperative construction process. H. H. Clark (1996) described a dialogue as a joint activity, a series of joint actions. The interleaved dialogue makes this joint activity visible. Later, Brandle (1998) found Clark's joint actions to be an ideal framework for the analysis of acknowledgments in our dialogues.

17.2.2 Procedure Names Versus Procedure Descriptions

The change from using procedure names in Version 2 to using procedure descriptions in Version 3 started with an inspiration on the part of Byung-In Cho (2000). He set out to calibrate his new formula for Global Assessment (described in Section 14.5). By happenstance, he chose 10 log files collected in April 1998 from students in the alternative (problem-based learning) curriculum at Rush Medical College. He calculated their Global Assessment scores and discovered that these students consistently improved their scores from the second problem to the third, but then dropped back down going from the third problem to the fourth. The values can be found in Table 17.2 and a plot appears in Fig. 17.3.

When Cho examined the detailed log files, he realized that the students had found it difficult to determine the primary variable (the first variable in the Prediction Table affected by the perturbation) in the fourth problem. Further analysis of the log files showed that the students had been able to identify the primary variable easily in the earlier problems. What made the difference? The name of the primary variable was included in the name of the earlier procedures but not in the name of the fourth one. Our primary goal here is not to make things easy for the student, but to help the student learn how to identify the primary variable correctly, since this is an important part of the problem-solving process. So, Cho's analysis convinced us that we should use the full problem descriptions instead of problem names. Thus, in Version 3, we are replacing the kind of menu shown in Table 2.4 with a new screen like that in Figure 17.4—a screen with a choice of up to five procedure descriptions and no procedure names appearing (although we still store the names in the system for the convenience of the experts working on adding procedures to the system).

TABLE 17.2

Cho's Global Assessment Values

(From Table 5.1, p. 59, of Cho, 2000; Copied with Permission of the Author)

Student Codename	*Procedure No.*	*PTS (Prediction Table Score)*	*LA (Local Assessment)*	*GA (Global Assessment)*
bycx	2	0.142857	0.12374	0.12374
	3	0.333333	0.43186	0.27780
ev	2	0.809524	0.83894	0.83894
	3	0.904762	0.94398	0.89146
fugt	2	0.333333	0.41176	0.41176
	3	0.714286	0.81232	0.61204
	4	0.904762	0.91947	0.76576
irufgt	2	0.809524	0.86345	0.86345
	3		0.94888	0.90616
	4	0.714286	0.81723	0.86169
jqxcwd	2	0.809524	0.87325	0.87325
	3	0.904762	0.91506	0.89415
	4	0.809524	0.86835	0.88125
kp	3	1.0	1.0	1.0
	4	0.904762	0.919547	0.95973
olaz	2	0.714286	0.79272	0.79272
	3	0.904762	0.94888	0.87080
	4	0.714286	0.75840	0.81460
pknm	2	0.57143	0.87185	0.87185
	1	0.904762	0.91947	0.89566
	3	1.0	1.0	0.94783
	4	0.714286	0.78782	0.85913
rishqj	2	0.619048	0.62395	0.62395
	3	0.904762	0.94888	0.78641
	4	0.619048	0.72689	0.75665
vehs	2	0.428571	0.53151	0.53151
	3	0.619048	0.66317	0.59734
	4	0.238095	0.38025	0.48880

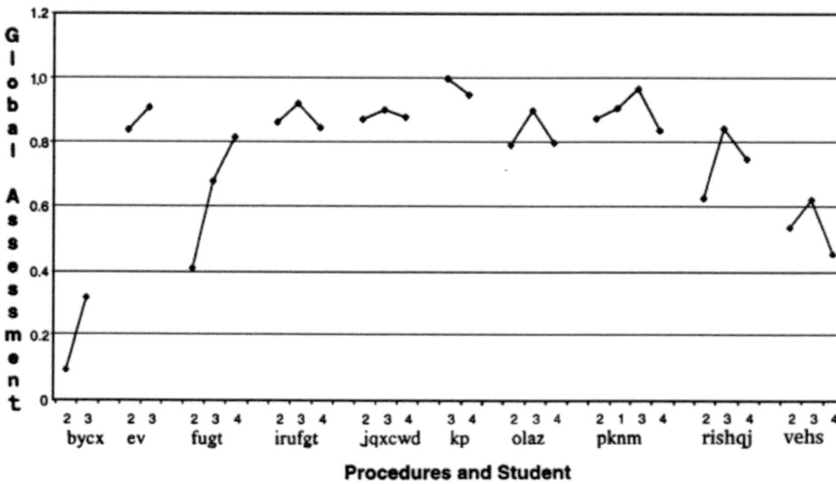

FIG. 17.3. Plot of student performance from Procedure 2 to Procedure 4, showing the decline from Procedure 3 to Procedure 4 (adapted from Cho, 2000, p. 62).

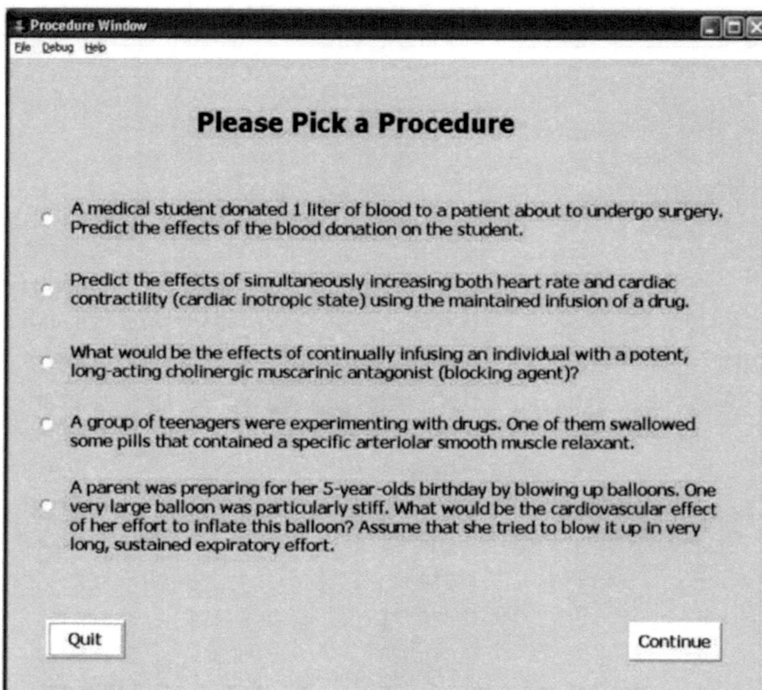

FIG. 17.4. New procedure selection window in Version 3 (new Screen Manager by Hyun Seok Roh, written in Allegro Lisp 6.2).

17.2.3 Providing Genuinely Helpful Help

The problem of determining how much "help" is really most helpful for the student and when to give that help is a pervasive one both in tutoring systems and in textbooks. Mathematics texts too often group problems about a particular solution technique together at the end of the chapter. This helps students solve those particular problems, but fails to give them practice in figuring out which solution techniques apply to a given problem. This is a problem that we have not really solved. We have dodged it instead by giving more detailed instructions and by inviting the students to put problems into words.

Kurt VanLehn (VanLehn, Lynch, et al., 2002) has come up with an excellent solution to this interface problem, using an idea that never occurred to us because we are terrified of tape. The ANDES/ATLAS team has obtained useful information by audiotaping students while they are using the ANDES physics tutor. To avoid synchronization problems, they store the audiotape contents in the log file using a commercial product called ScreenCAM. These tapes revealed student problems in figuring out what to do next that were not addressed by the low-level "Help" available and which did not show up in their original log file. After listening to the confusion expressed on the tapes, VanLehn's team added a dialogue on global problem-solving strategies to the system, based on the solution graph. This dialogue asks questions like "What quantity does the problem seek?" and "What principle should be used to find it?" which address high-level problem solving ideas that are often left tacit in formal lectures.

17.2.4 Additional Screens for Version 3

We were distressed to discover that the Version 2 Screen Manager did not work well with the emerging Version 3 of CIRCSIM-Tutor. In the summer of 2004, two master's students (H. S. Roh and Y. W. Kim) built two new Screen Managers for Version 3, one in Allegro Lisp 6.2, which includes the new screen standard, and one in Java, which would allow us to produce a Web-enabled version of the system comparatively easily. We are still experimenting with both of these new components and connecting them to the new database. Figure 17.4

shows one of the new screens written by Roh and Kim to support Cho's curriculum planning.

17.2.5 A Separate Window for Student Notes

Several years ago, Joel Michael and Allen Rovick suggested that we add a window for student notes across the bottom of the screen. We hoped that students would use this window to record any unanswered questions or points of confusion for later study. We used the window extensively in debugging the system but no student ever entered any notes. So we recently removed the window. This change gave us more space for the dialogue window and the procedure descriptions.

We believe that the window for student notes was a good idea before its time. Students might indeed make effective use of a window of this type, if it were available across the board in the software systems that they use, and if they had a special-purpose editor to date these notes automatically, collect them, and organize them effectively for later use.

17.3 TAKE-HOME MESSAGE

Among the lessons that we have learned about screen design, the one most useful to other system implementers is likely to be the value of interleaving the tutor and the student contributions to the dialogue. The switch from separate dialogue screens for student input and tutor output to one dialogue screen with interleaved input and output made a material difference to our users.

We have included our experience with procedure names and procedure descriptions in the hope that it may help us all think more carefully about the communicative power of labels. We have certainly tried to take advantage of this power in writing this book, by putting labels on lots of small sections and appealing to the readers' talents for integration. Names in windows on a screen are probably even more important in promoting the comfort and understanding on the part of the user.

Although we ultimately gave up on the window for student notes, we are still convinced that there is the germ of a good idea there. We would like to write a suite of tools for medical students that provides a window like this in all of the school software, involving knowledge sources of every kind from Web browsing to text to educational systems, that includes an automatic means for putting this material in files on a laptop, and an editor for organizing it, storing it, and retrieving it.

The effort of implementing the Screen Manager has made us more aware than ever of the importance of standards—the emergence of Common Lisp as we were implementing the current version of the system made a big difference to our work. The first version was implemented on Xerox Lisp machines in Interlisp. Conversion of the system to Common Lisp was a huge effort but much of the code written at that time is still running. The fact that the initial version of Common Lisp that we used did not yet contain the standard for screen commands has meant that the changes in the screen described here have all required major implementation efforts.

This page intentionally left blank

PART IV: What Have We Learned?

In this final part we talk about what happens when we use CIRCSIM-Tutor in the classroom, what works and what does not, what we want to fix and how we plan to go about it. We try to provide a sense of current research in this area and describe some of the hot topics. Then we discuss what research we hope to do next and what we hope that other people will do. Finally, we recapitulate the take home lessons that we sprinkled through the book.

Chapter 18 describes our experiments with CIRCSIM-Tutor in the classroom, pretests, posttests, and what happened in between. Chapter 19 talks about other current research in dialogue-based tutoring. Chapter 20 points to some directions for new research. Chapter 21 reveals the secrets of our success.

This page intentionally left blank

18

CIRCSIM-Tutor in the Classroom

18.0 GOALS OF THE CIRCSIM-TUTOR PROJECT

When we began the CIRCSIM-Tutor project in 1987, we had two goals clearly in mind: (a) learn enough about expert human tutoring so that we could build a model for a computer tutor capable of carrying out one-on-one tutoring using a natural language dialogue, and (b) actually build such a tutor and use it in the classroom with students. In the preceding chapters, we have described what we needed to learn about human tutoring, how we learned it, and what we have been able to implement. Now we want to tell you about our experiences using CIRCSIM-Tutor in the classroom.

18.1 DETERMINING THE EFFECTS OF USING CIRCSIM-TUTOR

There are various ways of looking at the effects of using a piece of teaching software. One can ask about changes in the attitudes of the students to the educational content (e.g., "I think it's relevant to my career goals," or "I like the subject matter."). One can ask whether the program has helped students acquire new or additional knowledge about the domain. Finally, one can ask if the program has helped students learn to apply their knowledge to solve certain kinds of problems. Whichever question is of interest, a pretest–posttest paradigm is an appropriate and useful approach to answering it (Dimitrov & Rumrill, 2003; Ravid, 2000).

Our interest has always been in the effect of using CIRCSIM or CIRCSIM-Tutor on the students' ability to apply their knowledge of the baroreceptor reflex to solve problems about the regulation of blood pressure. Neither program is intended to convey new information about the cardiovascular system, although when students use programs like these, they do learn things they failed to learn in prior learning experiences (as pointed out by VanLehn, 1996). Thus, we needed to measure changes in student problem-solving behavior as a consequence of working with CIRCSIM-Tutor.

What should we attempt to measure? It would be insufficient to determine *only* whether students can solve baroreceptor prediction problems better after using CIRCSIM-Tutor. We also want to know whether the use of the program increases the students' understanding of the individual relationships that make up the baroreceptor reflex. Finally, we want to know whether the students can apply their understanding of blood pressure regulation to problems that are presented in a context or format very different than CIRCSIM-Tutor problems.

Thus, we usually employed a three part pretest and posttest: (a) a test of student knowledge of the individual relationships between cardiovascular variables making up the baroreceptor reflex, (b) a baroreceptor reflex problem to be solved using a Prediction Table, and (c) a set of multiple choice questions posed in a clinical context requiring application of the same understanding of the system. The pretest and posttest were always administered as paper-and-pencil exercises. Samples 18.1, 18.2, and 18.3 (to be found at the end of the chapter) contain examples of each of the three tests that we used.

The relationship test listed eight cardiovascular variables in alphabetical order and asked the students to define 12 causal relationships between appropriate pairs of variables. They were also asked to identify whether the relationship was a "direct" one or an "inverse" one (these terms were defined on the test page). A correct answer, then, had to specify a correct immediate causal relationship between two variables (1 point was awarded) and it had to correctly identify the nature of the relationship (direct or inverse, a second point was awarded). The maximum score for the Relationship Test was therefore 24. In some experiments, we were also interested in how many correct relationships were identified (the maximum number is 12) and how many incorrect relationships were listed (there is no maximum). These scores are clearly not fully independent of one another, but they do examine somewhat different aspects of the students' knowledge.

In all of these experiments, we presented the students with a description of a disturbance to the cardiovascular system and a Prediction Table (see Sample 18.2) to be filled in. The definitions of the DR, RR, and SS phases of the response were provided on the page. In some of the experiments, the primary variable, the first variable in the Prediction Table that changes, was identified and its direction of change was indicated. In other experiments, the students were not given the correct prediction for the primary variable. One measure of performance is simply the number of correct predictions that are made. Therefore, the maximum score for this measure is 20 or 21, depending on which version of the Prediction Table was used.

There is, however, another way to think about the effect of using CIRCSIM-Tutor. Each of the 20 predictions made on the pretest is either correct (C) or wrong (W). We can then ask whether using CIRCSIM-Tutor results in changes in the correctness of these predictions. Is a W prediction on the pretest changed to a C prediction (W-C) on the posttest or is a pretest C prediction changed to a W prediction (C-W)? If CIRCSIM-Tutor is effective, one would expect that the number of (W-C) changes would be greater than the number of (C-W) changes. The McNemar change test (a nonparametric test that is a form of the Sign Test; Siegel & Castellan, 1988) can be used to determine the statistical significance of the differences obtained, and this analysis was used in some experiments.

There is another aspect of performance on a baroreceptor Prediction Table problem that is of interest. Particular prediction errors, or patterns of errors, are diagnostic for certain conceptual difficulties or misconceptions (Michael et al., 2002). We have in the past (Rovick & Michael, 1992) referred to such errors as "bugs." We have identified four different bug categories and a total of 17 different bugs. In some experiments reported here, we scored the number of bug categories present and the total number of bugs present.

In our experiments with CIRCSIM-Tutor, we used two different sets of disturbances in the paper-and-pencil pretests and posttests. One was either an increase or a decrease in HR due to a malfunctioning electronic cardiac pacemaker. The other was an increase or decrease of arteriolar resistance (Ra, the major component of TPR, the Total Peripheral Resistance) caused by administration of a drug. The pairs of disturbances (increase or decrease) ought to be of comparable difficulty, and the results reported below demonstrate that, in fact, they are equivalent problems.

It can be argued that the ability to predict correctly the changes in system behavior that are the focus of CIRCSIM and CIRCSIM-Tutor need not reflect any deep understanding (Michael, 2001) of cardiovascular function. Indeed, one of the IIT graduate students participating in the CIRCSIM-Tutor project quickly learned to make correct predictions for any disturbance whose primary variable he could identify while having essentially no understanding of cardiovascular physiology as could be assessed by any other measure (for example, the ability to explain the mechanisms underlying the casual relationship between two variables). Thus, we thought it important to demonstrate that students could apply their understanding of the baroreceptor reflex to novel situations. This is why we wrote eight multiple choice questions (MCQs) that required students to use their understanding of the baroreceptor reflex to select the correct choice and used four of them in the pretest and four in the posttest. As we described in Chapter 10, analysis of the results after the experiments in 1999 showed that the two sets of multiple choice questions that we wrote are not entirely comparable, and so we do not report the MCQ results.

The statistical significance of the pretest–posttest differences (learning gains) was routinely determined with one-tailed *t* tests (assuming equal variance). In addition, we generally calculated the effect size (J. Cohen, 1988; Coe, 2000) to determine whether the learning gains were large or small. The size of the learning effects (ES = effect size) was calculated using the following formula:

ES = (Posttest mean–Pretest mean)/standard deviation of the gain scores

Finally, when it appeared that the pretest scores of the control and treatment groups being tested were different, we dealt with this by performing an analysis of covariance (Becker, 2000; Wildt & Ahtola, 1978) on this data using SPSS®.

In addition to determining the learning effects of using CIRCSIM-Tutor, we wanted to determine the student response to use of this program. We wrote a survey made up of 10 questions employing a 5-point Likert-type scale (*definitely YES* = 1 to *definitely NO* = 5) and 1 free response question, which asked the following: "Please comment on any of the preceding questions or any other issue (problems using the system, help that wasn't provided but should have been, changes you would like to see in the system)." This survey can be seen in Sample 18.4 at the end of the chapter.

18.2 THE PILOT EXPERIMENT (APRIL 1998)

The first test of CIRCSIM-Tutor with a significant number of students took place in April 1998. Twenty-three 1st-year Rush Medical College medical students in the Alternative Curriculum, a problem-based learning curriculum, used CIRCSIM-Tutor in a regularly scheduled computer laboratory (students in previous years had used CIRCSIM). This laboratory was the culminating exercise in a 4-week block during which the students had been learning cardiovascular and respiratory physiology. Students worked in groups of two to three at a computer with an instructor (Joel Michael) circulating and available to answer questions. Two students did not complete the posttests. Hence we have data from 21 students.

A 30-min three-part pretest was administered. The students then worked with CIRCSIM-Tutor for 1 hr. Finally, a 30-min posttest and survey were administered. This protocol is similar to the one used in the CIRCSIM experiment (see Section 1.1; Rovick & Michael, 1992). The pretests and posttests differed somewhat from the tests described in the previous section.

The first part of the pretest asked the students to define the relationships between seven cardiovascular parameters by filling in the blanks in nine different statements; the maximum score for "relationship questions" (the number of completely correct statements) is 9. There are 16 possible correct parameters to complete the 9 statements; the maximum score for "relationship points" (total number of correct variables) is 16. Part 2 of the pretest presented 18 statements in the form of "if A increases/decreases, then B will increase, decrease, or be unchanged." The maximum score for "determinants" is therefore 18. The third part of the pretest presented a cardiovascular perturbation, a baroreceptor prediction problem, and asked the students to fill in the complete Prediction Table giving a maximum score of 21 for "correct predictions." Parts 1 and 2 of the pretest and posttest were different only in that the same set of relationships were tested by different statements of this same form. The problems to be solved described either an increased or a decreased HR due to a malfunctioning pacemaker. An attempt was made to administer one version of the pretest to half the students and the second version to the other half. However, because of the three dropouts from the experiment, the number of students in each group was not the same.

18.2.1 Version 2.6 of CIRCSIM-Tutor and What It Could Do

The version of CIRCSIM-Tutor used in this experiment, Version 2.6 (Table 11.1), was the first to incorporate Michael Glass's parser (see Chapter 13) and Stefan Brandle's Screen Manager (see Chapter 17). Only four of the eight standard procedures used in CIRCSIM were available for student use. The "I'm sorry, I don't understand you" message was replaced with a set of more helpful messages that tell the student what the system is expecting.

18.2.2 Learning Outcomes

We first examined the raw scores for the two versions of the pretest to determine whether they are, in fact, equivalent; our hypothesis was that the means would be the same. Hence, in this case, we applied two-tailed t tests to each pair of scores. Table 18.1 contains this data. The p values obtained show that there is no significant difference between the pretest scores on the two versions of the pretest.

Most important, we can now say that the two baroreceptor reflex problems we routinely use on our pretest and posttest, one involving an increase and the other a decrease in HR, are of equal difficulty.

Next we compared the pretest and posttest scores for all students to determine whether any learning occurred as a consequence of using CIRCSIM-Tutor. This data can be seen in Table 18.2. One-tailed t tests (assuming equal variance) were applied to the pretest and posttest scores for each variable. We also calculated the effect size (see Section 18.1). The mean relationship score improved from

TABLE 18.1

Comparison of the Two Versions of the Pretests Used to Assess Learning Gains from CIRCSIM-Tutor in April 1998

	Test Version 12 (N = 13)	*Test Version 21 (N = 8)*	*Gain*	p *Value* (12–21)*
Relationship points[a] (Mean/*SD*)	9.31 (2.84)	11.25 (1.16)	1.94	.083
Relationship questions[b] (Mean/*SD*)	3.54 (2.11)	4.75 (0.46)	1.21	.129
Determinants[c] (Mean/*SD*)	13.23 (1.79)	13.63 (2.13)	0.40	.653
Correct predictions[d] (Mean/*SD*)	13.31 (4.46)	10.75 (3.70)	–2.56	.183

[a]Maximum score = 16; [b]Maximum score = 9; [c]Maximum score = 18; [d]Maximum score = 21.
*2-tailed *t* test (assuming equal variance) was performed because our hypothesis was that the means were the same.

TABLE 18.2

Effects of CIRCSIM-Tutor on Learning in April 1998

	Pretest Mean (SD)	*Posttest Mean* (SD)	*Gain*	*(Pre–Post) p Value**	*Effect Size*
Relationship points[a]	10.05 (2.50)	11.81 (2.73)	1.76	< .05	0.88
Relation questions[b]	4.00 (1.76)	5.19 (1.83)	1.19	< .05	0.62
Determinants[c]	13.38 (1.88)	13.10 (1.87)	–0.28	ns	–0.16
Correct predictions[d]	12.33 (4.19)	16.62 (2.97)	4.29	< .05	1.04

[a]Maximum score = 16; [b]Maximum score = 9; [c]Maximum score = 18; [d]Maximum score = 21.
*One-tailed *t* test (assuming equal variance).

10.05 to 11.81 out of a maximum of 16, with $p = .017$ and an effect size of 0.88. The mean score on the relation questions improved from 4.00 to 5.19 out of a maximum of 9, with $p = .019$ and effect size of 0.62. There was no significant difference in the mean determinant scores, which actually dropped from 13.38 to 13.10 out of a maximum of 18 ($p = .312$). The number of correct predictions rose from 12.33 to 16.62 out of a maximum of 21, with $p < .001$ and a large effect size of 1.04.

The effect sizes seen here are surprisingly large; J. Cohen (1988) classified effects of 0.5 as moderate and 1.0 as large. We can claim that CIRCSIM-Tutor "worked" in its earliest test with a whole (small) class.

There is no doubt that using CIRCSIM-Tutor improved students' ability to predict the behavior of the cardiovascular system when blood pressure is perturbed ("correct predictions" scores improved significantly) and also improved the students' knowledge of the relationships between the cardiovascular variables involved in blood pressure regulation ("relationship points" and "relationship questions" scores are significantly improved). There was no significant difference in the pretest–posttest scores for "determinants."

18.2.3 Survey Results

Not all students wrote comments about CIRCSIM-Tutor, but those students who did write something were quite positive about their experience. They often produced helpful suggestions about improvements that they thought would make the program better. The students generally agreed that CIRCSIM-Tutor was easy to use (Sample 18.4, questions 1–5). Students were somewhat less positive about the dialogue being "varied and interesting" (question 6). The hints and explanations generated by CIRCSIM-Tutor were judged to be informative (question 7). Somewhat to our surprise, the students were relatively satisfied with the column by column protocol and did not express a strong interest in having the system respond immediately to each individual prediction error (question 8). It is also interesting to note, however, that question 8 generated responses with by far the highest standard deviation; students were more strongly divided in their opinions about this issue than for any of the other issues we sampled. Most important, the students expressed the opinion that CIRCSIM-Tutor had helped them understand the baroreceptor reflex and make predictions about its responses (questions 9 and10). These results can be seen in Fig. 18.1.

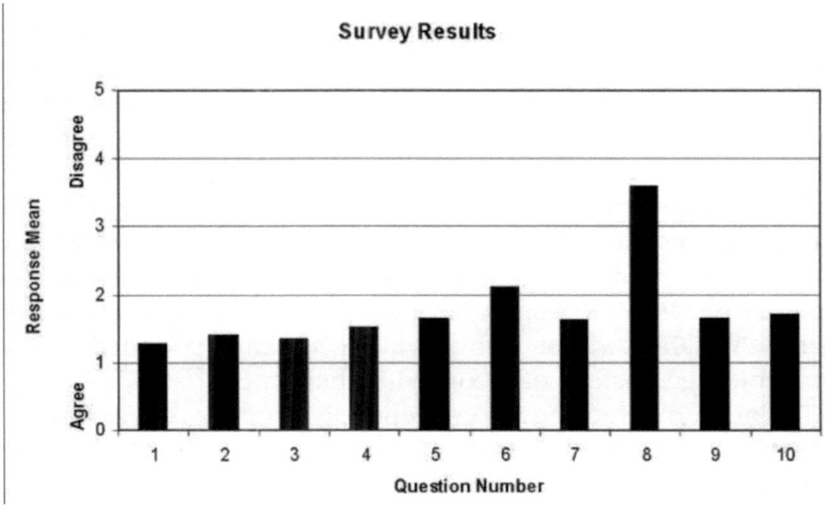

FIG. 18.1. Results of the CIRCSIM-Tutor Survey, April 1998 (the survey questions appear in Sample 18.4).

18.2.4 System Performance

One computer crashed, presumably reflecting a bug in the new parser. The student restarted the program without even telling us about it and finished all four procedures before the laboratory was over. Because the student erased the first log file in the process, we were never quite sure what had happened. Most of the other students also finished all four procedures, and we realized that we needed to add more procedures and also expand the amount of natural language interaction in all of them. When we read over the log files, the most glaring problem was the sparseness of the hints and the quality of those that the system asked. Although Gregory Hume (1995) had completed his analysis of the hints produced by expert tutors (see Chapter 8), none of his work had yet been implemented and all of the hints in the system were reminders of one type or another beginning with "Remember" or "Think about …."

One consequence of having a more robust parser is that the system did not crash when the students expressed annoyance during the dialog and we were able to collect a few examples and correlate them with what the system was doing to cause this reaction. We identified a number of places where the student's answer was a "near miss"—essentially correct but not what the system was expecting. The system told the students that they were wrong and attacked the problem as if the students were totally ignorant. For example, if the student answered "ANS" (Autonomic Nervous System) or "BR" (Baroreceptor Reflex) or "RA" (Arterial Resistance) instead of "CNS" or "nervous system" when asked for the mechanism controlling TPR, the system responded "Wrong" and gave an explanation. We also found some similar spelling correction problems. Four students typed a small letter "o" instead of a zero when they wanted to convey that the variable did not change and the system responded with an error message, instead of recognizing their intent.

The new error messages were generally a success, but a couple of them proved to be difficult to understand and the students appealed to the experimenters for explanations. The student who tried to type in two different answers to one question did not understand the message, "You can't have it both ways." The message, "That is not the variable under discussion," appeared when the student was asked to update a value in the Prediction Table to reflect the results of the tutoring dialogue, but updated another variable instead. It did not help in one of the two situations where it appeared, so we reworded the request to refer to the variable by name. There were fewer questions about the program overall during the experiment and we were convinced that the students found the new interface easier to use, but we immediately noticed one unexpected problem. The teaching laboratory at Rush Medical College had a variety of new computers with screens of different sizes. The system ran on all of them, but we had not thought to make the screen adjustable to the monitor size.

18.2.5 Conclusions Drawn

We were pleased by the results of this experiment. CIRCSIM-Tutor proved to be robust enough for student use in a classroom setting; the system only crashed once, and it functioned, in the broadest possible sense, effectively. Students using CIRCSIM-Tutor clearly learned about the baroreceptor reflex and how to predict the responses of the system to changes in blood pressure. Students liked the program and thought that they had learned something from it. On a more pragmatic note, we now had evidence that the "mirror-image" problems that we used in the prediction component of the pretest and posttest (increases or decreases of HR or TPR) are, in fact, of equal difficulty.

18.3 OUR FIRST LARGE-SCALE EXPERIMENT (NOVEMBER, 1998)

Fifty 1st-year medical students volunteered for the experiment and were paid a nominal amount for their participation. Twenty-six students worked alone at a computer and 24 worked in pairs, two to a computer, which gave us a total of 38 log files. Each student individually spent 30 min taking a pretest. All students then worked with CIRCSIM-Tutor for 1 hr. Finally, the students spent 30 min individually taking a posttest and completing a survey describing their reactions to CIRCSIM-Tutor. The pretest and posttest were identical to those described in Section 18.1 in this chapter. This experiment has been described in greater detail in Michael, Rovick, Glass, Zhou, and Evens (2003).

18.3.1 Version 2.7 of CIRCSIM-Tutor and What It Could Do

CIRCSIM-Tutor Version 2.7 (see Table 11.1) was used in this experiment. The major change between April 1998 and November 1998 was the addition of the remaining four problems originally used in CIRCSIM. Yujian Zhou added the frames needed to support the new knowledge required for the additional problems presented. She also generated the first classification of student errors into six categories, and generated a set of different appropriate responses for each. This classification allowed Zhou and Glass to take the first steps in the attack on the "near miss" problem. Zhou created some hints for use in these cases. Glass built the first version of the ontology described in Chapter 13 so that the system could recognize a wider range of correct ways of describing the nervous system in response to mechanism questions. Zhou and Glass also did a lot to make the system more robust by adding checks for illegal (non-ASCII) characters and stripping them out of the inputs. Glass rewrote the list of error messages that the system generated when it did not understand the student's input, making them more informative and thus assisting students to generate an answer that could be understood by the system. Stefan Brandle modified the Screen Manager so that the screen could be adapted to the monitor size on the system on which it was installed, thus enabling CIRCSIM-Tutor to run well on all the machines in the laboratory. The dialogue window was bigger and both the dialogue window and perturbation window were scrollable.

18.3.2 Learning Outcomes

All five of the measures that we obtained showed that significant increases in learning occurred as a result of using CIRCSIM-Tutor (see Table 18.3). The number of relationship points rose from a pretest mean of 13.64 to a posttest mean of 16.16 ($p = .016$). The number of correct predictions increased from a mean of 14.30 to a mean of 17.27 ($p < .001$). The number of different types of bugs went down significantly (2.67 to 1.28; $p < .001$), as did the total number of bugs (4.07 to 1.10; $p < .001$).

When we asked whether the use of CIRCSIM-Tutor enabled students to correct the particular prediction errors they had made on the pretest, the answer was yes. The McNemar change test, a type of Sign Test (Siegel & Castellan, 1988), clearly indicates that there were many more W-C changes in comparing pretest and posttest than there were C-W changes (see Table 18.4). We can therefore argue that use of CIRCSIM-Tutor helped students to correct the prediction er-

TABLE 18.3
Learning Gains From Using CIRCSIM-Tutor in November 1998
(data from Michael, Rovick, Glass, Zhou, & Evens, 2003, used with permission and reformatted)

	Pretest Mean (SD)	*Posttest Mean* (SD)	*Gain Scores*	*(Pre–Post)* p *Values**
Relationship points[a]	13.64 (6.13)	16.16 (5.25)	2.52	.016
Correct predictions[b]	14.31 (3.81)	17.27 (1.88)	2.96	< .001
Bug categories[c]	2.67 (1.50)	1.28 (183)	–1.39	< .001
Total no. of bugs[d]	4.07 (2.27)	1.10 (1.59)	–2.97	< .001

[a]Maximum score = 12; [b]Maximum score = 24; [c]Maximum score = 7; [d]Maximum score = 4.
*One-tailed *t* test (assuming equal variance).

TABLE 18.4

The Effect of CIRCSIM-Tutor on Correcting Prediction Errors Measured in Terms of Pretest–Posttest Changes in November, 1998

		PostTest *C*	PostTest *W*
Pretest	*C*	556	67
Pretest	*W*	197	104

There were 197 predictions that were wrong on the pretest but correct on the posttest, compared with 67 predictions that were correct on the pretest but wrong on the posttest. The difference between the number of (w-c) changes and the number of (c-w) changes is statistically significant.) *Note.* C = correct. W = wrong.
*Data from Michael et al. (1999).

rors that they made on the pretest. Thus, it is fair to say that CIRCSIM-Tutor produced definite learning gains.

18.3.3 Survey Results

Student responses on the survey were quite positive. They clearly felt that the program had helped them to learn something about the baroreceptor reflex. They were less positive about the natural language aspects of the program; the language being generated was recognized as being stilted, although the hints and explanations were useful, and there were still too many explanations and not enough hints. This definitely favorable review by the students was evident in both the numerical ratings (which appear in Fig. 18.2) and the written comments (which appear in Table 18.5).

18.3.4 System Performance

The system was much more robust than it had been in April. There were no system crashes this time and the system was able to respond to a much larger percentage of its inputs. There were 1,801 inputs typed by the students. All but 10 of these (a total of 1,791) received a more or less reasonable response from the system. None of the 10 unusable inputs was more than five characters long and we could not understand what the student intended in any of them.

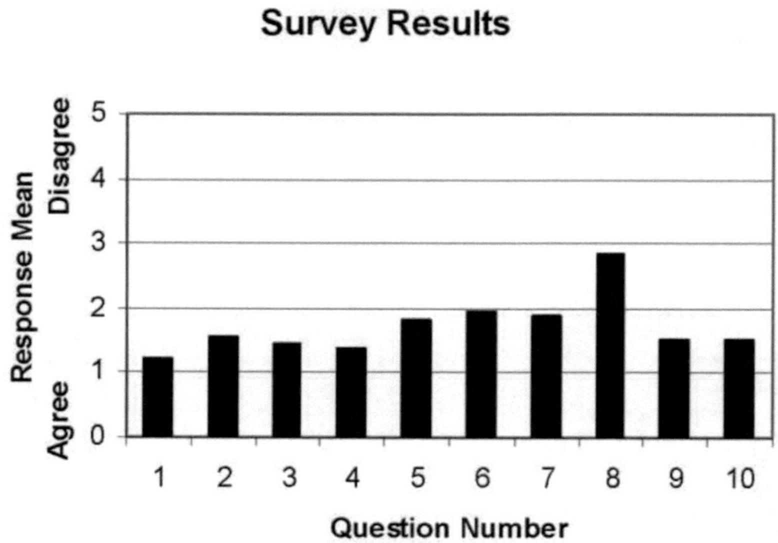

FIG. 18.2. Results of the CIRCSIM-Tutor Survey, November 1998 (from Michael, Rovick, Glass, Zhou, & Evens, 2003, p. 251). The survey questions appear in Sample 18.4.

For example, one student typed the answer "93," another typed "h"; we could not determine any relationship between these responses and the question asked. Of these 1,791 turns, three were bare question marks, presumably requests for help; 393 were a single symbol (+, –, or 0) or symbols like "o" which the system mapped into one of these. These were interpreted as meaning "increase," "decrease," and "unchanged," and tutoring proceeded along normal lines. Thus, there were 1,395 alphabetic turns. Thirty of these needed spelling correction and they were ultimately recognized, but 19 were not recognized at all by the system, although a human tutor could certainly make sense of them. That left 1,376 turns. About 5% of these were greeted with one of the error messages because the system could not understand how they related to the question asked by the system. The others received a response as part of a continuing tutoring dialogue. No student tried a student initiative, as far as we could tell; all of these student inputs were directed at trying to answer the questions.

TABLE 18.5

A Sample of Written Student Responses to the Survey in November, 1998 (copied from Michael et al., 2003, p. 252, with permission from http://www.tandf.co.uk)

There are a few instances when the dialogue appeared contradictory, yet one couldn't ask questions or further explore it, so in those cases I remained unclear on the particular situation. Otherwise very helpful program.

It would be helpful if the system provided a little more explanation about my wrong answers. I felt I corrected my errors because it told me to, but I didn't always understand the explanation. For example, I made a mistake in the SS segment. The system told me that SS followed RR and therefore the answer would be similar to DR.

The fact that one could use abbreviations was pretty ????? and helpful; specific word format was not an issue. The explanation for steady state answers and how it followed the direct response of baroreceptor response was a little weak, Otherwise, excellent program!

I enjoyed using this program—it was fun and it helped clarify certain things for me.

I thought the program was excellent—especially the way it responded to individual responses precisely. I think it would be very helpful.

It may be only my personal view, but whenever information, particularly when there is a lot of it, appearing on a computer screen, I tend not to read any of it. If you use simple short phrases for responses I might read them with more attention.

A deeper explanation of why answers are incorrect should be given. The print of the scenario described was too small. Overall it was an easy to follow program with concise answers.

Somewhat hard to answer questions presented because I didn't understand what was being asked.

The questions asked by the tutor are not phrased clearly and acceptable answers should be displayed along with the question. Too many questions not enough explanation.

Very good—I would like to have more of these situations (more than the 4 we covered). Please make this available before the exam. This is the best way to understand cardiovascular physiology.

A flow chart would have been helpful.

The explanations could be a little more detail & informative. Otherwise, great program.

BRAVO! Will it [the program] be available before the final exam?

Note. SS - Steady State; RR = Reflex Response; DR = Direct Response.

The spelling correction program had been enhanced to handle typographical errors found in the April log files, so by November 1998, it was able to map "rh" into "hr" and "trp" into "tpr." It also figured out that "inotrphic" was really "inotropic" and that "cariac" was intended to be "cardiac."

We spent a lot of time analyzing the 19 inputs that made sense to humans but that the system could not recognize (see Table 18.6), because we felt that these were places where we could and should make improvements. We discovered that the spelling correction program failed to recognize "increaseed" as "increase," and "in" as "inverse," and it could not break down "istpr" into "is" and "tpr." The system failed to recognize "neurological" properly because of an error in the lexicon, and "central venous volume" turned out to be missing from the lexicon completely, although it was in the knowledge base. The system also failed to recognize "metabolic factors," which is still not part of the system, because we decided that this concept was outside the domain. More seriously, the system had no way to respond to the word "help."

18.3.5 Conclusions Drawn

The results of this experiment were also quite satisfying for us: (a) Students clearly learned about the baroreceptor reflex from CIRCSIM-Tutor, their knowledge of important relationships increased, they were better able to predict the responses of the system,

TABLE 18.6
Inputs Not Recognized by CIRCSIM-Tutor in November 1998

Type of Input	***Frequency***
Spelling or typing errors ("istpr")	6
Missing or incomplete lexical entry ("neurological")	5
Expressions of frustration ("Kiss my ass")	2
Abbreviations ("in" for "inverse")	2
"Help"	2
Concepts outside the domain ("metabolic factors")	2
Total	19

and they reduced the bugs or misconceptions that were present when they started the program; (b) students continued to like using the program; and (c) CIRCSIM-Tutor was more robust and basically did a better job in its interaction with the student.

18.4 A COMPARISON OF CIRCSIM AND CIRCSIM-TUTOR (NOVEMBER 1999)

In November 1999, we conducted an experiment that was intended to answer several questions about student learning about the baroreceptor reflex: (a) Does being tutored by an expert human tutor help? (b) Does use of either CIRCSIM or CIRCSIM-Tutor help, and (c) is there any difference in the effectiveness of CIRCSIM and CIRCSIM-Tutor? The results of the tutoring experiment (question 1) have already been described in Chapter 10. Here we discuss only student use of CIRCSIM and CIRCSIM-Tutor.

18.4.1 Version 2.8 of CIRCSIM-Tutor and What It Could Do

Zhou and Glass made a vigorous attack on the problems in natural language understanding and in the generation of hints in the year between November 1998 and November 1999. Glass (1999) expanded the ontology and added a number of new terms to the lexicon, so that the system could recognize the inputs that had been missed in 1998. He (Glass, 2000) rewrote the approach to handling ambiguity so that the system could recognize "i" and "in" as meaning "increase" when the system is asking about a parameter change, but then recognize those same inputs as meaning "inverse" when the system is asking about the nature of a relationship. Glass and Zhou together made changes in the understander and the modeler to allow the system to recognize "Help" and "I don't understand" as being like "I don't know," so that the system would stop and explain and then carry on with the existing tutoring plan. Glass (2001) made a number of additions to the grammar as described in Chapter 13, so that the system could handle inputs with algebraic symbols in the midst of an English sentence. He worried about how to get the students to recognize this capability and finally suggested to Zhou that she add expressions of this type to some of the hints in the hope that the students would pick up this usage from the system.

Meanwhile, Zhou (2000) talked to Hume about hints and read and reread his thesis and papers and then implemented a large number of hints of different types. She realized that to do this, she needed to build a much more complete classification of student errors and a much more detailed student model to represent the state of the student's knowledge. She refined the 6 categories of student errors into 24 (see Section 13.5). Then she implemented a four-layer student model, as described in Chapter 17, to keep track of these errors (Zhou & Evens, 1999). Then, with a series of machine learning experiments using Hume's markup of hints in the transcripts and a lot of manual searching as well, she discovered what hints the experts used to match particular situations. She implemented all of this in terms of APE operators for use in Version 3 and then rewrote it in Lisp so that it would run in Version 2 (Zhou et al., 1999a, 1999b).

18.4.2 Protocol for the Experiment

Two computer laboratory sessions are routinely scheduled in the part of the course that focuses on cardiovascular physiology, and the second has as its content the baroreceptor reflex. This computer laboratory is the culminating exercise in the cardiovascular block of the course. The Rush Medical College computer laboratory is not large enough to accommodate the full class at one session, so half the class (approximately 60 students) is typically scheduled for each of 2 successive days.

In the first computer laboratory session, all of the students worked with CIRCSIM-Tutor, some of them solo and the others in pairs. In the second computer session, all students used CIRCSIM. Before starting either program, all students took a pretest. After completing the use of the program, all students took a posttest and completed a survey about the particular program they had used (CIRCSIM-Tutor or CIRCSIM). The pretests and posttests have been described in Section 18.1. We collected data from 22 students who used CIRCSIM-Tutor and 23 students who used CIRCSIM.

In this experiment, we were able to arrange for a control group. Fifty-three students had been recruited to participate in a tutoring experiment conducted over the weekend preceding the scheduled baroreceptor reflex computer laboratory (see Chapter 10 for a discussion of this experiment). Twenty-eight of these students served as controls, reading a specially edited chapter on the baroreceptor reflex (see Chapter 10, Section 10.2.1), but not being tutored. All participants in this tutoring experiment, both those who were tutored and those in the control group, took the standard pretest and posttest. These students all participated in the regularly scheduled computer laboratory, taking the pretest and posttest, *but the results, reported later, did not include their performance.* Thus, none of the 45 students whose performance was included in the study comparing CIRCSIM and CIRCSIM-Tutor had participated in the weekend experiment.

18.4.3 Learning Outcomes

The results (see Table 18.7) show that learning occurred in the control group students (who read the text) as well in the groups that used CIRCSIM or CIRCSIM-Tutor. For the control group (who read a text), and for CIRCSIM-Tutor, the pretest–posttest differences are statistically significant for all three measures (scores). For CIRCSIM, the pretest–posttest differences for predictions are significant, but the difference for relationship points is not significant. The effect sizes range from 0.48 (moderate) to 1.27 (large). Both CIRCSIM and

TABLE 18.7
Effects of CIRCSIM and CIRCSIM-Tutor on Learning in November 1999

	Pretest Mean (SD)	*Posttest Mean (SD)*	*Gain*	*(Pre-Post) p value**	*Effect Size*
Control (N = 28)					
Relationship points[a]	14.1 (4.8)	19.9 (4.5)	5.8	< .001	1.27
Correct predictions[b]	12.2 (3.0)	13.8 (2.6)	1.6	.018	0.48
CIRCSIM-Tutor (N = 22)					
Relationship points[a]	10.9 (5.5)	14.2 (6.3)	3.3	.039	0.65
Correct predictions[b]	11.5 (4.8)	16.8 (1.8)	5.3	< .001	1.24
CIRCSIM (N = 23)					
Relationship points[a]	11.0 (5.5)	13.7 (6.8)	2.7	.071	0.54
Correct predictions[b]	11.5 (5.1)	16.4 (1.6)	4.9	< .001	1.05

[a]Maximum score = 24; [b]Maximum score = 20. *One-tailed *t* test assuming equal variance.

CIRCSIM-Tutor help students learn to solve problems about the baroreceptor reflex, as does reading a carefully edited text.

To determine whether there were differences in the effectiveness of the three treatments (reading text, using CIRCSIM or CIRCSIM-Tutor), we performed a univariate analysis of covariance on each outcome measure, with treatment as the independent variable, posttest scores as the dependent variable, and all three pretest scores as covariates (to control for possible differences in pretest scores across the three groups; see Table 18.7). For the relationship scores, the control group outperformed both computer tutors, $F(2, 65) = 4.799, p = .011$, but for the prediction scores, use of either computer program produced better posttest scores than did the control treatment of reading text, $F(2, 65) = 16.692, p < .001$. There were no significant differences between CIRCSIM-Tutor and CIRCSIM for any of the outcome measures.

Thus, we can say that both CIRCSIM and CIRCSIM-Tutor work, and that they work better than reading a carefully selected and edited text for helping students learn to predict the behavior of the system (although not for learning the relationships). However, the tests that were used do not show different learning outcomes from the use of the two different computer programs.

18.4.4 Survey Results

The responses to the survey continue to be quite positive (see Fig. 18.3). Students found the program easy to use and helpful (i.e., they thought it helped them improve their ability to predict the responses of the baroreceptor reflex). They indicated that they would recommend use of the program to other students.

18.4.5 System Performance

We wound up with 35 log files from CIRCSIM-Tutor, and, perhaps because some of these students had already been tutored over the weekend, 21 of these log files (60%) show all eight procedures completed. We would like to think that the improvements in the natural language modules had something to do with this as well. The total

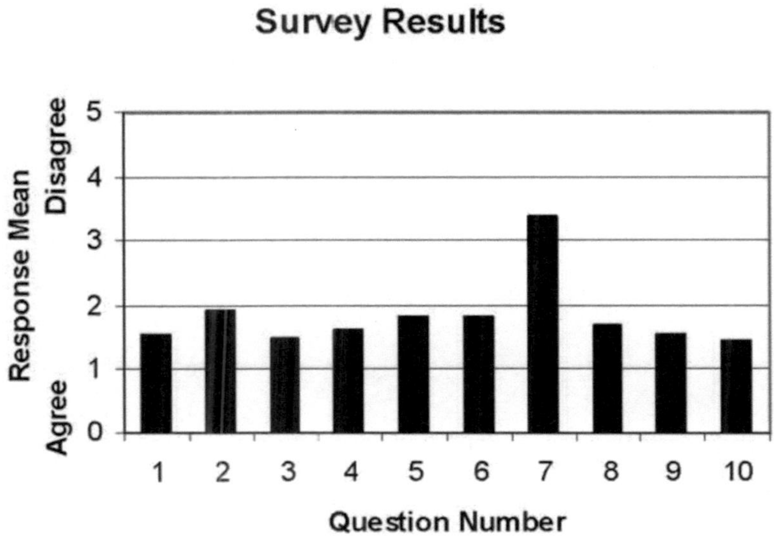

FIG. 18.3. Results of the CIRCSIM-Tutor Survey, November 1999 (the survey questions appear in Sample 18.4).

number of student inputs in the dialogue portions was 1,642; 86 were met with error messages. The students committed 96 spelling or typing errors and the system successfully corrected 91 of these. There were 449 nonalphabetic inputs (mostly "+" to indicate increase, "–" for decrease, and "0" for no change). (Table 18.8 shows these numbers for each student.) Given the large numbers of error messages, we decided to examine them carefully. Table 18.9 lists each message and the number of times that it occurred in the log file from November 1999.

Reading the log files in detail revealed two serious system errors and three more where the students figured out what to do in spite of the error and were able to continue working. One of these errors was created by an unforeseen problem with the error message module (Example 18.1) and the other by our spelling correction module (Example 18.2). In Example 18.1 we think that the student was so determined to correct his answer to the previous question that he did not even notice the error messages.

TABLE 18.8

Session by Session Counts for November, 1999 (For each log file we counted the number of procedures completed, the number of student inputs to the dialogue, the number of category error messages received by the student, the spelling errors and the errors corrected, and the number of inputs that consisted entirely of nonalphabetic symbols like + and 0)

Procedures Completed	*No. of Student Inputs*	*No. of Error Messages*	*No. of Spelling Errors*	*No. of Spelling Corrections*	*No. of Nonalphabetic Inputs*
8	33	1	5	5	0
8	31	0	0	0	12
3	48	6	1	1	0
7	37	4	1	0	12
8	9	0	0	0	4
8	19	0	0	0	9
8	48	0	0	0	2
8	19	3	7	7	0
4	56	3	1	1	28
8	21	0	8	8	0
8	82	4	3	3	39
8	9	1	0	0	0
8	52	1	3	3	20
8	29	2	13	12	1
8	54	1	1	1	21
8	79	3	0	0	36
8	49	1	1	1	18
8	59	0	6	6	0
8	38	3	1	1	12
7	75	7	2	2	28
7	69	4	4	4	25
8	94	5	2	2	34
6	45	5	0	0	17
8	79	5	8	6	0
5	21	1	1	1	0
5	55	6	0	0	26

Procedures Completed	No. of Student Inputs	No. of Error Messages	No. of Spelling Errors	No. of Spelling Corrections	No. of Nonalphabetic Inputs
3	32	2	10	9	0
5	69	4	0	0	30
8	74	2	3	3	1
8	38	3	1	1	17
4	16	1	0	0	0
5	37	3	0	0	1
8	62	3	1	1	27
6	59	2	0	0	27
7	45	0	13	13	2
Totals	1,642	86	96	91	449

TABLE 18.9

Error Messages Generated by CIRCSIM-Tutor in November 1999

Error Message	***Frequency***
Please respond with prediction table parameters.	28
Didn't recognize a stage: DR, RR or SS.	14
It should be increased, decreased, or unchanged.	13
Did not recognize directly or inversely related.	13
Is the mechanism of control neural or physical?	17
That is not the variable under discussion, please try again.	1
Total	86

Note. DR = Direct Response; RR = Reflex Response; SS = Steady State.

Example 18.1: The First of Two Serious System Errors in November 1999

T:	What stage must the value of Cardiac Output follow in SS?
S:	no change
T:	Didn't recognize a stage: DR, RR, or SS.
S:	decrease
T:	Didn't recognize a stage: DR, RR, or SS.
S:	0
T:	Didn't recognize a stage: DR, RR, or SS.
S:	no change in ss
T:	Nope, the value of Cardiac Output does not follow the value of Cardiac Output in SS.

The value of Cardiac Output must follow the value of Cardiac Output in DR.

In Example 18.2 the system changed "venour" to "veins" instead of to "venous" and then decided that "pressure" unqualified by any adjective it recognized must be Mean Arterial Pressure.

Example 18.2 The Second of Two Serious System Errors in November 1999

T:	Stroke Volume is determined by Central Venous Pressure and Inotropic State. Which determinant is dominant in this case?
S:	central venour pressure
T:	Nope, the important determinant of Stroke Volume in this case is not Mean Arterial Pressure. The important determinant of Stroke Volume in this case is Central Venous Pressure. The change in IS minimize the change in SV but does not reverse the direction of the change caused by CVP unless IS is the first variable been changed.

There were four more spelling correction errors. The most distressing example appears as Example 18.3. Here the spelling correction program, which had successfully corrected "storke" to "stroke" and "voulme" to "volume" elsewhere, collapsed when they appeared together. Fortunately, the student figured out the error and fixed it before there was any real trouble.

Example 18.3 Example of a Bad Spelling Correction Result in November 1999.

T:	Blood Volume determines CVP. However, no change in blood volume occurs in this situation. Think about another determinant.
S:	storke voulme
T:	Please respond with prediction table parameters.
S:	stroke volume

In a similar example, the student stepped in and made the correction when the system failed to correct "cop" to "co." Two other failures involved missing words. A student answered "initial" in response to the question, "What stage must the value of Stroke Volume follow in SS?" and we decided that "initial stage" was indeed a reasonable synonym for "DR." We also decided to add "clueless" to our synonyms for "help" because of the sad episode in Example 18.4.

Example 18.4. CIRCSIM-Tutor Fails to Understand in November 1999

T:	What is the other determinant of Mean Arterial Pressure?
S:	reflex
T:	Please respond with prediction table parameters.
S:	-
T:	Please respond with prediction table parameters.
S:	clueless
T:	Please respond with prediction table parameters.
S:	heart rate

In Example 18.4 "heart rate" is the wrong answer but it is a Prediction Table parameter, so CIRCSIM-Tutor is able to carry on with a tutoring plan from there.

There were also two embarrassing errors in the text generation program, one in a combination of a negative acknowledgment and a hint: "Nope, Inotropic State is not controlled by physical." The other (which appears at the end of Example 18.2) produced a sick "unless" clause: "The change in IS minimizes the change in SV but does not reverse the direction of the change caused by CVP unless IS is the first variable been changed."

The students did not complain about any of these embarrassing failures in the parser and the language generator, but they complained bitterly when the system made a bad dialogue move. In particular, the system told them the following:

> *You will now be asked questions regarding the subject matter. Click on the button or press <ENTER> when you have finished typing the answer.*

but then failed to ask them any questions at the end of the SS phase whenever the student had made a complete set of perfect predictions. The students found this error infuriating. Another problem that became clear as we read the log files is that good students could get through the whole set of eight procedures with very few text inputs. (A careful look at Table 18.8 shows that it was possible for a student to finish all eight procedures and only enter nine text inputs.) We resolved to add open questions to the system at the next opportunity and ask one of these questions whenever a student completed a set of perfect predictions.

18.4.6 Conclusions Drawn

We have shown that CIRCSIM-Tutor is more effective than reading a comparable text in helping students learn to solve problems. We believe that this is because active learning resources that foster the development of problem-solving skills, like CIRCSIM or CIRCSIM-Tutor, are more effective than a more passive resource, such as a text, at helping students correctly predict the responses of the baroreceptor reflex. However, we were not able to show any difference between the learning outcomes from CIRCSIM and CIRCSIM-Tutor.

On a more positive note, the continued development of CIRCSIM-Tutor resulted in a program whose robustness continues to improve. And students continued to be pleased with the program and perceived that it did help them understand the baroreceptor reflex.

18.5 OUR LAST EXPERIMENT (NOVEMBER 2002)

18.5.1 Version 2.9 of CIRCSIM-Tutor and What It Could Do

We made four major changes in the system between November 1999 and November 2002, in addition to some routine corrections and the removal of a very slight Chinese accent. We changed the error message routine so that if the student did not respond correctly to the second message in a row, it gave the student the correct answer and went on to another topic. Glass rewrote the spelling correction program so that it looked for phrases before it looked for single words. Zhou (2000) added some hints and changed some others that seemed not quite right to the experts. Then we invented open-ended questions and answers for them and added them to the system.

The addition of open-ended questions required the greatest effort, although the system makes no attempt to understand the students' answers, but just outputs a canned explanation. Our goal was to give more stimulation to the good students and to collect as many answers as possible, so that we could try to understand and eventually respond in a cogent manner. The experts commonly ask such questions when the students are doing really well, in an attempt to probe for misconceptions, to check whether the students have understood some important points, and to help them form some useful generalizations about the physiology and about the problem-solving process. Evens collected a large number of open questions from the expert transcripts. Then she wrote some possible answers based on explanations provided by the expert tutors in response to student answers to these questions. Finally, Michael edited both the questions and the answers and made the final decision about which to use in the experiment. These questions are listed in Table 18.10. Glass made the actual changes to the system: he inserted the questions so that they would appear only when the student had made a complete set of correct predictions, and made sure that no student saw a particular question more than once.

TABLE 18.10
Open Questions Used in November 2002

DR	Why did you predict that IS would not change? Can you explain why HR did not change? Why did you enter 'no change' for TPR?
RR	Why did you predict that IS would increase? Why did you predict that HR would increase? Why did you predict that TPR would increase? Why did you predict that CVP would decrease? Why did MAP change in the manner that you predicted?
SS	SV increased in DR and decreased in RR. Why did you predict that it would increase in SS? CO decreased in DR and increased in RR. Why did you predict that it would decrease in SS? Why is MAP still decreased/increased? <whichever applies> What does the baroreceptor reflex do? CVP increased in DR and decreased in RR. Why did you predict that it would increase in SS?

Note. IS = Inotropic State; HR = Heart Rate; TPR = Total Peripheral Resistance; CVP = Central Venous Pressure; MAP = Mean Arterial Pressure; SV = Stroke Volume; DR = Direct Response; RR = Reflex Response; SS = Steady State; CO = Cardiac Output.

18.5.2 Protocol for the Experiment

In this experiment, we employed a control group, 33 students, who, over the weekend prior to the scheduled CIRCSIM-Tutor laboratory, took a pretest, read a chapter about the regulation of blood pressure (Heller & Mohrman, 1981) that had been edited by Michael and Rovick to facilitate student learning about the baroreceptor reflex, and then took a posttest. The learning gains that resulted from this control treatment were then compared with the learning gains that occurred in 40 students who spent 1 hr doing CIRCSIM-Tutor, but who had not participated in the control group. The pretests and posttests have previously been described (Section 18.1).

18.5.3 Learning Outcomes

The results (Table 18.11) show learning gains for both the control group (which read a text) and the treatment group (which worked

TABLE 18.11
Effects of CIRCSIM-Tutor on Learning in November 2002

	Pretest Mean (SD)	*Posttest Mean* (SD)	*Gain*	*Pre–Post* p *Value**	*Effect Size*
Control (N = 33)					
Relationship points[a]	18.61 (5.1)	21.33 (4.4)	2.72	.012	0.64
Correct predictions[b]	15.55 (3.5)	17.55 (1.4)	2.00	.002	0.64
CIRCSIM-Tutor (N = 40)					
Relationship points[a]	13.95 (6.7)	18.05 (5.9)	4.10	.002	0.96
Correct predictions[b]	13.30 (4.1)	16.88 (3.4)	3.58	< .001	0.80

[a]Maximum score = 24; [b]Maximum score = 20; [c]Maximum score = 4.
*One-tailed *t* test assuming equal variance.

with CIRCSIM-Tutor). All pre–post gains are statistically significant (*p* values are all < .05). The effect sizes for the control group were in the medium range, whereas the effect sizes for the CIRCSIM-Tutor group ranged from medium to large, according to J. Cohen's classification (1988). These effect sizes clearly represent a "worthwhile" consequence of students either reading a specially prepared text or doing CIRCSIM-Tutor.

Examination of the data suggests that the control and treatment groups may have started from a different level of performance (the members of the control group were volunteers and there was no random assignment of students to control or treatment group). We therefore performed an analysis of covariance test on the data to control for the differences in pretest scores (for this purpose, all scores were converted to percentages of the maximum possible score).

The results of the analysis of covariance tell us several things. When the differences between the pretest scores of the control and treatment groups are taken into account, there is no significant difference between the gains of the control and treatment groups. However, there is a significant interaction between the group (control or CIRCSIM-Tutor) and the test (relationship points, correct predictions), such that the control group outperformed the CIRCSIM-Tutor group on the relationship test, but the CIRCSIM-Tutor group outperformed the control group on correct predictions, $F(2, 67) = 3.668, p < .05$.

Again, it appears that CIRCSIM-Tutor is more effective than reading a text in helping students learn to predict the behavior of the baroreceptor reflex. However, CIRCSIM-Tutor is not as effective as reading the text in helping students acquire a knowledge of the relevant cardiovascular relationships (although it clearly does help).

18.5.4 Survey Results

Student responses to CIRCSIM-Tutor were again quite positive. The results of the survey administered following use of the program can be seen in Fig. 18.4. A 5-point Likert-type scale was used with 1 = *definitely YES* to 5 = *definitely NO*.

Students provided many written comments, and a sampling of both the positive and negative comments can be seen in Table 18.12.

18.5.5 System Performance

There were 2,980 student inputs in 66 sessions, so an average of 45.2 per session, only a little above the previous figure from 1999. But it

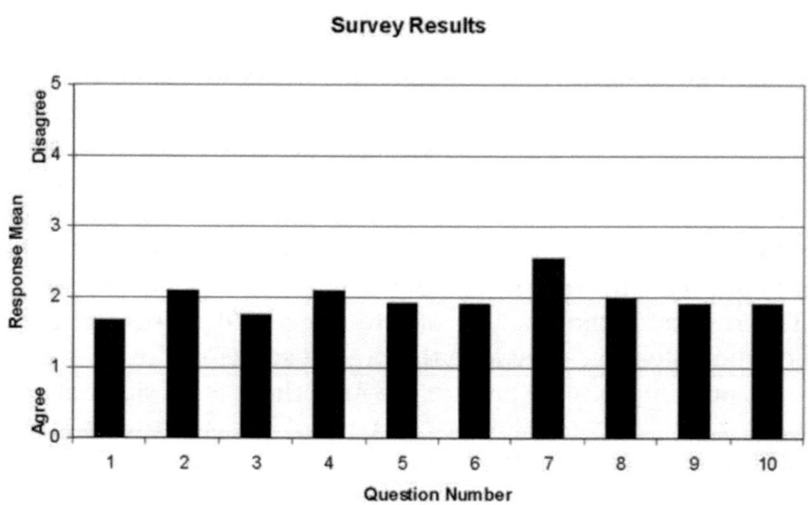

FIG. 18.4. Results of the CIRCSIM-Tutor Survey, November 2002 (the survey questions appear in Sample 18.4).

TABLE 18.12

A Sample of Comments From the Student Survey in November 2002

the program is somewhat frustrating to use in terms of having to enter a specific prediction first in the DR. However, overall it's a great program. I like the summaries @ the end of each section.

GREAT PROGRAM—MAKE AVAILABLE FOR STUDENTS HOME USE—check a disk out.

when entering in data (in the tables) be able to use the mouse and keyboard, depending on student preference. Overall I thought it was helpful.

Telling my mistakes immediately would be helpful. Also, I felt sometimes I had to "read the computer's mind" to answer the questions – better prompts would have been helpful.

It would be helpful if for some questions there was a list of answers to choose from—oftentimes, I did not know how the program wanted me to respond.

Overall, very good. would like to see a more complicated model taking all receptors into account. I would benefit more from integrating these concepts. Also, I think charts displaying the relationships of the variables would be helpful. E.g. <followed by an arrow and a graph mapping CVP against CO> This would jive w/ lecture.

perhaps a graph or some other type of visual aid would be nice to help illustrate the fact the direction that the reflex + SS are moving the parameters to. Just putting +, –, or 0 is sometimes confusing.

Much more helpful than previous program—the questions of the system were a little hard to get used to (i.e. the answer the system was looking for) but were tailored to the concepts well.

I thought it was really good and I usually don't like these types of things.

This program was much more helpful then receiving packets of information.

was no longer possible for a student to complete eight procedures and only type nine dialogue inputs—even the student who made perfect scores everywhere would encounter 11 open questions.

All but 12 of the 66 log files (82%) showed eight completed procedures, as opposed to 60% in 1999. What is more, five students went on to repeat one or more procedures—a phenomenon that we had never seen before.

The students made only 106 spelling or typing errors and the system corrected all but 2 of them without making any of the embarrassing miscorrections that we had seen before. On the other hand, it failed to correct "soconstriction" to "vasoconstriction" and "lood volume" to "blood volume." Obviously, we need to drop the assumption that the student will make sure that the first letter is correct, however incorrect the rest of the word may be. This assumption saved us a lot of time when every microsecond was precious, but now that PCs run so much faster, we should consider dropping it.

CIRCSIM-Tutor was not perfect, however. The tutor rejected two answers that should have been recognized as correct, because of a lack of vocabulary. The system turned down "calcium" as a mechanism, when, in fact, calcium ions are the mechanism by which the IS is increased. We have now added "calcium" to the ontology of neural mechanisms. The tutor also turned down "less" as a description of change—we have now added it as yet another synonym of "decrease" —and we have also added "more" as a synonym of "increase," although we have not observed it in a session, just to make sure that the system behaves in a logical way from the user's point of view.

We expected the number of category messages to fall slightly; the drop actually exceeded our expectations. There were 130 category error messages in 66 log files, as opposed to 86 in 35 sessions in 1999, so the number of these category errors dropped from 2.5 per session to an average of just less than 2 per session. (The messages are listed in Table 18.9.) Best of all, there were no serious system errors of the kind that we saw in 1999. In fact, there were no inputs that the system could not respond to in some appropriate way, so we feel justified in believing that the system must be easier to use and the hints must be more successful, as well.

We were most anxious to see what would happen with the open questions. Would students try to answer them or would they immediately recognize that the system was not attempting to understand their answers and just blow them off? Because the system did not present the student with an open question until that student had entered a complete set of correct predictions, many students did not see their first open question until fairly late in the hour. The maximum number of open questions that a student could see without repeating a procedure was 11. The students saw 535 open questions (an average of 8.1 per student) and answered 390 (an average of 5.9), but there was a large amount of variation. Most of the students took these questions seriously at first and tried to answer them. Only two students did not answer any at all. Some students gave up answering these questions when they realized that the system was not parsing this part of their input. Others continued to answer these questions to the end. In most cases, we do not know whether the student figured out that the system was not parsing the answer and just returning a canned explanation, because during the rest of the dialogue, the system parses the student input and will not let a student proceed without answering the system question. A handful of students were clearly testing the system to verify that it was not paying attention to these particular responses.

We were very excited when we looked at the answers themselves (C. H. Lee, Evens, & Glass, 2004). To give you a flavor, Example 18.5 shows four answers from log file M48. Like most other students, M48 made a serious attempt to answer these open questions. (The first, second, and fourth answers are rather good; the third is not. Note that in the session, these questions were separated by at least one stage of tutoring, usually more.)

Example 18.5 Four Answers to Open Questions from November 2002 (Log File M48)

T: What does the baroreceptor reflex do?
S: try and maintain MAP {{*good answer*}}

T: Why did you enter 'no change' for TPR?
S: it is under autonomic control {{*another good answer*}}

T: Why did MAP change in the manner that you predicted?
S: cardiac output and hr increase3d {{*not so good*}}

T: Why did you predict that CVP would decrease?
S: co increased {{*very good*}}

These answers are far from verbose; they are certainly shorter than the canned answers reeled out by the system. They definitely display more syntactic sophistication (three sentences and a verb phrase) than this student's answers to routine questions, however. More important, they have the potential to reveal much more about the student's thought processes.

A brief look at the answers to the last question in Example 18.5 over the whole range of students may give you a better picture.

There were 40 responses to this question. There were 23 complete sentences ("co increased,." "cardiac output and cvp are inversely related,." "hr is a major det of co, co increased and has an inverse relationship with cvp."). There were 7 because clauses ("Because CO is increased and the heart is pumping out more than it's getting," "because co goes up"). There were 6 noun phrases ("Inverse relationship with co," "loss of blood volume"). There was 1 verb phrase ("decrease CO"). There were 2 adjective phrases ("inversely related to cardiac output") and 1 other fragment ("indirect relationship with CO, which went up"). There were definitely more good answers than we expected, and we have reason to hope that we can parse many of them.

18.5.6 Conclusions Drawn

We were able to demonstrate again that CIRCSIM-Tutor aids student learning about the baroreceptor reflex and helps them learn to make more correct predictions about the responses of the system. More students were able to complete all eight of the procedures than in the past and the system was able to handle all of the language inputs it received. For the first time, we asked some open-ended questions and received answers, although the feedback provided by the system consisted of canned text, not a tutorial dialogue. As work continues on the project, we will attempt to understand student answers to such questions and actually respond in a specific manner to each student.

18.6 DISCUSSION OF THE RESULTS

We can say several things about CIRCSIM-Tutor based on the results of our experiments with it. First, it works; that is, it functions in a classroom setting in an acceptable manner. It responds to student prediction errors in a manner that helps the students correct their errors. It generates hints and questions that students can respond to appropriately. It understands student responses, and when it does not, it can explain what kind of answer it is expecting in a way that allows the student to generate an understandable response.

We can also say that CIRCSIM-Tutor works in the sense that students using it exhibit significant learning. This increase in performance is most striking for their ability to solve Prediction Table problems; the effect sizes seen are large and the improvement is clearly educationally significant. CIRCSIM-Tutor does help students learn relationships, although not necessarily as well as reading a carefully edited text. However, it is important to keep in mind that CIRCSIM-Tutor was never specifically intended to convey this kind of knowledge to its users.

We can also say that students like CIRCSIM-Tutor and they feel that they learn something from using it. In and of itself, this belief that they have learned from using CIRCSIM-Tutor may not mean much, but their conclusion is certainly meaningful when combined with the actual measured learning gains.

We can say that CIRCSIM-Tutor works better than reading an edited text in helping students learn to solve problems.

What is less clear is whether CIRCSIM-Tutor works "better" than using CIRCSIM. The comparisons that we were able to make are inconclusive. It is fair to say that CIRCSIM-Tutor works at least as well as CIRCSIM. Our inability to be more definitive about this issue is to a large extent a consequence of the difficulty of doing the kinds of experiments that would be required to obtain statistically meaningful results.

18.7 DOING RESEARCH ON TEACHING/LEARNING IS DIFFERENT THAN DOING RESEARCH IN PHYSICS

In his article, "Educational Research: The Hardest Science of Them All," Berliner (2002) briefly discussed some of the factors that make educational research so hard to do (and much harder than doing physics). E. Murray (2002) offered a very similar set of observations.

The experiments that we have described in this book suffer from all the problems identified by Berliner and by E. Murray. To appreciate these difficulties, it is useful to compare the research paradigm observed in studies of physical systems with what occurs in studies of teaching and learning. In studying the behavior of a physical system like a pendulum, it is possible to do the following:

1. Reach agreement among researchers about what parameter is the dependent variable of interest (the frequency of the pendulum).

2. Identify all of the possible independent variables (length, mass or weight, density, color of the pendulum, etc.).
3. Isolate and manipulate each independent variable of interest.
4. Measure the effect of varying an independent variable on the dependent variable.

In studying the behavior of humans who are engaged in teaching or learning, we are faced with significant limitations on our ability to carry out the experimental paradigm just described:

1. In studying learning, there are many possible outcome measures that can be selected as the "critical" dependent variable ("amount" learned, length of retention, extent of transfer, etc.), and it is not always obvious which one should be selected. As a consequence, there is not always agreement among researchers about what the dependent variable of interest ought to be.

2. It is often difficult to measure whatever dependent variable we have identified as being of interest, or there may be significant disagreement about how to do this most appropriately.

3. Most often we cannot identify all of the possible independent variables either before or after doing the experiment. Individual students have complex histories, interests, and desires that may affect the behavior we want to understand. The educational context in which the student operates is also incredibly complex, and we simply do not know what features of that context are relevant to the research question being pursued. In addition, the reasons for participating in the experiment can be highly varied from study to study and may affect the outcomes obtained. Finally, all of these factors described here probably interact with with one another in ways that we cannot identify.

4. To the extent that we identify a set of possible independent variables, we are usually limited (either practically, ethically, or both) in our ability to isolate and manipulate some or all of them.

We have attempted to carry out two different (but clearly related) research programs as part of the CIRCSIM-Tutor project. First (chronologically and logically), we studied human one-on-one tutoring, asking two different kinds of questions (discussed later). Second, we studied the consequences of using CIRCSIM-Tutor in the classroom, asking questions about the program itself and the responses of the students (learning and otherwise) using the program. Each of these kinds of experiments suffered from certain inherent limitations in doing experiments involving human participants.

Perhaps the most serious problem (problem 1) that we faced is that for most of our studies, our student participants were volunteers, not a randomly selected subset of students from the population of interest (first-year medical students at Rush Medical College). Our volunteers clearly differ in their level of understanding of cardiovascular physiology at the point in time when we conduct our experiments (after all didactic experiences have been completed, except for doing CIRCSIM or CIRCSIM-Tutor). However, we do not know if we recruited the better students eager to extend their knowledge and gain a few points on the next exam, or whether we recruited poorer students looking for help in mastering the material, or some of each. The consequences of this are different for different experiments we did, and we attempt to describe these effects later.

A second problem (problem 2) is that the total educational context in which our experiments took place changed from year to year over the duration of the project for two different reasons: (a) the students admitted to Rush Medical College got "better" over the years (higher MCAT scores, higher grade point averages; personal communications with Jan Schmidt, Director of the Office of Admissions), and (b) how cardiovascular physiology was taught changed (what was included in the syllabus, what was lectured on, what was emphasized), in large part as a direct result of the CIRCSIM-Tutor project.

Research on Human One-on-One Tutoring

We did two fundamentally different kinds of studies. Our first studies of tutoring looked at what happened during a one-on-one tutoring session. That is, we were interested in what the tutor and the student did in response to each other's input to the dialogue. Do expert and novice tutors behave differently? The left side of Table 18.13 lists some of the specific questions that we sought to address in these studies. However, we later pursued a quite different set of questions. Is one-on-one tutoring by a tutor better than some other educational intervention, and do expert tutors produce a larger effect than novice tutors? The right side of Table 18.13 lists some of the questions that we investigated.

TABLE 18.13
Experimental Questions About Human Tutoring Pursued in the CIRCSIM-Tutor Project

What happens in a one-on-one tutoring session?	*Does one-on-one tutoring work and is it "better" than something else?*
What language is used by student and tutor?	Does tutoring result in a learning gain even when the students are mature, highly motivated, intelligent learners?
What knowledge is used by student and tutor?	Does tutoring result in more learning than something else (reading a text)?
What tactics does the tutor employ?	Do expert tutors produce a larger gain than novice tutors?
Do novice tutors do things differently than expert tutors?	

The use of domain knowledge by student and tutors is determined more by the domain than it is by the state of the students or the tutors. But the presentation of that knowledge in the syllabus, in lectures, and in available textbooks certainly changed. Students using CIRCSIM-Tutor in the experiments in 1999 and 2002 made active use of the concept map in their syllabus. Michael and Rovick started to put much more emphasis on the concept map in their course after we launched the CIRCSIM-Tutor project and they discovered how helpful the developers found it in our representation of knowledge. Thus, our study of domain knowledge is certainly affected by Problem 2.

Tutor "tactics" clearly evolved over the course of the project (Problem 2), but such changes were, in fact, incorporated into our planning and implementation of CIRCSIM-Tutor.

The study of novice tutors did not obviously suffer from Problem 1. Although we did use volunteer tutors, they were selected for inclusion in the study by virtue of certain relevant characteristics.

All of the studies that looked at the learning gains of tutoring certainly suffered from both Problems 1 and 2. If the student volunteers had a better understanding of cardiovascular physiology than the overall cohort, the learning gains that could be demonstrated would necessarily be limited (the "ceiling effect"). In addition, this problem may have been compounded by Problem 2; as the educational context changed, more student volunteers are likely to be functioning already at a high level when they participate in the experiments.

Overall then, our studies of human one-on-one tutoring suffered in only a limited way from the problems of doing research with human participants identified earlier. This is the case because these studies, by their very nature, were attempts to observe what specific individuals did in a more or less specifiable context. The issues here called for careful observation and description, not a hypothesis testing experiment. Perhaps the most serious problem with these experiments was the small number of tutors (expert and novice) whose behaviors and outcomes we studied.

Research on CIRCSIM-Tutor

Our studies of CIRCSIM-Tutor in the classroom focused on two different things: how well did CIRCSIM-Tutor, the computer program, function, and what was the response of students to CIRCSIM-Tutor? Table 18.14 lists the questions that concerned us. Clearly, the most important question was whether students learned something from their use of CIRCSIM-Tutor.

Studies of how CIRCSIM-Tutor worked did not suffer from either of the research problems identified because the studies did not involve human behavior. Our studies of student interactions with CIRCSIM-Tutor were very much affected by the two research problems described earlier.

TABLE 18.14

Experimental Questions About CIRCSIM-Tutor Explored in the CIRCSIM-Tutor Project

How did CIRCSIM-Tutor work?	*How did students respond to CIRCSIM-Tutor?*
How often did it "crash"?	What, and how much, did the students learn?
How well did it understand student inputs?	Did they learn more or less than students doing some control procedure?
How well did it respond to student errors and problems?	What did they like and dislike about CIRCSIM-Tutor?

For example, consider the 2002 CIRCSIM-Tutor experiment in which we had a control group. The context for the experiment we were conducting did not allow us to randomly assign students to the control or treatment groups. Perhaps as a consequence, the control group pretest scores were significantly higher than the pretest scores of the students doing CIRCSIM-Tutor, potentially creating a number of problems in interpreting our results. We can only speculate that the students who volunteered for the control experiment were ones who felt most prepared (had already learned the most) and thus did better on the pretest. Although the use of an analysis of covariance enabled us to partially deal with this problem, it would have been preferable not to have the problem in the first place.

18.8 TAKE-HOME MESSAGE

CIRCSIM-Tutor "works." Actually, it "works" in three different senses of that term: (a) The program is robust. It understands most of the student input (and when it fails to understand something it tells the student what kind of input it is expecting). Its output is appropriate and intelligible. (b) Use of CIRCSIM-Tutor produces measurable learning gains; student performance on all three components of the posttest is better than performance on the pretest. Further, the effect size is educationally of great significance; using CIRCSIM-Tutor truly makes a difference to students' development of problem-solving skills in this domain. (c) Students enjoy working with the program and feel that it is contributing to their learning about the baroreceptor reflex; they are clearly willing to accept the obvious limitations of language understanding and generation that are evident in using CIRCSIM-Tutor.

SAMPLE 18.1

The Relationship Test Used in Determining the Learning Effects of CIRCSIM-Tutor

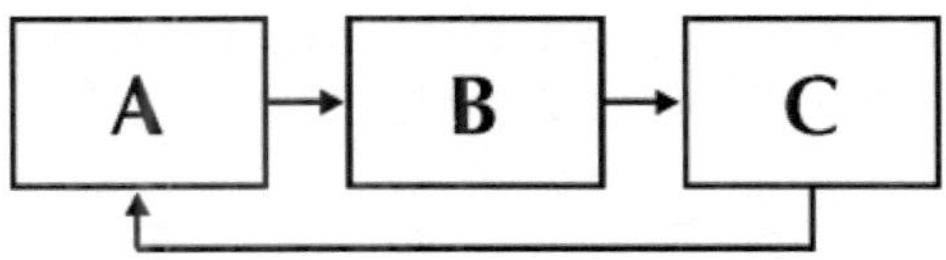

In the system shown above
A|B, B | C and C | A are *IMMEDIATE CAUSAL RELATIONSHIPS*
while A | C is NOT an immediate causal relations.
If A increases and B increases (or A decreases and B decreases)
the relationship is said to be a *DIRECT* one
If A increases and B decreases (or A decreases and A increases)
the relationship is said to be an *INVERSE* one
List all the *IMMEDIATE CAUSAL* relationship between pairs of variables below
and indicate whether each relationship is a *DIRECT* or *INVERSE* one

inotropic state (IS)
total peripheral resistance (TPR)
cardiac output (CO)
baroreceptor firing rate (BR)
stroke volume (SV)
mean arterial pressure (MAP)
heart rate (HR)
central venous pressure (CVP)

	Variable 1	*Immediate Causal Relationship DIRECT/INVERSE?*	*Variable 2*
1			
2			
3			
4			
5			
6			
7			
8			
9			
10			
11			
12			

SAMPLE 18.2

The CIRCSIM Problem Used to Determine the Effectiveness of CIRCSIM-Tutor

Mr. X has an implanted electronic pacemaker which is the *sole determinant of his heart rate*. A sudden failure of the pacemaker causes his heart rate to decrease from 70/min to 50/min.

1. In the DR column predict the DIRECT RESPONSE (DR) of the seven parameters listed in the table below caused by the change in Mr. X's heart rate. The DR occurs before any reflex change can occur. DR is the immediate, physical consequence of the heart rate change. Indicate the direction of change from the normal value of each parameter (+ means increase, – means decrease, 0 means no change) as a consequence of the change in heart rate.
2. Next, in the RR column predict the REFLEX RESPONSE (RR) that will occur. Indicate the direction of change (+ means increase, – means decrease, 0 means no change) relative to the value of each parameter at the end of the DR.
3. Finally, in the SS column predict the new STEADY STATE (SS) that will be present in the system. Indicate, relative to the parameter values before the pacemaker failure, whether the parameter will be +, –, or 0.

Parameter	***DR***	***RR***	***SS***
Inotropic state (IS)			
Central venous pressure (CVP)			
Stroke volume (SV)			
Heart rate (HR)	–		
Cardiac output (CO)			
Total peripheral resistance (TPR)			
Mean arterial pressure (MAP)			

SAMPLE 18.3

Examples of the Multiple Choice Questions Used to Determine the Effectiveness of CIRCSIM-Tutor

1. Mr. Haddock is being treated with digitalis. One night he accidentally ingests several pills simultaneously, a serious overdose. As a consequence his inotropic state is greatly elevated and his cardiac output therefore increases. Compared with the period before he took the digitalis, Mr. Haddock's central venous pressure will be:
   a. increased
   b. decreased
   c. still normal
2. Phentolamine is an alpha-adrenergic blocking agent. As a result of administering this drug, total peripheral resistance will:
   a. increase
   b. decrease
   c. remain unchanged
3. Administration of digitalis increases the inotropic state of the heart and hence increases stroke volume. As a consequence the cardiovascular changes that result there will be a reflex ______________ in heart rate.
   a. increase
   b. decrease
   c. no change
4. A student donates a pint of blood at the Blood Bank and experiences a fall in mean arterial pressure (MAP) as a result. Which of the following statements correctly describes the reflex response that will result from the fall in MAP:
   a. CVP decreases but CO is nevertheless increased
   b. IS, HR, and TPR will change reflexly and will result in MAP being restored completely to its pre-donation value
   c. CVP and IS will both increase
   d. all of the above are correct

Note. CVP = Central Venous Pressure; CO = Cardiac Output; IS = Inotropic State; HR = Heart Rate; TRP = Total Peripheral Resistance. We eventually discovered that the questions in two of the four pairs of multiple choice questions were not comparable, so we do report the results in Chapter 18, but we thought that the questions might be of interest.

SAMPLE 18.4

Survey of Student Attitudes About the CIRCSIM-Tutor System (copied from Michael et al., 2003, p. 262, http://www.tandf.co.uk)

YOUR VIEWS ON CIRCSIM-TUTOR

1 = definitely YES ... 2 ... 3 ... 4 ... 5 = definitely NO

1.	The system was easy to use.	1	2	3	4	5
2.	The introductory screens were helpful.	1	2	3	4	5
3.	Entering predictions into the table was easy.	1	2	3	4	5
4.	Entering answers to the tutor's questions was easy.	1	2	3	4	5
5.	The system's use of language seemed varied and helpful.	1	2	3	4	5
6.	The tutor's hints and explanations were informative.	1	2	3	4	5
7.	I would prefer that the system always tell me about my mistakes immediately.	1	2	3	4	5
8.	CIRCSIM-tutor helped me to understand the behavior of the baroreceptor reflex.					
9.	CIRCSIM-tutor improved my ability to predict the cardiovascular responses to disturbances in blood pressure.	1	2	3	4	5
10.	I would recommend the program to friends taking physiology.	1	2	3	4	5

Please comment on any of the preceding questions or any other issue (problems using the system, help that wasn't provided but should have been, changes you would like to see in the system).

____

____

____

____

____

____

(You may continue on the back if you have more to say.)

H:/CSTexp2002/cstsurvey.wpd

19

Machine Tutors and Natural Language

In this chapter, we attempt to give a brief description of some of the most important Intelligent Tutoring Systems based on natural language dialogue with an emphasis on current research systems. Then we summarize the state of some current major issues in dialogue-based ITS. We begin with the first round of systems developed by Carbonell and Collins and Stevens, by Burton and Brown, and by Woolf and McDonald. Then we describe some of the second round of systems developed in the late 1980s and 1990s: Lesgold's SHERLOCK II, Wilensky's UNIX Consultant, Cawsey's EDGE, VanLehn's ANDES/ATLAS, and Kevin Ashley's CATO. Finally, we describe the current research systems: AutoTutor, Why2-Atlas and ITSpoke, BEETLE, CATO, CyclePad, and SCoT.

We are especially interested in how this work addresses questions of learning the sublanguage of the domain being taught, the self-explanation effect, dialogue issues and the dialectic effect, and Socratic versus didactic approaches to tutoring. We are also, of course, interested in tutoring strategies and scaffolding or fading. Our coverage is necessarily brief and idiosyncratic—these are the systems that we have found most exciting and inspiring, and from which we have learned the most.

19.0 EARLY DIALOGUE-BASED TUTORING SYSTEMS

19.0.1 SCHOLAR and WHY

The story of Intelligent Tutoring Systems (Barr & Feigenbaum, 1982; Wenger, 1987; Woolf, 1988) begins with J. R. Carbonell's (1970) SCHOLAR program. SCHOLAR was designed from the beginning to conduct a natural language dialogue with the student. The language generation was entirely template-driven, but the parsing was more sophisticated, based on Fillmore's (1968) case grammar. (The case information is very much like the case frames that we show in Table 13.1.) The system asked the student some questions to build a model and pick an appropriate problem for this particular student. It then tried to help the student solve the problem. The domain, the weather and geography of South America, was represented as a semantic net, following the approach of Collins and Quillian (1972). The system pursued an agenda, but there was very little long-range planning, which made the dialogue seem a little lacking in focus.

Collins carried on after Carbonell's untimely death and built a system called WHY (Stevens & Collins, 1977) with the same domain. WHY used Socratic principles, as formulated in well-stated "if-then" rules, to try to teach the student to reason about weather using important basic principles. Collins (1977) based much of this work on his own brilliant study of human tutorial dialogues, which describes the interactive nature of expert tutoring and the strategies that expert tutors used to get students to solve problems for themselves (Collins & Stevens, 1980, 1982, 1991). Collins and Stevens (Stevens & Collins, 1977, 1980) also added scripts to the knowledge base to help organize knowledge at a higher level. These scripts were then used to guide the Socratic tutoring (Collins, Brown, & Newman, 1989). The parser kept the case frames but used a more explicit semantic grammar with word classes defined in terms of semantic categories like "precipitation" instead of parts of speech. The natural language generation was still template-driven.

Collins also led the way in recognizing the importance of entrenched misconceptions as opposed to simple errors, the importance of diagnosing these misconceptions, and the need for special scripts (or schemas or algorithms) to help students recognize these errors and acquire better models (Stevens, Collins, & Goldin, 1982). These issues are still of serious concern to ITS developers.

19.0.2 SOPHIE and BUGGY

Burton and Brown built SOPHIE (Burton & Brown, 1979, 1982; J. S. Brown, Burton, & deKleer, 1982) to tutor problem-solving skills in a simulated electronics laboratory. The system selected a fault, inserted it into a model of a circuit, and told the student how the controls were set. The student was shown a schematic diagram of the circuit and the tutoring dialogue began. The student had to decide what to measure, and where, to find the fault.

From the natural language processing point of view, this system represented a big step forward. When the student asked: "What is the output?" the system understood that output meant "output voltage," a significant piece of disambiguation guided by the information attached to the schematic, and answered the following: "The output voltage is 11.7 volts." If the student then asked, "What is it in a working system?" the system understood that "it" referred to the output voltage and responded as follows: "In a working circuit the output voltage is 19.9 volts." The generation was also significantly improved. The system stored alternative ways of referring to concepts and so the dialogue is much less repetitive. This system also used a semantic grammar. It was one of the first systems to look for expected concepts in the input and skip words that it did not understand. Glass's parser in CIRCSIM-Tutor (Section 13.5) uses the same approach. We learned from SOPHIE (Burton & Brown, 1979) to avoid some of the negative consequences of misunderstanding the student by phrasing the tutor response in terms of a full sentence, so the student can tell what the system understood.

SOPHIE also represented a step forward in reasoning about possible student misconceptions. It generated hypotheses to explore and then explored them. SOPHIE had trouble, however, in following up appropriately on the student errors that it found.

Brown and Burton went on to build SOPHIE II (J. S. Brown et al., 1982) to provide better explanations. They also included a troubleshooting game that two teams of students could play with the goal of motivating students to stick with the system long enough to take thorough advantage of it.

Burton and Brown also built a computer coach for a computer game called "How the West Was Won" (nicknamed "West" by its friends) that is designed to teach elementary arithmetic (Burton & Brown, 1982). A coach, as opposed to a tutor, is designed to look over the learner's shoulder and provide occasional criticisms and suggestions for improvement. The research for this project focused on two problems: (a) identifying the diagnostic strategies needed to figure out the misconceptions, and (b) developing explicit tutoring strategies for figuring out how and when to interrupt and how to phrase those interruptions. The system had a separate natural language generation module that made use of a collection of tutoring strategies and a separate collection of explanation strategies (Barr & Feigenbaum, 1982; Burton & Brown, 1979; J. S. Brown & VanLehn, 1980). Another important first for Burton and Brown was an actual classroom experiment in which elementary school students who used the coach were compared with those who played the game without the coach. Students who used the coach not only did significantly better, they chose to play again later with much more enthusiasm.

J. S. Brown and Burton (1978) are probably even better known for their work on diagnosis of misconceptions in the BUGGY system than they are for their work on natural language explanations. They did an exhaustive study of erroneous algorithms for subtraction used by the children with whom they worked and implemented these alternative algorithms to discover what kinds of errors they produce. They then made a catalogue of errors, so that whenever the user made a subtraction error, they could figure out which bugs produce that particular error. One of the biggest difficulties in student modeling is caused by the fact that students rarely express just one misconception at a time. Burton and Brown figured out how to combine two faulty algorithms into one and check for combinations of bugs. Burton later developed DEBUGGY (1982), which was able to execute up to four faulty algorithms dynamically and determine which combinations of bugs could produce a particular error. VanLehn (1988) stated that this work laid the foundation for model-tracing and issue-tracing tutoring systems.

19.0.3 Meno-Tutor

Beverly Woolf's Meno-Tutor (1984) paid homage to Socrates not just in its name but in its whole approach to tutoring. Woolf did a serious study of dialogue issues and the dialectic effect. She studied and implemented a host of tutoring strategies in the framework of a natural language dialogue. Her thesis advisor was David McDonald, one of the leading figures in natural language generation. Most important of all, she recognized that generating an instructional plan and generating a tutoring dialogue are planning problems, different from planning other kinds of natural language text, although they also require sophisticated planning capabilities (Woolf & McDonald, 1985).

We now move on to a later group of systems, those under development when we started to work on CIRCSIM-Tutor.

19.1 THE SECOND ROUND

19.1.1 SHERLOCK II and Reflective Tutoring

The development of Sherlock II (Lesgold, 1988, 1992; Lesgold, Eggan, Katz, & Rao, 1992, Lesgold, Katz, Greenberg, Hughes, & Eggan, 1992; Lesgold, Lajoie, Bunzo, & Eggan, 1992) and the experiments carried out using this system are especially important to the history of Intelligent Tutoring Systems in a number of ways. Lesgold did pioneering work in curriculum design, in tutoring strategies, in student modeling, and in system evaluation. The evaluation of SHERLOCK II showed that technicians learned more about electronics troubleshooting from using this system for 24 hr than from 4 years of informal learning in the field.

The same talents that made Alan Lesgold a leading figure at the Learning and Development Research Center at the University of Pittsburgh (and now Dean of the School of Education) enabled him to collect a stellar research team to build SHERLOCK II. He persuaded Johanna Moore, who had just completed a book (1995) about text generation, to take the template-driven textual output and regenerate it using her system. The template-driven text was full of repetitions, because the original SHERLOCK II output messages were triggered every time a particular error was seen. Moore's generation module organized the output in a logical order, added an introduction, and included discourse markers to emphasize the important points and indicate transitions (Moser & Moore, 1995). A later version of Sherlock II (Moore, Lemaire, & Rosenblum, 1996) included references to earlier problems where the student had made the same mistake. It then asked the student to consider how the problem had been corrected before.

Barbara Di Eugenio worked with Moore at Pittsburgh on discourse planning and then moved to the University of Illinois at Chicago to set up a research program of her own in natural language generation (Van der Linden & Di Eugenio, 1996a, 1996b). She (Di Eugenio, 2001) has recently carried out an ingenious experiment to demonstrate the advantages of using natural language generation in a tutoring system. She took an existing CAI tutor and added a natural language generation component to take the original output of canned error messages and generate organized and cohesive natural language text. A comparative evaluation showed that the new version of the tutor was significantly more effective.

Sandra Katz of the Learning Research and Development Center at the University of Pittsburgh was recruited to help analyze human tutoring data for the SHERLOCK task, to design the original experiment with SHERLOCK II, and to perform the data analysis (Katz, Lesgold, Eggan, & Gordin, 1993; Katz, Lesgold, Eggan, Gordin, & Greenberg, 1992; Katz, Lesgold, Eggan, & Greenberg, 1996; Katz, Lesgold, Hughes, Peters, Eggan, Gordin, et al., 1988). Katz (2003; Katz & Allbritton, 2002) has more recently carried out a study of physics tutoring with and without an added period for reflection on the session, which also gives an opportunity to generalize about the earlier work the student has done. These experiments have shown that this kind of reflective tutoring produces significant improvements, and they have inspired reflective tutoring in a number of current tutoring systems. Her insightful analysis of the tutoring strategies and the language used provides an opportunity for others to try to simulate this kind of tutoring in a variety of problem-solving environments (Katz, O'Donnell, & Kay, 2000; Rosé & Torrey, 2004).

19.1.2 UC (the Unix Consultant)

Robert Wilensky did extensive research on planning (1983) before he started to build UC, the Unix Consultant (Wilensky et al., 1988), so it is not surprising that he treated planning as a central issue. UC is really a coach and not a tutor. It waits until the user asks for help in dealing with Unix, to offer advice. UC does magnificent opportunistic dynamic planning, and it also made significant forward leaps in natural language understanding and generation.

The original UC parser was named PHRAN (short for Phrasal Analyzer) because the Unix sublanguage, like our own, is full of multiword expressions. PHRAN was written by Yigal Arens (Wilensky, Arens, & Chin, 1984). It recognized patterns in answers, using a lexicon that associated patterns and concepts. This is basically a semantic grammar approach, but of a highly sophisticated kind. The pattern development was based on an extensive analysis of user transcripts, which was carried out by David Chin (1984).

The UC natural language generation system, PHRED, written by Paul Jacobs (1988), also used patterns extensively for generation purposes. The resulting output integrated phrases into the generated text in a smooth and elegant way. The phrases used in generation were also derived from analysis of user transcripts.

19.1.3 EDGE

Alison Cawsey's (1992) book, *Explanation and Interaction,* takes a Conversational Analysis approach to tutoring electronics that extends the work of Sinclair and Coulthard (1975) on educational dialogue in the classroom. In the process, she describes the way that expert tutors make an explanation interactive by turning it into a series of questions and then provides sequences of rules for planning discourse that implement the tutoring strategies that she observed. Although the actual dialogue produced by EDGE (Explanatory Discourse GEnerate) is template-driven, it is still a faithful simulation of the dialogue generated by expert human tutors. Cawsey's (1992, 1993) work has had a major impact on the CIRCSIM-Tutor project.

19.1.4 Discourse Planners—Longbow and APE

Johanna Moore had already completed a series of ground-breaking papers in Text Generation when she and Michael Young decided to write a special purpose discourse planner called Longbow (Young, 1994; Young & Moore 1994a, 1994b; Young, Moore, & Pollack, 1994). They named it Longbow in honor of its revolutionary nature. Longbow does dynamic, hierarchical, opportunistic, unification-based planning.

Long before she went to Pittsburgh to work with Moore, Reva Freedman sat in a laboratory at Illinois Institute of Technology and struggled with a planning engine from the University of Washington called UCPOP (Penberthy & Weld, 1992). Freedman had obtained UCPOP because it fit her list of abstract good qualities needed in a planner, but she discovered that it did not really work well with discourse. When she moved to Pittsburgh, she found Longbow and became an enthusiast, but then decided that she could do even better, especially when it came time to express preconditions. She wrote the Atlas Planning Environment or APE to improve on Longbow (Freedman 2000a, 2000b; 2001). APE does the planning for the Atlas Physics Tutor at Pittsburgh (Freedman, Rosé, Ringenberg, & VanLehn, 2000) and for Freedman's own CAPE Tutor (Freedman et al., 2004). Lane and VanLehn (in press) have also used APE to do all of the tutorial planning for ProPL, a very attractive new tutor that uses natural language dialogue to teach beginning programmers how to design programs. We were delighted when Freedman agreed that we could use APE for our Version 3 (Mills, 2001; Mills, Evens, & Freedman, 2004).

19.1.5 Andes and Atlas

Kurt VanLehn's Andes system (Schulze et al., 2000), an excellent model-tracing tutor for teaching physics, has been one of the major successes in the ITS field. It has been used at the Naval Academy in Annapolis and extensively tested in the Pittsburgh school system. With encouragement from ONR and from the NSF Circle program, Kurt VanLehn headed a team to build a natural language tutor that covers the same material in physics as Andes. The resulting Atlas system (Freedman, 2000a, 2000b; Rosé, Jordan, Ringenberg, Siler, VanLehn, & Weinstein, 2001) carries on a natural language dialogue using Rosé's parser, the COMLEX lexicon (Grishman, Macleod, & Meyers, 1994), Freedman's APE for discourse planning, and Jordan's collection of knowledge-based tutoring strategies (Freedman et al., 2000). Comparisons between Andes and Atlas (Rosé et al., 2001) have shown that Atlas is even more effective than Andes (VanLehn, Jordan, et al., 2002; VanLehn, Lynch, et al., 2002).

19.1.6 AutoTutor

Graesser's group at the University of Memphis has produced some of the best research on human tutoring (Graesser, Lang, & Horgan, 1988; Graesser & Person, 1994; Graesser, Person, & Huber, 1993; Graesser, Person, & Magliano, 1995; Person, Graesser, Magliano, & Kreuz, 1994; Person, Kreuz, Zwaan, & Graesser, 1995). Now this group has made use of their research to build a conversational tutor with the natural language processing components based on Latent Semantic Analysis (LSA). The first version (Graesser, Franklin, & Wiemer-Hastings, 1998) was implemented in the domain of computer literacy and the LSA analysis was surprisingly successful at recognizing poor student explanations and providing suggestions about how to improve them (Graesser, Wiemer-Hastings, Wiemer-Hastings, Kreuz, & Tutoring Research Group, 1999; Graesser et al., 2000; Person, Graesser, Harter, Mathews, & Tutoring Research Group, 2000). The AutoTutor approach has been used to build several other tutors, including one for advising students on English compositions (Wiemer-Hastings & Graesser, 2000a, 2000b) and another for research methods in psychology (Wiemer-Hastings, 2004). Latent Semantic Analysis provides a pathway to rapid development of tutors that carry on a simple natural language dialogue. There seem to be some problems, however, when that tutor needs to analyze a complex argument presented by the student (Wiemer-Hastings, 2000; Wiemer-Hastings & Zipitria, 2001). When these capabilities are needed, qualitative reasoning seems to be more effective.

19.2 CURRENT RESEARCH SYSTEMS

We now move on to discuss some current ongoing work, including new developments in the systems that we have already described and some new research teams.

19.2.1 Why2-AutoTutor

When the Office of Naval Research funded a Multidisciplinary Research Initiative to compare the LSA approach used in Memphis with the more symbolic approach to natural language understanding used in Pittsburgh, Graesser and VanLehn agreed to build two qualitative physics tutors to facilitate the comparison: the result was Why-AutoTutor and Why-Atlas, now revamped as Why2-AutoTutor (Jackson, Person, & Graesser, 2004; Jackson, Ventura, Chewle, Graesser, & Tutoring Research Group, 2004) and Why2-Atlas (VanLehn, Jordan, et al., 2002; VanLehn, Lynch, et al., 2002). Both systems pose a problem in qualitative physics and then ask the student to provide a short essay answer.

Then they analyze the essay and use it as a basis for a tutorial dialogue that attacks any misconceptions revealed, produce a critique of the essay, and help the student rewrite it.

One advantage of the LSA approach is that it is easier to retarget to another tutoring domain. The Memphis group has now developed a formal methodology for retargeting, which specifies the kind of text to be collected and the parameters of the LSA system that does the analysis. They have also added a number of tutoring strategies identified in earlier research on human tutoring (Person, Bautista, Graesser, Mathews, & Tutoring Research Group, 2001).

19.2.2 Why2-Atlas

Kurt VanLehn (VanLehn et al., 2004; VanLehn, Jordan, et al., 2002a; VanLehn, Lynch, et al., 2002b) has assembled a superb team in Pittsburgh to build the natural language processing components of the Why2-Atlas system. Carolyn Rosé's parser (Rosé, 1997a,b; 2000a,b; Rosé & Lavie, 2001) handles extended essays as well as student inputs to the follow-up dialogue and produces detailed output in the form of a series of propositions. Pamela Jordan's inferencing and generation system (Jordan, 2004; Jordan, Makatchev, & VanLehn, 2003, 2004; Jordan, Rosé, & VanLehn, 2000) produces fluent questions and critiques, and also diagnoses misconceptions by exploring the logical consequences of the reasoning process extracted from the essay. Jordan uses a theorem prover (Tacitus-Lite) to probe the faulty inferences in the student's explanation. If it finds a serious error, Why2-Atlas provides the student with a simpler problem to solve that uses the same kind of reasoning (Jordan, 2004). Then it moves back to the original problem and gives the student a chance to recognize the errors and correct them before launching into a tutorial dialogue to help the student to make appropriate revisions.

What can Why2-Atlas do that Why2-AutoTutor cannot? Presented with the often-observed impetus misconception, "If there is no force on a moving object, it slows down," Why2-AutoTutor treats this statement as a bag of words (paying no attention to the word order so it cannot distinguish between "A causes B" and "B causes A") and judges it in terms of its similarity to known sentences containing the same words. Why2-Atlas parses the sentence, analyzes it, and deduces its logical consequences, to see whether it is consistent with the correct answer and whether it covers the complete argument. As a result, it can recognize both missing concepts and misconceptions.

Wiemer-Hastings and Zipitria (2001) have analyzed the weaknesses of the LSA approach and have proposed methods of adding some syntactic and semantic information to the Auto-Tutor analysis. Rosé, Gaydos, Hall, Roque, and VanLehn (2003) have now constructed a suite of tools for building a robust sublanguage parser that begins with corpus analysis and carries the user through the construction of the grammar for the new sublanguage. These tools were used in an ITS summer school run by Aleven and Rosé (2004) in Pittsburgh in 2004.

19.2.3 CyclePad

The experience that Rovick and Michael had with MacMan almost 30 years ago was not unique—other experimenters have found that students need constant support from an instructor in order to learn effectively from simulation programs. Forbus (1997, 2001) built CyclePad to function as a computer coach for students learning to solve design and analysis problems in thermodynamics in a simulation environment. CyclePad does routine calculations for the student. It makes modeling assumptions explicit. It critiques student designs, looking for errors and contradictions by arguing from constraints; students often propose impossible designs. Both the modeling and simulation software and the system explanations make use of Forbus's (1988) well-known work on qualitative reasoning. The system is already being widely used because it gets good results with students, but it is still more effective if the students carry on a reflective dialogue with the instructor about the designs they have just developed. This experience prompted Forbus to collaborate with a team from Carnegie-Mellon to add a natural language dialogue system to CyclePad (Rosé, Torrey, & Aleven, 2004; Rosé, Torrey, Aleven, et al., 2004). These dialogues are designed to help students identify problems and use qualitative reasoning to work through principled improvements to their designs.

19.2.4 BEETLE

Some of the most exciting research on tutoring systems is coming from Johanna Moore's group at Edinburgh. Group members are building a tutor for basic electronics called BEETLE that combines Moore's own expertise in planning and text generation with Rosé's work on parsing and Core's work on dialogue management (Core, Moore, & Zinn, 2000, 2001, 2003; Rosé, Di Eugenio, & Moore, 1999). They are also doing significant work on system architecture (Zinn, Moore, & Core, 2002) and on recognizing, understanding, and responding to student initiatives (Core, Moore, & Zinn, 2000, 2001, 2003). The quality of the generated text is especially impressive (Moore, Foster, Lemon, & White, 2004; Moore, Porayska-Pomsta, Varges, & Zinn, 2004).

Recently they have come up with a new approach to make Rosé's Carmel parser still more robust (Core & Moore, 2004; Rosé et al., 2002). The semantic analysis assigns a confidence score to competing interpretations of the student input and then determines which one is most appropriate to the context. The same confidence score approach is used with the spelling correction component, which is otherwise based on our earlier work (Elmi & Evens, 1998). Alternative spelling corrections are each given a score and then the system decides which one makes more sense. BEETLE does a better job by postponing the final choice until the syntactic and semantic analyses are complete. In our older version, that decision is made at the very beginning of the analysis and all alternatives are thrown away.

19.2.5 CATO and Student Explanations

Ever since he finished his dissertation with Edwina Rissland 15 years ago, Kevin Ashley has been a leader in applications of artificial intelligence to law. Ashley and his students have been working for several years on CATO, a tutor that uses a natural language dialogue to help students learn to make better legal arguments. This system went through a large-scale classroom evaluation in 1997 (Aleven & Ashley, 1997a, 1997b) and has been in active use ever since at the University of Pittsburgh, where Ashley has a joint appointment between the College of Law and the Learning Research and Development Center. CATO is also being used actively in a long sequence of research projects in case-based reasoning, in tutoring, and in natural language understanding (Aleven & Koedinger, 2000a, 2000b).

Aleven (2003) has made a number of extensions to CATO's natural language understanding capabilities, so that it can better understand the legal argument that the student is trying to make. Working with Koedinger, he has also rebuilt the natural language component of the Geometry Explanation Tutor, so that it can understand student self-explanations and respond to them (Aleven, Koedinger, & Popescu, 2003).

19.2.6 Spoken Language Tutors—SCoT and ITSpoke

There is a widespread feeling that the future of tutoring using natural language lies with spoken language tutors, but at this point, the problems of understanding spoken language are still quite serious—so serious that they have scared researchers away from trying to confront the problems of tutoring at the same time.

The tremendous advantages of using spoken language in the Computer Aided Language Learning (CALL) domain have made these folks braver than the rest (Holland, Kaplan, & Sams, 1995). Spoken language has some clear advantages of speed and bandwidth in all domains. It is also clear that it is easier to recognize user frustration in spoken language because of the available prosodic cues (Kirchhoff, 2001; Litman, Hirschberg, & Swerts, 2000).

Speech also has tremendous advantages in training people to respond to stressful situations where hands and eyes are busy. A team at the Center for the Study of Language and Information (CSLI) at Stanford University led by Stanley Peters is building a spoken language tutor (SCoT) for naval damage control. It combines David Wilkins's DC-TRAIN (Bulitko & Wilkins, 1999) system for naval damage control assistants with knowledge about tutoring and knowledge about speech interaction into an effective tutorial. By building an extensive semantic model, including a detailed representation of the ship in question, and a sophisticated representation of the navy sublanguage, they have succeeded in providing appropriate tutorial responses to almost all of the student utterances. The speech technology is provided by Nuance and the natural language understanding component uses SRI's Gemini system. The system has been tested on Stanford undergraduates (after a short tutorial on ships and their parts) and in a small course at the Naval Postgraduate School (Bratt et al., 2002; B. Z. Clark et al., 2003; Pon-Barry, Clark, Schultz, Bratt, & Peters, 2004a, 2004b, 2004c).

Diane Litman has produced a functioning speech-enabled ITS called TTSpoke by adding a speech interface to Atlas (Forbes-Riley & Litman, 2004; Litman & Forbes-Riley, 2004). The student still types in an essay, as in Atlas, but the tutoring interaction in which the system critiques the student's essay is entirely spoken in the new system. Although the system typically misunderstands more than 10% of the student's words, it uses the tutoring context so effectively that it almost always obtains a correct logic form. Litman has also produced two other dramatic results. The spoken language system speeds up the tutorial interaction and it is also successful in using prosodic information to assess the emotional state of the student.

Litman has also carried out a fundamental experiment (in conjunction with VanLehn, Rosé, and Jordan) comparing the spoken modality with keyboard modality in human tutoring sessions, showing that spoken tutoring has significant advantages in learning gains (Litman et al., 2004).

19.3 INTELLIGENT TUTORING SYSTEMS AND THE POWER OF NATURAL LANGUAGE

19.3.1 Learning the Language and Learning the Domain

We are convinced that learning physiology is inextricably involved with learning the language of physiology, learning how to talk physiology. Frawley (1988, p. 356) argued that learning the language is learning the domain, that "scientific knowledge is a lexical structure." Hobbs and Moore (1985) argued for this point of view as part of their "theories of the commonsense world." Michael McCloskey

(1983) made the same kind of argument; for him, mental models are full of words.

The current emphasis in the field of knowledge acquisition on ontology, on acquiring a taxonomy or ISA hierarchy of some domain of interest, as the basis of knowledge base construction, suggests that we are not alone in this belief. The Association for Computing Machinery is currently collecting philosophers and computer scientists together for a series of conferences on the Formal Ontology of Information Systems, and a new standard Ontology Information Layer (called OIL) has just been defined for Web semantics.

19.3.2 The Self-Explanation Effect

Michelene Chi and her colleagues at the University of Pittsburgh (Chi, Bassok, Lewis, Reimann, & Glaser, 1989; Chi, de Leeuw, Chiu, & LaVancher, 1994; Hausmann & Chi, 2002) have demonstrated convincingly that constructing self-explanations of new material as it is digested is an extremely effective learning strategy, that this strategy is widely used by effective learners, and that pushing students to use this strategy produces a significant improvement in learning gains. McNamara (2004) has shown similar results in studies of students reading scientific texts. George Miller, father of WordNet (Miller, Beckwith, Fellbaum, Gross, & Miller, 1991) and many other important areas in cognitive psychology, told Evens (personal communication, September 19, 1996) that he believes that Chi's research offers the best reason known for the success of human tutoring, and we have come to agree with this assessment.

Our own experience of how much student attempts at explanations improve student learning was one of the factors that convinced us to undertake the CIRCSIM-Tutor project. It is the reason for our current focus on open questions and student initiatives.

Aleven, Koedinger, and Cross (1999) demonstrated that this self-explanation effect carries over to tutoring systems. The problem is that students tend to stop producing explanations when they discover that the system cannot understand them (Aleven & Koedinger, 2000b). Aleven and Koedinger are now trying to add natural language understanding to their tutor to keep the explanations coming (Aleven, Popescu, & Koedinger, 2001).

19.3.3 The Dialectic Effect

Although Hegel and his followers effectively co-opted the word *dialectic,* we are using it in the original sense—in the words of *Webster's Seventh New Collegiate Dictionary* (G. & C. Merriam Company, 1963, p. 229): "discussion and reasoning by dialogue as a method of intellectual investigation." Herbert Clark (H. H. Clark & Brennan, 1991; H. H. Clark & Schaefer, 1989) has argued for a "collaborative theory" of conversation in which conversational participants work together to create the meaning of their joint utterances until they reach mutual understanding. We are convinced that participation in a dialogue creates a level of shared understanding beyond that obtainable from a monologue, whether that monologue takes the form of a classroom lecture or a chapter in a textbook. This conviction implies that the next experiment that we plan should attempt to discover whether students remember what they learned about the baroreceptor reflex for a longer period of time after a session with CIRCSIM-Tutor than after reading text about the system.

Jean Fox Tree (1999) has carried out an ingenious experiment to confirm this theory about the efficacy of dialogue. She taped 10 task-oriented dialogues, then she concocted monologues with the same content and taped them also, and finally she arranged for 160 university students to listen to one version or another. She then tested their ability to perform the task. The students who listened to the dialogue did significantly better at the task. Kevin Ashley (Ashley, Desai, & Levine, 2002) has demonstrated the dialectic advantage with educational software as well. People learn better from dialogues than from monologues.

Rickel, Lesh, Rich, Sidner, and Gertner (2002) argued for the use of "collaborative discourse theory as a foundation for tutorial dialogue" (p. 542) as embodied in Rich and Sidner's Collagen system (C. Rich & Sidner, 1998). Collagen, which is based on the work of Grosz and Sidner (1986), tracks the attentional state as well as the intentional state of the discourse participants. In other words, the system tries to keep track of the plans and the focus of attention of both participants in the dialogue. Tutoring systems that make use of this approach may indeed be better able to understand and respond to student initiatives. Perhaps CIRCSIM-Tutor could profit from adding attentional information to the student model—it might help the system recognize initiatives and interpret answers to open questions.

19.3.4 The Socratic Effect

Two experiments have been carried out with ITS that show that larger learning gains occur with Socratic tutoring than with didactic tutoring. One experiment is described in Rosé, Moore, VanLehn, and Allbritton (2001). The other study was conducted by Aleven as part of the evaluation of alternative forms of a tutoring system, one more didactic and one more Socratic (Aleven et al., 2003). Both studies suggest that Socratic Tutoring works better. Neither is really conclusive. Aleven clearly believes that the main virtue of the Socratic mode is that it forces students to give explanations themselves.

It is clearly important that more experiments of this kind should be carried out with larger and more diverse groups of students. We suspect that some kind of Socratic tutoring within a fairly directive system with a tutor agenda and enough tutor control to prevent wandering will turn out to give the best results for medical students, but this is our own highly subjective opinion. Results may easily vary for students at different ages and in different stages of learning.

19.4 PROVIDING SCAFFOLDING AND FADING

There are still a couple of other unresolved issues for those involved in dialogue-based ITSs that seek to emulate the performance of human tutors: (a) How can we provide the same scaffolding and fading, cognitive and emotional, without the same bandwidth available for judging the student response that is immediately available in face-to-face tutoring? (b) How can we provide the kind of back-channel responses that human tutors give face-to-face? and (c) How can we develop the same kind of approach to co-construction of the solution that human tutors can provide by writing on the same piece of paper or the same blackboard with the student?

One of the many strengths of Atlas/Andes, inherited by Why-2 Atlas, is the way that these systems handle scaffolding and fading. VanLehn et al. (2000) have developed a number of interesting ideas about implementing these abilities in natural language systems. New work by Reiser and his group at Northwestern University studies various approaches to scaffolding and how students respond to it (Quintana et al., 2004; Reiser, 2004; Reiser et al., 2001; Sherin, Reiser, & Edelson, 2004; Tabak, 2004).

Vasandani and Govindaraj (1994, 1995) have demonstrated that fading is just as important as scaffolding. ROTC students learning about boilers in ship engine rooms learned significantly more when they were informed that the scaffolding would disappear than when it was provided throughout the session.

Neil Heffernan and Ken Koedinger (2000a, 2000b, 2001, 2002; Heffernan, 2001) have implemented a tutoring dialogue for word problems in algebra using many of the same tutoring strategies that we have described. This dialogue uses rather rudimentary language generation and menu input from the student, but it embodies many good dialogue strategies and appropriate tactics to carry them out. Heffernan's (2001) experiments with his algebra tutor, Ms. Lindquist, have shown that adding even a little natural language to the tutoring process helps to increase both learning and motivation in algebra students. Further experiments with Ms. Lindquist (Croteau, Heffernan, & Koedinger, 2004; Heffernan, 2003; Heffernan & Croteau, 2004) have shown that students learn more and continue to use the tutor longer, when the tutor uses strategies that force them to induce the answer from examples and verbalize the algorithm.

In moving from face-to-face tutoring to an ITS with a keyboard interface, there is a real loss of bandwidth and of nonverbal cues to what the student is thinking and feeling. Along with that loss has come the loss of the back-channel language feedback that Fox (1993b) described as very important in student decisions about whether to go ahead with what he or she is saying or break off and start over (see also Duncan, 1974). AutoTutor is attempting to introduce a version of that feedback using approving or disapproving facial expressions. Rush Medical College students have suggested that CIRCSIM-Tutor might use happy faces and other emoticons from e-mail to obtain some of that expressiveness.

Michael and Rovick work hard at coconstructing the answer with the student, but when the answer involves an equation or a diagram, it becomes really difficult on a keyboard. Fox (1993b) discussed the significant communication that goes on when the student and the tutor are building the same equation on the same piece of paper or altering the same diagram. Jung Hee Kim and Michael Glass (2004) have developed a way to preserve this process of coconstruction in collecting human tutorial dialogues for an algebra tutoring project. Their system for capturing algebra tutoring sessions (Patel, Glass, &

Kim, 2003) has an interface that supports and records cooperative construction of a diagram or an equation by the tutor and the student. Diagrams and equations are displayed on the screens of the tutor and the student simultaneously and either one can edit the screen display when holding the turn. This becomes part of the session transcript.

J. H. Kim and Glass (2004) have also developed a Wooz (Wizard of Oz) Tutor that provides an effective method for implementing a variety of natural language tutoring strategies and studying their effectiveness. A human tutor sits at a keyboard and carries out an algebra tutoring session with a student located somewhere else. Whenever the tutor is ready to select a new tutoring strategy, the system presents a list of strategies it believes to be appropriate at that point in the session. The tutor picks one and starts typing or rejects them all to strike out on his or her own. The first experiments suggest that the system-aided sessions cover more material in the same amount of time and that the students cannot distinguish system strategies from human strategies.

19.5 SUMMARY

The take-home message from this chapter is a mixed one, combining much progress with many problems. For many years, CIRCSIM-Tutor was the one and only natural language based ITS, but CIRCSIM-Tutor is not so lonely anymore. There are now at least six other systems that carry on a natural language dialogue with their students: BEETLE, Why2-Atlas, Why2-Autotutor, SCoT, and ITSpoke, with CATO hovering on the threshold. (Both UC, the Unix-Consultant, and CyclePad have impressive language abilities, but they function as coaches so they do not need to generate the same kind of interactive dialogue, and we have therefore decided to leave them out of this discussion.) Even these six ITSs differ in the portion of the natural language dialogue spectrum that they attack. BEETLE, like CIRCSIM-Tutor, is designed to carry on a complete truly interactive Socratic dialogue, beginning with predictions from the student, focused on the problem-solving process. Both systems are faced with the problem of interpreting a wide range of short answers; they must generate questions, hints, acknowledgments, and explanations.

Why2-Atlas and Why2-AutoTutor describe a physics problem and then ask their students to write a short essay that explains what happens in terms of qualitative physics. The system then critiques the essay and asks the student to rewrite it. Thus, their primary area of natural language understanding is really written language, not spoken language, but they also find their input to be terser than they expected. Why2-AutoTutor uses LSA to assess the essay and to identify some appropriate comments. Why2-Atlas produces a logical representation of the text entered by the student and uses a state-of-the-art logical analysis to assess the relationship between the essay and the system's store of knowledge of physics to determine how to critique it.

ITSpoke and SCoT use speech to communicate with their students. ITSpoke is a speech-enabled version of Why2-Atlas. Litman et al. (2004) have shown that the spoken version can cover the material faster and it also has an advantage in recognizing student emotional states. SCoT carries on a reflective tutoring session after a student encounters Wilkins's Damage Control Assistant simulation. It provides an important first step toward ITSs for emergency management.

CATO has added natural language interaction to respond to student self-explanation after a series of experiments that demonstrate that self-explanation in an ITS context is also extremely beneficial to student learning, but that students will not continue the self-explanation process unless the system can understand and comment on what the student has to say.

All of these projects are concerned with ways to represent and deploy a wide range of tutoring strategies and tactics. The Wooz Tutor of Kim and Glass provides a useful tool to test alternative strategies; Heffernan's work with Ms. Lindquist suggests a methodology for this kind of analysis. Domain knowledge and linguistic knowledge language also present problems in knowledge acquisition, representation, evaluation, and storage for all of these systems. All of these projects are trying out different approaches to student modeling and starting to look at ways to represent student affect and confidence as well as student knowledge levels.

20

Where Do We All Go From Here?

20.0 POSSIBLE RESEARCH DIRECTIONS

Enticing paths for future research lead off in all directions, but we list only a few that seem most vital, attractive, and manageable. Much of this agenda is of interest to the much broader research community interested in teaching, learning, or tutoring, or to the community of ITS developers. Many items on this agenda are of general applicability, whereas others reflect our interest in continuing the development of CIRCSIM-Tutor itself.

We start with a discussion of issues related to human tutoring. Next we discuss some educational experiments. Then we describe some additions that we would like to make in CIRCSIM-Tutor. Finally, we mention some other language-based tutors that we would like to build ourselves or see others build.

20.1 FINDING OUT MORE ABOUT HUMAN TUTORING

Our understanding of human tutoring is still incomplete—finding out more would add to our collective understanding of this important education phenomenon and also help us improve CIRCSIM-Tutor and other computer tutors. In this section, we summarize some areas where we feel that much work remains to be done, especially in the generation of analogies, dealing with misconceptions, responding to pathic expressions and hedging, and examining differences between novice and expert tutors.

20.1.1 Use of Analogies by Tutors and Students

A number of studies have shown that analogy is a very effective teaching strategy (Gentner, 1983; Goldblum, 2001; Holyoak & Thagard, 1995). Several ITSs have made use of analogies using "canned" or template-driven language generation (T. Murray, Schultz, Brown, & Clement, 1990; Winkels & Breuker, 1990; Woolf, 1984). As we described in Section 7.2.7, we are starting to try to understand how expert tutors use analogies or respond to analogies proposed by students (Lulis, Evens, & Michael, 2003) with the hope of making CIRCSIM-Tutor capable of generating and repairing analogies.

Analysis of the bases used by tutors show that some are abstract (Ohm's Law; see Example 7.10), whereas others are concrete (balloon; see Example 7.7). Some involve comparisons with entities from outside the session (balloon and Ohm's Law); others with entities within the session (an earlier procedure or another neural variable; Lulis, Michael, & Evens, 2004a, 2004b, 2004c). Both Moore (Moore, Lemaire, & Rosenblum, 1996) and Katz (Katz, O'Donnell, & Kay, 2000) have studied tutor comparisons between the current event and earlier events and found them very useful to the student. (See Section 20.3.4 for more about our plans to incorporate analogies in CIRCSIM-Tutor.)

There are many open questions. When, under what conditions, do tutors offer an analogy to help the student solve a problem? What analogies do they use? When there is more than one base corresponding to the target the student needs to understand, how does the tutor chose the one to use? When the student does not respond appropriately, how does the tutor attempt to repair the situation? How do tutors respond when the student offers an analogy?

20.1.2 Diagnosing and Responding to Student Misconceptions

Misconceptions are ingrained beliefs that are, in fact, wrong. Michael (1998, 2002) has described them as faulty mental models of the phenomena in question or as conceptual difficulties. The question of how misconceptions are formed and how to change them is still a problem not just for human and machine tutors but for all teachers.

We have found that, although students are usually very willing to fill gaps in their knowledge, they are usually very resistant to giving up their misconceptions, especially when they have based their understanding of other phenomena on those explanations. Chi and Roscoe (2002) have similar results.

Michael and Rovick have identified certain patterns of prediction errors that predict particular misconceptions and there are some conversational clues that cause them to pursue one or another of these issues. They have developed a set of special tutoring strategies to deal with particular misconceptions; we discussed some examples in Chapter 7. They believe that other kinds of errors are truly vanquished after the student has gotten that material correct three times in a row, but they are not nearly so optimistic about misconceptions. They regard a student who has ever betrayed a given misconception as more likely to suffer from it later than not, no matter how many times that student has given correct answers. Feltovich, Spiro, and Coulson (1989) have given us reason to believe that this pessimism may be well-founded. Their research shows that even practicing physicians suffer from some of the same misconceptions as our first-year medical students.

Misconceptions are a serious problem for all teachers and learners, not just human and machine tutors. It seems to us that there are three fundamental issues here: Where do misconceptions come from and how they are formed? The work by Feltovich, Coulson, and Spiro (2001) and the current studies by Gwendolyn Campbell at the Naval Air Warfare Center Training Systems Division are making inroads in this new territory. As tutors and developers of ITS, we are even more interested in the second issue: How do tutors, and by extension ITSs, diagnose the presence of misconceptions held by the student? Finally, there is an issue of very general interest: How can we correct misconceptions and bring about conceptual change?

20.1.3 Understanding and Responding to Affective or Pathic Expressions

Recent research on making computers understand emotions has prompted the ITS community to start to investigate how to provide emotional scaffolding and to respond to affective expressions, especially indications of confusion, rage, and frustration, from the user. Our initial investigations (Bhatt, 2004; Bhatt, Evens, & Argamon, 2004) suggest that the kind of affect that students express to human tutors (mostly gratitude and apologies for errors) is totally different from the expressions of affect received by our ITS (mostly rage and frustration), mostly buried in answers to open questions. Some of these expressions seemed to be aimed at testing the system. Log files from November 1998 and 1999 reveal several expressions of confusion, rage, and frustration, also.

The CIRCSIM-Tutor log files from November 2002 contain 20 expressions of student affect, all in response to open questions. Some were clearly probing the system to confirm their correct suspicions that the system was not parsing that portion of the input. Some expressed frustration with the system. When CIRCSIM-Tutor asked, "Why did you enter 'no change' for TPR?" Student T48 answered, "you know why." When the system asked, "Why is MAP still decreased?" T48 answered, "I don't want to tell you." T74 answered this same question with "blalaal."

20.1.4 Understanding and Responding to Student Hedges

Hedging has been discussed at several ONR Grantees' Meetings and at a SIGDIAL Workshop at the Annual Meeting of the Association for Computational Linguistics in Pittsburgh in 2001. The suggestion was made that ITSs should record hedging and use it as a general measure of the student level of confidence and also an indicator of whether the student actually knew the content that was hedged.

During the first eight tutoring sessions in 1989, Michael and Rovick often commented on hedges. In their discussion and debriefing after those eight sessions were completed, they decided to stop doing so because they felt that hedging was not a good clue to student knowledge but instead a matter of student style and self-presentation. They concluded that commenting on hedges is a waste of tutor time. They did, however, continue to respond to those few hedges that seemed to indicate real student distress.

This experience made us doubt whether it was appropriate to treat hedging primarily as an expression of student lack of confidence. Robin Lakoff (1975) described hedging as principally a politeness strategy, an expression of deference. It has also been suggested that students may find it more "scientific" to hedge, especially when the tutor is an expert in the field. We were also interested in this question for practical reasons; we had spent a considerable amount of time thinking about how to parse hedges in CIRCSIM-Tutor (Glass, 1999). These considerations prompted a preliminary study of hedging in the 25 most recent expert human tutoring sessions, K52 to K76, carried out in November 1999 (Bhatt, 2004; Bhatt, Evens, & Argamon, 2004).

As we reported in Section 7.6, we found that all 25 of the students hedged, but in amounts varying from twice to 22 times in an hour. When we compared the correctness of hedged answers to unhedged ones, we found that hedged answers to tutor questions are more likely to be wrong than unhedged answers. Nevertheless, hedged answers are more likely to be right than wrong. It would take a very sensitive student modeler to make effective use of this information. It is clear that we need to study more sessions to come to firm conclusions.

Armed with our list of hedges found in human tutoring sessions, we looked at the student input to CIRCSIM-Tutor. There were no hedges in the log files from November 1998 and November 1999, and one marginal hedge in the 66 log files from November 2002, included in an answer to an open question. Carolyn Penstein Rosé (personal communication, December 26, 2003) told us that Atlas does not see hedging either. These results seem to suggest that student hedging is a conscious expression of deference and politeness, which students use with human tutors, and not an unconscious expression of lack of knowledge or lack of confidence in that knowledge. But it is, of course, conceivable, that if CIRCSIM-Tutor were a better conversationalist, students would hedge to it more often. We remain convinced that if our ITS sounded smarter, students would ask questions and indulge in other initiatives.

There are a number of open questions here. Do students hedge as often in other domains? Do they hedge in the same way in all domains? Do they hedge in the same way in spoken and in keyboard contexts? Do they hedge to some ITSs and not to others?

20.1.5 Similarities and Differences between Novice and Expert Tutors

What we know about tutoring has come from studies that have looked at the behavior or the outcomes of tutors ranging from experts to novices (see Chapter 10). But we still have only a partial understanding of how tutors accomplish whatever they accomplish. One approach to gaining the needed knowledge is to compare the behavior of novice and expert tutors and determine how those differences impact the learning outcomes that result.

In Chapter 10, we described the results of our studies of novice and expert tutors. For a variety of reasons, we were only able to come to a few limited conclusions. The behavior of novice tutors is quite different from that of expert tutors. We present some evidence that expert tutors achieve significantly better learning gains but further experiments with more students should be carried out to confirm these results.

More studies of this type clearly need to be done with more tutors and more students. We need to ask the following questions: What do novice and expert tutors do and how do they do it? We need as fine-grained an analysis of tutor behaviors as possible and we need to study many more tutors. What learning outcomes result from tutoring by novices or experts? Do novices and tutors produce different results? What are the most appropriate measures of the learning outcomes that result from one-on-one tutoring? We need to look for evidence of meaningful learning and we need to ask whether the learning outcomes are temporary or long lasting (see Section 20.1.4). Are there important differences between tutoring in different domains? Answers to these questions are needed to improve human tutoring and to enable us to build more effective computer tutors.

20.2 EXPERIMENTS ON EDUCATIONAL ISSUES

There are many questions about teaching and learning that are extremely difficult to answer, and we briefly discussed some of these difficulties in Section 18.7. One of the major problems with studying tutoring is the difficulty of scripting what is basically an opportunistic exercise. It is also difficult for a human tutor to follow a script while attempting to assist a student in learning something. On the other hand, a computer tutor can be programmed with a script defining some particular approach to tutoring. And the computer tutor will follow that script with each student who uses the system. Thus, if we want to find out whether immediate feedback is always the best course, or discover the effect of different approaches to teaching an algorithm, we may be able to get more reliable results with an ITS than with a human tutor.

Although CIRCSIM-Tutor and other current ITSs clearly do not make use of some of the more sophisticated tutoring strategies employed by expert human tutors, they can be a very useful research tool in attempts to find out more about tutoring. Different versions of a computer tutor can be programmed to carry out one of a set of alternative tactics or protocols and it can do so in a tireless and consistent way for hours. Thus, it would be possible to arrange for large numbers of student subjects to use different versions of the system and do a kind of controlled experiment that is almost impossible with human tutors. Some of the issues that we would like to see explored are described in the next few sections.

20.2.1 Exploring the Immediate Feedback Issue

One important educational issue that has also become an important design issue for CIRCSIM-Tutor and other ITSs is the question of immediate feedback. Although there are many arguments for immediate feedback, Michael and Rovick have always argued that it is more important that the tutor collect evidence for a detailed student model before beginning to tutor. That is why CIRCSIM-Tutor asks for a whole column of predictions before it starts its remedial dialogue. John Anderson (Schooler & Anderson, 1990) has made a similar argument.

We would like to see researchers address the following questions using a computer tutor able to function in alternative ways. Is there a difference in the learning outcomes (quantitative and qualitative) from receiving immediate feedback compared with delayed feedback? How does tutor behavior change when immediate feedback is provided and a less rich student model is available? Which approach results in the student building the most robust mental model?

Cho (2000; Cho, Michael, Rovick, & Evens, 2000) collected evidence that Michael and Rovick switch protocols themselves, when the student becomes seriously confused (as described in Section 7.1). He wrote APE rules for CIRCSIM-Tutor Version 3, providing for protocol switches on the basis of the state of the student model. We are eager to get Version 3 to a state where we can explore these alternative protocols in a controlled experiment.

20.2.2 Helping Students Learn an Algorithm or Problem-Solving Approach

Most of the time, the computer scientists on our team have found the human tutoring sessions carried out at Rush Medical College to be inspiring in their depth and sophistication. We have been critical of Michael and Rovick's approach to teaching the problem-solving algorithm, however. In general, as people who spend much of our time teaching algorithms, we (the IIT group) believe that it is an excellent idea to encourage people to figure out the algorithm for themselves. On the other hand, it is also essential to make an explicit statement of the algorithm before the lesson is over, even if it sometimes cuts down on the time that students have available to develop their intuition.

VanLehn has begun a series of experiments looking at this issue, comparing the new Pyrenees Tutor with the Andes Tutor. The Pyrenees Tutor provides the student with an explicit discussion of the problem-solving technique. Preliminary results show that the process of putting together an explicit description of the algorithm that the students find helpful and interesting is not easy and straightforward. But trials with the system suggest that students using Pyrenees are less likely to flounder around without figuring out what to do next than students using Andes (VanLehn et al., 2004).

There are a number of related questions that require investigation. How should tutors scaffold the students developing problem-solving skills? Do explicit descriptions of algorithms help? If so, what kinds? Does guided inquiry lead to the development of robust problem skills, or does it result in a frustrating experience with few learning gains? Using an ITS that can be programmed to utilize different approaches to teaching algorithms offers one experimental approach to addressing these questions.

20.2.3 How Much Time Does It Take to Have an Effect and How Long Does It Last?

There are at least two questions about time and tutoring that require further research from us and from other people with expert tutors and working ITS systems. One question is whether students who are tutored retain what they learned for longer than students who learn in some other way. There are few, if any, studies that have looked at long-term retention (weeks, months, years), and such studies are needed. If the effects of one-on-one tutoring, whether by human or machine tutors, are brief (days to weeks), such a finding would certainly call into question the cost effectiveness of such an approach to learning.

The other question is, if possible, even more important. It affects the design of curricula and of experiments in both human and machine tutoring. The question is how long does it take, how much time spent in one-on-one interaction with a tutor (human or computer), to produce a significant, and measurable, learning gain (Du Boulay, 2000)? The famous success stories of one-on-one tutoring involve tutoring spans much longer than those that we have used in our experiments. The students in Bloom's famous 2-sigma study (1984) were tutored for an hour every day for 3 weeks (15 weekdays). The students who worked with Lesgold's (1992) Sherlock II used the system for a total of 24 hr to achieve learning gains better than those obtained in 4 years of informal learning in the field. Part of the problem is that different approaches to tutoring may produce varying amounts of learning gains as well as varying retention results.

20.3 IMPROVING CIRCSIM-TUTOR

Throughout Part III of this book, we described a number of possible improvements and additions to CIRCSIM-Tutor. Once we have Version 3 working, we want to try to implement more of the novel tutoring strategies that we have seen in our studies of human tutors. We want to enable the system to understand student answers to open questions. We also want to make the system understand and respond to some of the pathic remarks, especially some of the expressions of confusion and frustration that it now receives. We hope that demonstrating these wider powers of the Input Understander will prompt the students to produce student initiatives, which are likely to present the system with the same kind of problems in parsing. If the system can understand these new types of input, then we need to be able to generate appropriate responses. This means adding additional plans to the Discourse Planner and even more complex changes to the Turn Planner, to integrate longer explanations into smooth and fluent turns.

During the span of the research described in this book, we have refrained from adding any visual components to the learning process, because the focus throughout has been on the power of natural language dialogue and our attempts to implement this kind of dialogue. We have built a separate system to tutor some of these same topics with concept maps (Jeong, Evens, & Kim, 1998; Y. C. Kim, 2003) and we would like to study the effects of combining these two approaches. Finally, we would like to try the system out with a wider range of students and find out how useful it is with different audiences.

20.3.1 Student Modeling

A number of different approaches to student modeling have been developed by the ITS community, but it is not clear which approaches are most effective in guiding computer tutors. We have implemented several different algorithms for student modeling in CIRCSIM-Tutor. We need to do a serious evaluation of these different approaches to see which gives us better results.

VanLehn has done some interesting work with Bayesian modeling (Conati, Gertner, VanLehn, & Druzdzel, 1997; Gertner, Conati, & VanLehn, 1998; Martin & VanLehn, 1995). More recently, David C. Wilkins has used a Bayesian approach in the Damage Control Assistant simulation program and in his work on tutors for decision making in crisis situations (Fried et al., 2003). This approach has become part of the SCoT Tutor (Bratt et al., 2002). The CIRCSIM-Tutor project team ought to implement a Bayesian modeling scheme and see if it predicts the student's performance in the next procedure or the student's results on the posttest better than the more ad hoc counts that we are now using. One reason that we have not done so already is that we now have four separate student models (Zhou & Evens, 1999), at four different levels (current variable, current phase, current procedure, overall), to provide input to four sets of rules, planning what to do immediately while tutoring the current variable, what to do during the current phase, what to do during the current procedure, and what to do throughout the whole curriculum (Cho, 2000), and it is hard to see how to integrate these levels in a Bayesian model.

There is another new approach that would be potentially easier to integrate with ours. Jim Minstrell, a master teacher of high school physics, has developed a methodology called FACETS to model student concepts, including misconceptions. Using Andrea diSessa's work as a theoretical framework (diSessa & Minstrell, 1998), and working with other teachers, he has developed an exhaustive inventory of physics concepts used in student explanations, including both correct and problematic responses (Minstrell & Kraus, 2001). Minstrell and the well-known artificial intelligence researcher, Earl Hunt, have obtained National Science Foundation Funding for a joint project called Diagnoser, a collection of diagnostic instructional tools for middle and high school students and teachers (Hunt & Minstrell, 1994; also online at http://tutor.psych.washington.edu).

If we could establish real confidence in our student model, then we could compare outcomes from different protocols or strategies or tactics and decide which worked better on the basis of the state of the model, rather than waiting until we can do a comparative study of learning outcomes. It not only takes a great deal of time to do such a study, it requires a big effect to make a difference in learning gains, and when it comes to individual tutoring strategies, it makes a lot more sense to look for multiple small effects.

20.3.2 Understanding and Responding to Open Questions

First of all, we want to extend the capabilities of the Input Understander so that it can deal with the answers to the open questions that we added to Version 2.9 (as described in Section 13.6). We obtained a lot of brief answers like the answers to our more directive questions generated during the tutoring phase, and we think that it should be relatively easy to understand many of these answers and match them to the "canned ideal answer" written by Joel Michael that the system reels out after it obtains an answer from the student. We need to figure out how to devise new discourse plans or schemas, like the multiturn schemas described in Chapters 7 and 8, created for the remediation of misconceptions. These schemas will provide a positive acknowledgment of the part that the student got right and then attempt to elicit the missing parts of the explanation. Then these schemas must be expressed as APE planning operators. Because they involve existing logic forms and concepts that the system can already handle, this seems feasible.

Although almost all of the student answers to the open questions are brief fragments of the kind that the students use elsewhere, there are a few longer more serious answers that our information extraction parser may not handle well. One possibility is to revert to our older, more conventional parser, when the count of words ignored by the current parser gets too large. We also want to try out the new parser now being written by Chung Hee Lee (C. H. Lee & Evens, 2004).

20.3.3 Understanding and Responding to Student Initiatives

We hope that if students see that the Input Understander can understand their answers to open questions, then they may generate more of the student initiatives studied by Shah (Shah, Evens, Michael, & Rovick, 2002). Students do not frequently generate spontaneous questions or propose explanations to CIRCSIM-Tutor as they do to human tutors. They do ask such questions of classmates in the room during the CIRCSIM or CIRCSIM-Tutor laboratories. We believe that they will generate these initiatives to the system if they have reason to believe that it can understand them.

There seem to be four major problems in recognizing and responding to student initiatives: (a) recognizing that the student is not answering the question asked by the system but instead taking the initiative, (b) handling the turn-taking and the return to the previous topic in a graceful fashion, (c) parsing the initiative, and (d) generating an appropriate response.

We are trying to use lexical cues to recognize student initiatives (cf. Chu-Carroll & Brown, 1997; Green & Carberry, 1999; Litman, 1996; Litman & Allen, 1987). McCawley (1988), Walker and Whittaker (1990), and Traum and Allen (1994) addressed the issues around turn-taking. Core, Moore, and Zinn (2001, 2003) have developed algorithms for handling initiatives in BEETLE.

Shah's work on student initiatives (Shah et al., 2002) includes a detailed analysis of the responses generated by expert tutors. These responses involve longer and more detailed explanations than the tutors usually provide to students. Unless students explicitly ask for an explanation or attempt to give one and ask the tutor to comment, expert tutors will usually attempt to get the students to create the explanation themselves (Cawsey, 1992; G. Sanders, 1995). Generating this discussion may require building some more extensive multiturn plans.

20.3.4 Generating and Understanding Analogies

To make CIRCSIM-Tutor support the kind of tutor–student interaction about analogies that we see in human tutoring sessions (see Section 7.2.7), we need some kind of model of analogy. In examining some of the recent literature, we discovered that Gentner's (1983) structured mapping model of analogies seems to describe rather clearly the processes that we see happening in these dialogues. After we explained what we were trying to do, Gentner and Forbus generously offered to allow us to use their Structure Mapping Engine (Forbus, Gentner, & Law, 1995) to store our analogies and plan the responses when the student fails to understand the analogy or to make appropriate inferences from it. This process typically involves making the structure mapping explicit as in Example 7.10.

Lulis and Michael have drawn up a list of the analogies that the experts would like the system to propose. Lulis has developed APE operators to express our schemas for the reflective analogies involving another neural variable or another procedure. She is now working on a formalism for the other bases (Lulis, Michael, & Evens, 2004c). The next step is to formulate instructional plans and discourse plans to implement these analogies.

20.3.5 Providing Encouragement As Needed

Bozena Thompson (1980) did the first analysis of pathic expressions in human–computer dialogues. Thompson's emphasis was on deleting this input to avoid parsing problems and most other research has focused on this same approach. But there is a new movement to try to understand what is troubling the student in these circumstances and to provide more direct help. The ITS community held its first session on dealing with affective input at ITS 2002. At that session, Vicente and Pain (2002) discussed some of the modeling issues, and Aist, Kort, Reilly, Mostow, and Picard (2002) offered evidence of the value of emotional scaffolding. Two sessions on targeting student affect were scheduled for ITS 2004.

We have done a preliminary study (Bhatt, 2004) of affective expressions in human tutoring sessions, again using the 25 human keyboard sessions from November, 1999. The majority of students, but not all of them, generate expressions of affect—where we are classifying as affective any input that does not discuss the problem-solving issues or the physiology of the baroreceptor reflex. When we look for expressions of affect in the machine tutoring log files, we find less affect (20 examples in 66 log files from the fall of 2002) and affect of a much more negative kind. The system has drawn a number of affective expressions of anger ("kiss my ass"), and frustration ("abcd," "asdf"") over the past few years.

The current version of CIRCSIM-Tutor, Version 2.9, responds to pathic expressions or inputs that consist of a question mark, as to other inputs that it cannot parse, by telling the student what kind of input it is expecting. The result is snippets of dialogue where the student says "Clueless," or "You stupid computer," or "kiss my ass," and the system answers, "Please respond with prediction table parameters." If the student still fails to produce an appropriate answer after two such messages, then the system gives the answer and goes on to the next topic. This approach is often successful in getting the student back on track, but it gives a rather unfriendly impression. We would like to try to understand and respond to some of these pathic inputs, and see whether this gives the system a better image—we would keep the old algorithm handy for those inputs we cannot recognize. (People are always inventing new obscenities.) Because our experts do not see inputs like this, we have no examples of good responses, and so we are somewhat confused about what kind of answer would be most helpful.

20.3.6 Improving the Reasoning Powers of CIRCSIM-Tutor

Human tutors definitely draw more inferences and better ones than CIRCSIM-Tutor. They use their reasoning powers especially often in the student modeling process, figuring out whether an error derives from a slip, a missing piece of information, or a real misconception. To consider a simple example, if a student predicts wrongly that the variable TPR will change in the DR period, it could be a slip, it could be that the student does not know that TPR is a neural variable or that neural variables do not change in DR, or the student could be confused about the meaning of DR (Hume, Michael, Rovick, & Evens, 1995; Webber, 2004). McRoy and Hirst (1995) used abductive inference to repair speech act misunderstandings. Jordan, Makatchev, and VanLehn (2003, 2004) use Tacitus-Lite in detecting contradictions in student essays. Freedman has outlined a number of ways to use inference processes (Freedman & Evens, 1997).

20.3.7 Combining Natural Language Techniques With Diagrams

During some of our initial meetings, Rovick and Michael drew us a concept map to explain the approach to causal reasoning that they want their students to internalize and to describe the relationships between specific variables (see Chapters 2 and 5). Such concept maps are now included in the syllabus of the physiology course at Rush Medical College, partly because we found them so helpful. During the last few years, we have built a Concept Map Tutorial System (Jeong, Evens, & Kim, 1998; Y. C. Kim, Evens, Michael, & Trace, 2002) and used it at Rush Medical College and with other students as described in the next section. We would like to discover the effects of using concept maps in combination with CIRCSIM-Tutor.

Rovick and Michael also draw diagrams of certain functional relationships after the keyboard-to-keyboard session is over, especially if the student seems particularly confused about some particular relationship. We would like to study the effect of displaying such drawings in CIRCSIM-Tutor.

20.3.8 Finding New Targets for CIRCSIM-Tutor

CIRCSIM, GASP, and ABASE, the three Prediction Table based computer-aided instruction programs written by Michael and Rovick, were designed for use by first-year medical students. CIRCSIM-Tutor was aimed at this same audience. We are now trying to discover whether there are other students who would benefit from using the system. The most obvious target is other medical schools. Michael and Rovick have sold many copies of their computer-aided instruction programs CIRCSIM, GASP, and ABASE to medical schools around the world. At this point, the Indiana University School of Medicine and the University of Vermont College of Medicine have copies of CIRCSIM-Tutor.

Another possible target is students in other professional schools, such as colleges of dentistry or veterinary medicine. Many undergraduate programs offer courses in physiology as well, and many have purchased copies of CIRCSIM; we are starting to talk to faculty at such schools in the Chicago area about trying CIRCSIM-Tutor.

We wonder how much background it really takes to learn something useful from CIRCSIM-Tutor. In pursuit of this question, we did an informal experiment with a group of high school girls in a summer program at Illinois Institute of Technology, called Women In Science and Technology (WISE). We gave them 15 min to play with the CIRCSIM Concept-Mapper and use it to build the top-level concept map that underlies CIRCSIM-Tutor. Then we turned them loose on the program. They were able to understand the questions and even answer some of them. Working in pairs, most of them completed one problem. Several went on to solve multiple problems. This group included a number of girls who are considering careers in biology and medicine. It is not at all clear whether this success reflects the improved self-explanatory abilities of CIRCSIM-Tutor or the power of the concept-mapping tool.

20.4 BUILDING MORE LANGUAGE-BASED TUTORS

Finally, we discuss our initial work on GASP-Tutor, an ITS for teaching students about the physiological control of respiration and the two interrelated negative feedback systems that control breathing. Then we briefly mention some of the other types of language-based ITSs that we would like to implement ourselves or that we hope to see implemented, tutors in mathematics, science, electronics, and second-language learning.

When we established that CIRCSIM-Tutor was an effective learning tool in our experiments in 1998 and 1999, we started to think about appropriate ways to generalize the system. Several years ago, Rovick and Michael wrote a computer-aided instruction program called GASP (Rovick & Michael, 1989, 1995), designed to help students master the two interacting negative feedback systems that control respiration in the human body. GASP, like CIRCSIM, presents a problem to the student and then asks for predictions about behavior of important physiological variables. A GASP-Tutor seems like the most feasible next step in our research.

Michael and Rovick carried out four human tutoring sessions in January 2000 so that we could collect some language samples. We proceeded to make vocabulary counts and a KeyWord in Context index in order to study the sublanguage. We were surprised to discover that there were only 139 words in the four dialogues (and 75 more in the text files that are part of GASP) that did not already appear somewhere in the human tutoring dialogues in the CIRCSIM domain. By contrast, when we added 25 new hour-long sessions to the 50 already obtained human tutoring sessions used as the basis for CIRCSIM-Tutor, we added over 600 new words.

Larger scale dialogue structures and tutoring strategies in the four GASP tutoring sessions seem to very closely resemble those already found in the CIRCSIM-Tutor domain. We have carried out some detailed semantic analyses and find that we can represent the dialogue with only half a dozen new logic forms to handle the discussions of the relevant chemistry, plus two for breathing (one for inspiration and one for expiration). Chung Hee Lee has developed methods for handling the problems of building an ontology and case frames automatically from the examples of language use in the four GASP sessions and the GASP program text (Lee & Evens, 2003; Lee, Seu, & Evens, 2002a, 2002b).

This analysis has led us to two conclusions. First, it may not be as difficult to build a GASP tutor as we feared. That said, it is important to note that the physiology content to be dealt with in a GASP tutor includes a significant number of chemistry concepts that will have to be tutored, something not present in CIRCSIM-Tutor. It also appears to be feasible to extend the tutor to work in domains like physics and electronics that require the same kind of causal reasoning. Second, it may be that the sublanguage that we have captured in our studies and implemented in our tutor should be labeled the language of qualitative, causal reasoning and not the language of cardiovascular physiology.

There are several other places in a standard course in Medical Physiology where students have similar difficulties in solving problems, especially those involving negative feedback systems. Two areas of need are the endocrine system and acid-base balance. Our ideas should generalize easily to these areas.

Solving problems in basic electronics, elementary physics, and the trouble-shooting of control systems involves the same kind of causal reasoning. This has made it possible for us to learn a great deal from the work of Kieras (1985), Fox (1993b), Cawsey (1992), Lesgold (1992; Lesgold, Lajoie, Bunzo, & Eggan, 1992), as well as from the work of the Circle project at Pittsburgh, led by VanLehn; the AutoTutor project at Memphis, led by Graesser; and the new work at Edinburgh, led by Moore and Pain.

There has been very little interaction between ITS researchers and the people who are building tutoring systems for Computer-Assisted Language Learning or CALL Tutors (Hamburger & Tecuci, 1998). Perhaps the new research at University of Southern California Information Science Institute (Johnson et al., 2004) is a signal that this wall is disappearing. We suspect that both sides have a lot to learn from the other. In particular, CIRCSIM-Tutor is too shy about explicit teaching of language, something that CALL tutors do all the time, as do Michael and Rovick.

21

What Have We Learned?

21.0 INTRODUCTION

We want to close with a summary of what we have learned over the many years of the CIRCSIM-Tutor project. First, we address the ideas we have developed about how to build an intelligent tutoring system. Then we describe some of the lessons that we have learned about tutoring and about intelligent tutoring systems. We hope that these ideas will contribute to the advancement of the research agenda of the ITS community.

21.1 HOW TO BUILD AN INTELLIGENT TUTORING SYSTEM

In this section, we look back at what we have done and how, and try to identify the factors that have contributed to our success in fielding a system that can sustain a tutorial dialogue.

21.1.1 Assemble a Team of Experts in Content, Tutoring, and Natural Language Processing

We succeeded in building an intelligent tutoring system that can carry on a natural language dialogue with the student largely because we were able to assemble a team of experts in the content of the domain (cardiovascular physiology), in tutoring in this domain, and in computers and natural language processing. Equally important, we evolved a way of working together effectively. Allen Rovick and Joel Michael were professors of physiology. They were content experts (on the baroreceptor reflex of the cardiovascular system). They were also experienced and expert tutors in this domain. Before we started, they had already spent years developing successful computer-aided instruction systems for their own courses and integrating them into student laboratories. Martha Evens is a professor of computer science and a former president of the Association for Computational Linguistics. She has spent years developing natural language applications in a variety of fields, including medicine.

The students at Illinois Institute of Technology who contributed to the research and who built the system were also heavily involved in teaching computer science. All but two or three are now teaching full time in a university. Many of them are also working on ITS research and development.

Another important factor in our success, we feel, is that we planned for and organized regular occasions for these different people to talk to each other, sometimes one-on-one, sometimes in a group. In particular, Michael and Rovick welcomed the computer scientists to Rush Medical College and spent a lot of time teaching them physiology—in the process providing us with a useful illustration of their teaching methods.

21.1.2 Recognize the Difference Between Tutoring and Teaching

The process of tutoring is quite different from the process of teaching. Often people who are excellent teachers, who are skilled at designing a curriculum, who recognize student misconceptions and give brilliant explanations, do not function effectively as tutors. Tutoring is a learnable skill, however, and we hope that this book will help others to acquire this skill.

Michael and Rovick really believe in Simon's (2001, p. 210) principle that "learning takes place inside the learner and only inside the learn," and, watching them tutor, the rest of us came to believe in it too. They do not solve the problem, they make sure that the student solves the problem. They do not lecture, they ask questions. They do not tell the student things, they get the student to tell them. If the student cannot answer the questions, they ask easier questions; they provide scaffolding. They sometimes provide half the answer, but they make sure that the student comes up with the other half. They push the student into activity in every conceivable way. In the process, they sometimes become contentious. They hint all the time; they keep the focus on the problem, and they generally brush off student attempts at small talk. They embrace the fact that good educational dialogue follows different precepts from ordinary conversation. They give up the chance to display their expertise and wit and charm in favor of eliciting some grain of truth from the student.

21.1.3 Find Students to Use the System As Early and Often As Possible

We became convinced as we started to work on this project that several excellent computer systems under development at the time suffered from lack of experience with real students—especially Dan Russell's IDE System (Russell, Moran, & Jordan, 1988) and Wilensky's Unix Consultant (Wilensky et al., 1988). We made a point of using our system with students as early and often as possible. Beginning in December 1991, we were able to field a working system and collect student comments. Even when we met with only one or two or three students at a time, we found that observing their experiences with the system was extremely informative, and their comments extremely useful—almost as useful as their errors and complaints.

These observations seem obvious, but their importance is great. It is almost impossible for the developers of an ITS to critique their product from the perspective of the ultimate users, the student audience that is being targeted for the application. Only with constant feedback from students can developers avoid some of the serious errors and shortcomings that have too often characterized software designed for the classroom.

21.1.4 Find Students Who Are Motivated to Learn What Your System Is Trying to Teach

Both the first-year medical students who were our original targets and the second-year students who have occasionally used the system to study for their licensing examinations have been extremely helpful. Medical students make wonderful experimental subjects because they are willing to work on anything that they believe will help them learn. Although we advertised our experiments as chances to "earn while you learn," it was clear that the opportunity to learn more about a subject that they believed to be important was a much stronger motivator than the modest monetary stipend that they earned. They worked hard at solving the CIRCSIM problem presented to them in tutoring sessions. Later, they worked hard to learn as much as possible from CIRCSIM-Tutor, and in the process, they worked the system hard as well. They spent a lot of time and thought on testing the system. If there was an error, they found it and told us about it. When they finished using CIRCSIM-Tutor, they took the time to make a lot of creative suggestions.

It would be hard to overestimate the importance of doing educational research with students who are highly motivated to learn, because that learning matters to them. Certainly, in the absence of such motivation, it may be very difficult to know how to interpret any results obtained.

21.1.5 Use the System in the Classroom

It is extremely helpful to take the system into the classroom and use it there as a regular part of a course. It is, of course, first necessary to demonstrate that the system is a valuable learning tool with small numbers of students in controlled experiments. But once the system has been validated, large numbers of students can use it and large controlled experiments can be performed.

This kind of usage provides a better test of the software and makes it easier to obtain statistically relevant results. In a classroom setting, the system is used repeatedly by a large number of students and any errors and interface problems rapidly become obvious. Our system is now available in an open laboratory at Rush Medical College so that students can use it whenever they please. This kind of usage uncovered several points where the system is not as self-explanatory as it appeared when groups of students were using it in a laboratory, able to prompt each other if someone got stuck.

21.1.6 Be Clear About Your Goals

Our ultimate goal was to produce a conversational resource that could be used by students to learn to solve problems about the baroreceptor reflex. We wanted to produce a program usable and useful in the classroom. We determined that the best approach was to learn how expert human tutors help students learn this material. Then we set out to simulate what our expert human tutors did.

We realized, however, that our final goal was not to simulate an expert tutor, it was to produce an effective learning resource within the bounds of natural language dialogue. We avoided using GUI and diagrams although we have used them in other systems and we believe that they can be effective. But to provide a working system with immediate and effective dialogue, we occasionally chose to abandon the human model. CIRCSIM-Tutor makes use of some of the strengths of the computer (the Student Modeler has a much better memory for past student responses than our human tutors have), while not attempting to incorporate everything that we know human tutors do. (CIRCSIM-Tutor cannot interpret student answers to truly open-ended questions.) We built a system to be an effective learning resource, as well as to test our theories about how human tutors function.

21.1.7 Go Public Early and Often

From the very beginning of the CIRCSIM-Tutor project, we have taken our ideas, and eventually our accomplishments, to every public forum available to us and our colleagues have responded generously with suggestions for how to do better. Michael and Rovick discussed the project with their colleagues in the computer-aided instruction and physiology education communities. Evens talked about our ideas for the implementation of CIRCSIM-Tutor with computer science and natural language program colleagues. As soon as we had enough work accomplished, we presented and published that work. When we started receiving funding from the Office of Naval Research, the grantees' workshops organized by Dr. Susan Chipman, Director of the Cognitive Science Program, proved to be invaluable sources of feedback and stimulation. Without this feedback, without the comments, suggestions, and criticisms of our colleagues, we would not have accomplished what we did.

21.2 LESSONS LEARNED ALONG THE WAY

21.2.1 Language Is the Tool That Makes Tutoring Work

When a human tutor and a student work together, a conversation ensues. This dialogue serves several important functions. For the tutor, the dialogue offers important clues about the knowledge state of the student, what the student knows and what the student still needs to learn, what the student can do and cannot do, what misconceptions are present that interfere with learning. In other words, it is through the dialogue that the tutor builds a model of the student that will be used in determining what the tutor will do next.

For the student, contributing to the dialogue requires practicing the language of the domain under discussion. Sustaining half of the dialogue requires the student to articulate an understanding of the domain in a way that successfully communicates ideas to someone else. The need to respond to questions, and to offer explanations, is a powerful aid to building a useful and correct mental model of the phenomena under discussion.

It should be noted that the power of language is not limited to human one-on-one tutoring. We and others have shown that intelligent tutoring systems that support natural language dialogue can be a very effective learning resource. This claim in no way disparages the large number of non-language-based ITSs that succeed at engaging students in ways that lead to learning.

21.2.2 Tutoring Works When the Student Is Encouraged to Do the Intellectual Work

Learning is done by the learner. A teacher, or a tutor, can, of course, help the learner in the learning process, but it is the learner who carries out the actual work of learning. The job of the tutor, then, is to create a context in which this work is explicitly the responsibility of the student. The tutor can deliver the information needed by the student to build a correct mental model, but it is the learner who must build the model.

One powerful tool with which the tutor keeps the student actively engaged in this work is hinting. By reminding students of things they should know without revealing the answer to the current question or piece of the problem, hints help students put the pieces together to arrive at an answer. Although hints are not always successful, they always force the student into engagement with the process of solving the problem.

The ability to keep the learner actively engaged in the process of learning undoubtedly accounts for the ability of a diverse array of computer-based learning resources (tutorials, simulations, intelligent tutoring systems) to promote learning.

21.2.3 Tutors Use a Lot of Many Different Kinds of Knowledge

Tutors (whether human or silicon-based) need to have a breadth and depth of domain knowledge that is adequate for the task at hand, and the amount of knowledge needed to help a student solve a problem is generally greater than the amount of knowledge needed to simply solve the problem. But tutors also need to know how to most effectively help the student learn what he or she needs to learn. This knowledge, pedagogical content knowledge, starts with an understanding of the domain but adds to it an understanding of what aspects of the domain are difficult for students and how to help them overcome these difficulties. Finally, all tutors need to understand some basic pedagogy, such as how to motivate students and keep them interested in the task at hand.

21.2.4 Tutors Do a Great Deal of Planning

Tutoring is fundamentally a process of planning on the fly. Tutoring starts with some kind of agenda and some starting point, whether provided by the student ("Dr. Michael, I don't understand why mean arterial pressure falls if ...") or by the tutor ("Can you tell me why mean arterial pressure falls if ..."). What happens next, what the tutor does, always depends in part on what the student does. In either case, the plans that the tutor develops must include choices about what to say, how to say it, what question or problem to pose next, when and how to hint, what analogies to offer by way of explanation, and so forth. These plans are the product of the tutor's own understanding of the domain, tutoring experience (pedagogical content knowledge), and the student's responses.

It is important to recognize that even experienced tutors find it difficult to explain (articulate) what they do and how they plan. This observation should not suggest that what tutors do is "unconscious" or that tutoring is an "art form" not subject to analysis. Neither conclusion is correct. It does mean, however, that to understand what the tutor does and how it is done requires a great deal of probing.

If you are building an intelligent tutoring system, or are intending to do so, you must keep in mind the need for multiple layers of modeling and planning and also figure out ways of extracting these plans and models from expert human tutors in your domain.

21.2.5 Expert Tutoring Is a Highly Complex Skill That Employs a Great Many Different Tactics

Experienced tutors have available to them a great many tactics that can be used to help the learner. One of the major planning tasks is to determine which element in this repertoire to use at which particular point in the dialogue. Some of these tactics are generic in the sense that they can be used in tutoring in any domain, some are specific to domains in which qualitative causal reasoning is a major feature, whereas still others may be specific to the particular domain being tutored.

21.2.6 Studying Tutors at Work Is Essential

There is no substitute for watching tutors and students during the process and asking them lots of questions. Then you go home and read the transcripts, make more hypotheses, and ask more questions. For substantiating hypotheses or sometimes disproving them, there seems to be no substitute for marking up transcripts.

Electronic markup of those transcripts, preferably with a markup tool, has a multitude of advantages. It makes it easier to find markup errors and correct them. It makes it easier to count the results and to compare markup done by different raters. It makes it easier to store, retrieve, and combine different kinds of markup. Most important, it turns your transcripts into data for machine learning programs.

21.2.7 Implications for the Implementation Process

Tutoring is, among other things, a very complicated dynamic planning process at many levels, so start with a planner or dialogue manager like APE or Longbow that provides dynamic, hierarchical, reactive, opportunistic planning capabilities.

Student modeling is an essential ingredient; expect that you will constantly discover more things to model and make it flexible.

Tutoring is a very knowledge-intensive process. Look for good tools for modeling and storing knowledge and make that knowledge accessible to every part of your system.

Learn everything you can about dialogue, because language understanding and generation in dialogue are different from monologues, from essays and textbooks. This is why foreign students that arrive reading and writing good English still have to learn to converse. Your system needs to converse.

Building an Intelligent Tutoring System is still a major enterprise, so think hard about the software engineering process, write system design documents, and agree on documentation and coding standards before you begin. Make everything modular so that it is easy to replace a piece that does not work.

21.3 SUMMING UP

Dialogue fosters learning (which is why Plato's *Dialogues* are still in print). Students remember dialogues better than monologues. Learning from tutorial dialogue is the best and fastest way to learn to solve problems (more effective than reading text even for intelligent and motivated students). Students learn from putting things into words. Understanding what they say and commenting intelligently is the only way to keep them talking—and comments that make them think about relevant issues help them learn faster. For all of these reasons, intelligent tutoring systems (or some of them, at least) should converse with their students. Even if our systems cannot handle natural language as well as expert tutors do, they are still good enough to promote learning (more learning than students can derive from textbooks).

Expert tutors push their students to think with hints, they challenge them with contradictions. They constantly try to figure out what the students know and what they are missing. They probe for misconceptions. They figure out what piece of the puzzle their students need next and push them in the right direction. They use this model in scaffolding, to produce a world where the student can succeed. They provide harder problems and fewer hints when students do well; they provide easier problems and more support when students do poorly.

Implementing a system is full of excitement. When the system says the wrong thing, you learn more about language. When the system does work, but the student does not learn anything new, you learn more about tutoring. When it works and the student does learn, everybody celebrates, and it is time to build a new system.

References

Abbas, H., & Evens, M. (2000). Domain knowledge base for an intelligent tutoring system: CIRCSIM-Tutor. In S. Y. Shin (Ed.), *Proceedings of the International Conference on Computers and Their Applications* (pp. 338–343). New Orleans, LA.

Aist, G., Kort, B., Reilly, R., Mostow, J., & Picard, R. (2002, June). Experimentally augmenting an intelligent tutoring system with human-supplied capabilities: Adding human-provided emotional scaffolding to an automated reading tutor that listens. In P. C. Yuen, Y. Y. Tong, & P. S. P. Wang (Eds.), *International Conference on Multimodal Interfaces* (pp. 483–490). Los Alamilos, CA: IEEE Computer Society.

Aleven, V. (2003). Using background knowledge in case-based legal reasoning: A computational model and an intelligent learning environment. *Artificial Intelligence, 150,* 183–237.

Aleven, V., & Ashley, K. (1997a). Teaching case-based argumentation through a model and examples: Empirical evaluation of an intelligent learning environment. In B. du Boulay & R. Mizoguchi (Eds.), *Proceedings of the Eighth World Conference of the Artificial Intelligence in Education Society*. (pp. 87–94). IOS Press: Amsterdam.

Aleven, V., & Ashley, K. (1997b). Evaluating a learning environment for case-based argumentation skills. In L. K. Branting (Ed.), *Proceedings of the Sixth International Conference on Artificial Intelligence and Law, ICAIL-97* (pp. 170–179). New York: Association for Computing Machinery.

Aleven, V., & Koedinger, K. (2000a). Limitations of student control: Do students know when they need help? In G. Gauthier, C. Frasson, & K. VanLehn (Eds.), *Proceedings of ITS 2000* (pp. 292–303). Berlin, Germany: Springer.

Aleven, V., & Koedinger, K. (2000b). The need for natural language dialogue to support explanation. In C.P. Rosé & R. Freedman (Eds.), *Proceedings of the AAAI Fall Symposium on Building Dialogue Systems for Tutorial Applications* (pp. 65–73). Menlo Park, CA: AAAI Press.

Aleven, V., Koedinger, K., & Cross, K. (1999). Tutoring answer explanation fosters learning with understanding. In S. P. Lajoie & M. Vivet (Eds.), *Proceedings of AI-ED '99* (pp. 199–206). Amsterdam: IOS Press.

Aleven, V., Koedinger, K., & Popescu, O. (2003). A tutorial dialogue system to support self-explanation: Evaluation and open questions. In U. Hoppe, F. Verdejo, & J. Kay (Eds.), *Proceedings of Artificial Intelligence in Education* (pp. 39–46). Amsterdam: IOS Press.

Aleven, V., Ogan, A., Popescu, O., Torrey, C., & Koedinger, K. (2004). Evaluating the effectiveness of a tutorial dialogue system for self-explanation. In J. C. Lester, R. M. Vicari, & F. Paraguaçu (Eds.), *ITS 2004* (pp. 443–454). Berlin, Germany: Springer-Verlag.

Aleven, V., Popescu, O., & Koedinger, K. (2001). Towards tutorial dialogue to support self- explanation: Adding natural language understanding to a cognitive tutor. In J. D. Moore, C. L. Redfield, & W. L. Johnson (Eds.), *Proceedings of Artificial Intelligence in Education* (pp. 246–255). Amsterdam: IOS Press.

Aleven, V., & Rosé, C. P. (2004). Towards easier creation of tutorial dialogue systems: Integration of authoring environments for tutoring and dialogue systems. In N. Heffernan & P. Wiemer-Hastings (Eds), *Proceedings of the Workshop on Dialog-Based Intelligent Tutoring Systems, ITS 2004* (pp. 1–7). Berlin, Germany: Springer.

Allen, J. (1987). *Natural language understanding.* Menlo Park, CA: Benjamin/Cummings.

Allen, J., & Core, M. (1997). *Draft of DAMSL (Dialog Markup in Several Layers)* (Report of the Multiparty Discourse Group at the DRI Meeting at Schloss Dagstuhl). Retrieved April 14, 1998, from www.cs.rochester.edu/research/csid/resources/damsl/

Anderson, J. R., Conrad, F. G., & Corbett, A. T. (1989). Skill acquisition and the lisp tutor. *Cognitive Science, 13,* 467–505.

Anderson, J. R., Corbett, A. T., Koedinger, K., & Pelletier, R. (1995). Cognitive tutors, lessons learned. *Journal of the Learning Sciences, 4,* 167–207.

Anderson, J. R., & Reiser, B. J. (1985). The lisp tutor. *Byte,* 159–175.

Appelt, D. E. (1985). *Planning English referring expressions.* Cambridge, England: Cambridge University Press.

Ashley, K., Desai, R., & Levine, J. M. (2002). Teaching case-based argumentation concepts using dialectic arguments vs. didactic explanations. In S. Cem, G. Gouardères, & F. Paraguaçu (Eds.), *Proceedings of Intelligent Tutoring Systems 2002* (pp. 585–595). Berlin, Germany: Springer-Verlag.

Bangerter, A., & Clark, H. H. (2003). Navigating joint projects with dialogue. *Cognitive Science, 27,* 195–225.

Bangerter, A., Clark, H. H., & Katz, A. R. (2004). Navigating joint projects in telephone conversations. *Discourse Processes, 37,* 1–23.

Barfield, L. (1993). *The user interface: Concept and design.* Reading, MA: Addison-Wesley.

Barnard, D., Burnard, L., Gaspart, J., Price, L., & Sperberg-McQueen, C. M. (1995). Hierarchical encoding of text: Technical problems and SGML solutions. *Computers and the Humanities, 29,* 211–231.

Barr, A., & Feigenbaum, E. A. (1982). *The handbook of artificial intelligence. Vol. II.* Los Altos, CA: Kaufmann.

Barrett, A., & Weld, D. (1994). Partial order planning: Evaluating possible efficiency gains. *Artificial Intelligence, 67,* 71–112.

Bateman, J. A., & Rondhuis, K. J. (1997). Coherence relations: Toward a general specification. *Discourse Processes, 24,* 23–50.

Becker, L. (2000). *Post-hoc statistical procedures: Analyses of covariance*. Syllabus, Psychology 590, University of Colorado, Boulder, CO. http://web.uccs.edu/becker/Psy590/ancova2.htm#Possible%20Outcomes%20in%20ANCOVA

Berliner, D. C. (1986). In pursuit of the expert pedagogue. *Educational Researcher, 15*(7), 5–13.

Berliner, D. C. (2002). Educational research: The hardest science of them all. *Educational Researcher, 31*(8), 18–20.

Berne, R. M., & Levy, M. N. (Eds.). (1998). *Physiology* (4th ed.) . St. Louis, MO: Mosby.

Bhatt, K. S. (2004). *Classifying student hedges and affect in human tutoring sessions for the CIRCSIM-Tutor intelligent tutoring system.* Unpublished master's thesis, Illinois Institute of Technology, Chicago.

Bhatt, K. S., Evens, M. W., & Argamon, S. (2004). Hedged responses and expressions of affect in human/human and human/computer tutorial interactions. In K. Forbus, D. Gentner, & T. Regier (Eds.), *Proceedings of the Cognitive Science Society 2004* (pp. 114–119). Mahwah, NJ: Lawrence Erlbaum Associates.

Bloom, B. S. (1984). The 2 sigma problem: The search for methods of group instruction as effective as one-to-one tutoring. *Educational Researcher, 13*(6), 4–16.

Bovair, S., & Kieras, D. E. (1985). A guide to propositional analysis for research on technical prose. In B. K. Britton & J. B. Black (Eds.), *Understanding expository text* (pp. 315–361). Hillsdale, NJ: Lawrence Erlbaum Associates.

Brandle, S. S. (1998). *Using joint actions to explain acknowledgments in tutorial discourse: Application to intelligent tutoring systems.* Unpublished doctoral dissertation, Illinois Institute of Technology, Chicago.

Bransford, J. D., Brown, A. L., & Cocking, R. R. (Eds.). (1999). *How people learn: Brain, mind, experience, and school*. Washington, DC: National Academy Press.

Bratt, E. O., Clark, B., Thomsen-Gray, Z., Peters, S., Treeratpituk, P., Pon-Barry, H., et al. (2002). Model-based reasoning for tutorial dialogue in shipboard damage control. In S. Cerri, G. Gouardères, & F. Paraguaçu (Eds.), *Proceedings of ITS 2002* (pp. 63–69). Berlin, Germany: Springer-Verlag.

Brecht, B., McCalla, G., Greer, J., & Jones, M. (1989). Planning the content of instruction. In D. Biermann, J. Breuker, & J. Sandberg (Eds.), *Proceedings of the 4th International Conference on AI and Education* (pp. 32–41). Amsterdam: IOS Press.

Brennan, S. E., & Clark, H. H. (1996). Conceptual pacts and lexical choice in conversation. *The Journal of Experimental Psychology: Learning, Memory, and Cognition, 22,* 1482–1493.

Bresnan, J. (1982). *The mental representation of grammatical relations.* Cambridge, MA: MIT Press.

Breuker, J. A. (Ed.). (1990). *EUROHELP: Developing intelligent help systems.* Copenhagen, Denmark: European Community.

Brown, J. S., & Burton, R. R. (1978). Diagnostic models for procedural bugs in basic mathematical skills. *Cognitive Science 2,* 155–192.

Brown, J. S., Burton, R. R., & deKleer, J. (1982). Pedagogical, natural language, and knowledge engineering techniques in SOPHIE I, II, and III. In D. H. Sleeman. & J. S. Brown (Eds.), *Intelligent tutoring systems* (pp. 227–282). New York: Academic.

Brown, J. S., & VanLehn, K. (1980). Repair theory: A generative theory of bugs in procedural skills. *Cognitive Science, 4,* 379–426.

Brown, P., & Levinson, S. (1987). *Politeness: Universals in language usage.* Cambridge, England: Cambridge University Press.

Bulitko, V. V., & Wilkins, D. C. (1999), Automated instructor assistant for ship damage control. *Proceedings of the Eleventh Conference on Innovative Applications of Artificial Intelligence, IAAI-99* (pp. 778–785). Menlo Park, CA: AAAI Press.

Burton, R. R. (1982). DEBUGGY: Diagnosis of errors in basic mathematical skills. In D. H. Sleeman & J. S. Brown (Eds.), *Intelligent tutoring systems* (pp. 157–183). New York: Academic.

Burton, R. R., & Brown, J. S. (1979). Toward a natural language capability for computer-assisted instruction. In H. O'Neill (Ed.), *Procedures for instructional systems development* (pp. 272–313). New York: Academic. Reprinted in B. Grosz, (Ed.), 1986, *Readings in natural language understanding* (pp. 605–625). Palo Alto, CA: Kaufmann.

Burton, R. R., & Brown, J. S. (1982). An investigation of computer coaching for information learning activities. In D. H. Sleeman & J. S. Brown (Eds.), *Intelligent tutoring systems* (pp. 79–98), New York: Academic.

Caramaza, A., McCloskey, M., & Green, B. (1981). Naive beliefs in "sophisticated" subjects: Misconceptions about trajectories of objects. *Cognition, 9,* 117–123.

Carberry, S. (1989). A pragmatics-based approach to ellipsis resolution. *Computational Linguistics, 15,* 75–96.

Carberry, S. (1990). Incorporating default inferences into plan recognition. In *Proceedings of the Eighth National Conference on Artificial Intelligence* (pp. 471–478). Menlo Park, CA: AAAI Press.

Carberry, S. (1991). *Plan recognition in natural language dialogue.* Cambridge, MA: MIT Press.

Carbonell, J. G., & Hayes, P. J. (1983). Recovery strategies for parsing extragrammatical language. *American Journal of Computational Linguistics, 9,* 123–146.

Carbonell, J. R. (1970). AI in CAI: An artificial intelligence approach to computer-aided instruction. *IEEE Transactions on Man–Machine Systems, 11,* 190–202.

Cawsey, A. (1992). *Explanation and interaction: The computer generation of explanatory dialogues.* Cambridge, MA: MIT Press.

Cawsey, A. (1993). Planning interactive explanations. *International Journal of Man–Machine Studies, 38,* 169–200.

Chang, R. C. (1992). *Surface level generation of tutorial dialogue using a specially developed lexical functional grammar and lexicon.* Unpublished doctoral dissertation, Illinois Institute of Technology, Chicago.

Chang, R. C., Evens, M. W., Michael, J. A., & Rovick, A. A. (1994). Surface generation in tutorial dialogues based on a sublanguage study. In Y. F. Chang (Ed.), *International Conference on Advanced Science and Technology* (pp. 113–119). Chicago: CAPAMA.

Chen, H. (1999). *Using an object-oriented methodology to build a graphical user interface for a medical tutoring system.* Unpublished doctoral dissertation, Illinois Institute of Technology, Chicago.

Chi, M. T. H., Bassok, M., Lewis, M. W., Reimann, P., & Glaser, R. (1989). Self-explanation: How students study and use examples in learning to solve problems. *Cognitive Science, 13,* 145–182.

Chi, M.T. H., de Leeuw, N., Chiu, M. H., & LaVancher, C. (1994). Eliciting self-explanations improves understanding. *Cognitive Science, 18,* 439–477.

Chi, M. T. H., & Roscoe, R. (2002). The processes and challenges of conceptual change. In M. Limon & L. Mason (Eds.), *Reconsidering conceptual change: Issues in theory and practice* (pp. 3–27). Dordrecht, The Netherlands: Kluwer.

Chi, M. T. H., Siler, S. A., Jeong, H., Yamauchi, T., & Hausmann, R. G. (2001). Learning from human tutoring. *Cognitive Science, 25,* 471–533.

Chi, M. T. H., Siler, S., & Jeong, H. (2004). Can tutors monitor students' understanding accurately? *Cognition and Instruction, 22,* 363–387.

Chin, D. N. (1984). Analysis of scripts between users and consultants. In D. J. Frailey (Ed.), *Proceedings of the National Computer Conference* (pp. 638–642). Reston, VA: AFIPS Press.

Cho, B. I. (2000). *Dynamic planning models to support curriculum planning and multiple tutoring protocols in intelligent tutoring systems.* Unpublished doctoral dissertation, Illinois Institute of Technology, Chicago.

Cho, B. I., Michael, J. A., Rovick, A. A., & Evens, M. W. (1999). A curriculum planning model for an intelligent tutoring system. In A. Kumar & J. Russell (Eds.), *Proceedings of the 12th Florida Artificial Intelligence Symposium (FLAIRS-99)* (pp. 197–201). Menlo Park, CA: AAAI Press.

Cho, B. I., Michael, J. A., Rovick, A. A., & Evens, M. W. (2000). An analysis of multiple tutoring protocols. In G. Gauthier, C. Frasson, & K. VanLehn (Eds.), *Proceedings of Intelligent Tutoring Systems 2000* (pp. 212–221). Berlin, Germany: Springer.

Chu-Carroll, J., & Brown, M. (1997). Tracking initiative in collaborative dialogue interactions. *Annual Meeting of the Association for Computational Linguistics* (pp. 262–270). East Stroudsburg, PA: Association for Computational Linguistics.

Clancey, W. J. (1982). Tutoring rules for guiding a case method dialogue. In D. Sleeman & J. S. Brown (Eds.), *Intelligent tutoring systems* (pp. 201–225). New York: Academic.

Clancey, W. J. (1987). *Knowledge-based tutoring: The GUIDON Program.* Cambridge, MA: MIT Press.

Clark, B. Z., Bratt, E., Schultz, K., Peters, S., & Evens, M. W. (2003). SCoT: A model of conversational and tutorial intelligence. In R. Alterman & D. Kirsh (Eds.), *Proceedings of the Cognitive Science Conference* (p. 1331). Mahwah, NJ: Lawrence Erlbaum Associates.

Clark, H. H. (1996). *Using language.* Cambridge, England: Cambridge University Press.

Clark, H. H., & Brennan, S. E. (1991). Grounding in communication. In L. B. Resnick, J. M. Levine, & S. D. Teasley (Eds.), *Perspectives on socially shared cognition* (pp. 127–149). Washington, DC: APA Books.

Clark, H. H., & Schaefer, E. F. (1989). Contributing to discourse. *Cognitive Science, 13,* 259–294.

Coe, R. (2000). *What is an "effect size"? A guide for users.* Retrieved November 17, 2004, from http://davidmlane.com/hyperstat/effect_size.html

Cohen, J. (1988). *Statistical power analysis for the behavioral sciences* (2nd ed.). Hillsdale, NJ: Lawrence Erlbaum Associates.

Cohen, P., Kulik, J., & Kulik, C. (1982). Educational outcomes of tutoring. *American Educational Research Journal, 19,* 237–248.

Collier, J., Evens, M. W., Hier, D., & Li, P.-Y. (1988). Generating case reports for a medical expert system. *International Journal of Expert Systems, 1,* 307–328.

Collins, A. M. (1977). Processes in acquiring knowledge. In R. C. Anderson, R. J. Spiro, & W. E. Montague (Eds.), *Schooling and the acquisition of knowledge* (pp. 339–363). Hillsdale, NJ: Lawrence Erlbaum Associates.

Collins, A. M., Brown, J. S., & Newman, S. E. (1989). Cognitive apprenticeship: Teaching the crafts of reading, writing, and mathematics. In L. B. Resnick (Ed.), *Knowing, learning, and instruction* (pp. 453–494). Hillsdale, NJ: Lawrence Erlbaum Associates.

Collins, A. M., & Quillian, M. R. (1972). How to make a language user. In E. Tulving & R. Donaldson (Eds.), *Organization and memory* (pp. 310–374). New York: Academic.

Collins, A. M., & Stevens, A. L. (1980). *Goals and strategies of interactive teachers* (Report No. 4345). Cambridge, MA: Bolt Beranek and Newman, Inc.

Collins, A. M., & Stevens, A. L. (1982). Goals and strategies of inquiry teachers. In R. Glaser (Ed.), *Advances in instructional psychology* (Vol. 2, pp. 65–119). Hillsdale, NJ: Lawrence Erlbaum Associates.

Collins, A. M., & Stevens, A. L. (1991). A cognitive theory of inquiry teaching. In P. Goodyear (Ed.), *Teaching knowledge and intelligent tutoring* (pp. 203–230). Norwood, NJ: Ablex.

Conati, C., Gertner, A., VanLehn, K., & Druzdzel, M. (1997). On-line student modeling for coached problem solving using Bayesian networks. In A. Jameson, C. Paris, & C. Tasso (Eds.), *Proceedings of UM-97, Sixth Interna-*

tional Conference on User Modeling (pp. 231–242). West Newton, MA: User Modeling Inc.

Conlon, S. P., Dardaine, J., D'Souza, A., Evens, M., Haynes, S., Kim, J. S., et al. (1994). The IIT lexical database: Dream and reality. (Current issues in computational linguistics: In honour of Don Walker). In A. Zampolli, N. Calzolari, & M. Palmer (Eds.), *Linguistica computazionale* (Vol. IX, pp. 201–225). Norwell, MA: Academic.

Conlon, S. P., & Evens, M. W. (1994a). A lexical database for nouns to support parsing, generation, and information retrieval. In S. Hockey & N. Ide (Eds.), *Research in humanities computing 3* (pp. 74–87). Oxford, England: Oxford University Press.

Conlon, S. P., & Evens, M. W. (1994b). An adverbial lexicon for natural language processing systems. *International Journal of Lexicography, 7,* 197–221.

Conlon, S. P., Evens, M. W., Ahlswede, T., & Strutz, R. (1993). Developing a large lexical database for information retrieval, parsing, and text generation systems. *Journal of Information Processing and Management, 29,* 415–431.

Corbett, A. T., & Anderson, J. R. (1992). The Lisp intelligent tutoring system: Research in skill acquisition. In J. Larkin, R. Chabay, & C. Scheftic (Eds.), *Computer assisted instruction and intelligent tutoring systems: Establishing communication and collaboration* (pp. 73–109). Hillsdale, NJ: Lawrence Erlbaum Associates.

Corbett, A. T., & Trask, H. (2000). Instructional interventions in computer-based tutoring: Differential impact on learning time and accuracy. *Proceedings of ACM CHI'2000 Conference on Human Factors in Computing Systems* (pp. 97–104). New York: ACM Press.

Core, M., Moore, J. D., & Zinn, C. (2000). Supporting constructive learning with a feedback planner. In C. P. Rosé & R. Freedman (Eds.), *Proceedings of the AAAI Fall Symposium on Building Dialogue Systems for Tutorial Applications* (pp. 1–9). Menlo Park, CA: AAAI Press.

Core, M., Moore, J. D., & Zinn, C. (2001). Initiative management for tutorial dialogue. *Proceedings of the NAACL Workshop on Adaptation in Dialogue Systems, ACL 2001* (pp. 9–16). East Stroudsburg, PA: Association for Computational Linguistics.

Core, M. G., & Moore, J. D. (2004). Robustness vs. fidelity in natural language understanding. Proceedings of the Workshop on Scalable Natural Language Understanding. *HLT-NAACL 2004* (pp. 1–8). Cambridge, MA: East Stroudsburg, PA: Association for Computational Linguistics.

Core, M. G., Moore, J. D., & Zinn, C. (2003). The role of initiative in tutorial dialogue. *Proceedings of the 10th Conference of the European Chapter of the ACL* (pp. 67–74). East Stroudsburg, PA: Association for Computational Linguistics.

Croteau, E. A., Heffernan, N. T., & Koedinger, K. (2004). Why are algebra word problems difficult? Using tutorial log files and the power law of learning to select the best fitting cognitive model. In J. C. Lester, R. M. Vicari, & F.

Paraguaçu (Eds.), *Proceedings of ITS 2004* (pp. 240–250). Berlin, Germany: Springer.

Dahlback, N., & Jonsson, A. (1989). Empirical studies of discourse representations for natural language interfaces. *Proceedings of the Fourth European ACL* (pp. 191–198). East Stroudsburg, PA: Association for Computational Linguistics.

Dale, R. (1992). *Generating referring expressions.* Cambridge, MA: MIT Press.

DAMSL. (1997). *DAMSL: Dialogue act markup in several layers*. Retrieved May 5, 1997, from http://www.georgetown.edu/luperfoy/Discourse-treebank/dri-home.html

Dardaine, J. (1992). Case frames for a lexical database. In M. Evens (Ed.), *Proceedings of the Third Midwest Artificial Intelligence and Cognitive Science Conference* (pp. 102–106). Carbondale, IL: Southern Illinois University.

De Jong, T., & van Joolingen, W. R. (1998). Scientific discovery learning with computer simulations of conceptual domains. *Review of Educational Research, 68,* 179–201.

Derry, S. J., Hawkes, L. W., & Ziegler, U. (1988). A plan-based opportunistic architecture for intelligent tutoring. In B. Goettl, H. Halff, C. Redfield, & V. J. Shute (Eds.), *Proceedings of Intelligent Tutoring Systems. ITS-88* (pp. 116–123). Berlin, Germany: Springer-Verlag.

Dickinson, C. J., Goldsmith, C. H., & Sackett, D. L. (1973). MACMAN: A digital computer model for teaching some basic principles of hemodynamics. *Journal of Clinical Computing, 2,* 42–50.

Di Eugenio, B. (2000). On the usage of Kappa to evaluate agreement on coding tasks. In M. Garrilidou (Ed.), *Proceedings of LREC* (pp. 441–444). Athens, Greece: International Association for Language Resources.

Di Eugenio, B. (2001). Natural language processing for computer-supported instruction. *ACM Intelligence, 12,* 22–32.

Di Eugenio, B., Jordan, P. W., Moore, J. D., & Thomason, R. H. (1998). An empirical investigation of collaborative dialogues. *Proceedings of COLING98* (pp. 325–329). East Stroudsburg, PA: Association for Computational Linguistics.

Di Eugenio, B., Jordan, P. W., Moore, J. D., & Thomason, R. H. (2000). The agreement process: An empirical investigation of computer-mediated collaborative dialogues. *International Journal of Human Computer Studies, 53,* 1017–1076.

Di Eugenio, B., Moore, J. D., & Paolucci, M. (1997). Learning features that predict cue usage. *35th Annual Meeting of the Association for Computational Linguistics* (pp. 80–87). East Stroudsburg, PA: Association for Computational Linguistics.

Di Eugenio, B., & Trolio, M. (2000). Can simple sentence planning improve the interaction between learners and intelligent tutoring systems? In R. Freedman & P. Jordan (Eds.), *Building dialogue systems for tutorial applications. AAAI Fall Symposium* (pp. 96–104). Menlo Park, CA: AAAI Press.

Dimitrov, D., & Rumrill, P. (2003). Pretest–posttest designs and the measurement of change. *Work: A Journal of Prevention, Assessment, and Rehabilitation, 20,* 159–165.

diSessa, A. (1983). Phenomenology and the evolution of intuition. In D. Gentner & A. L. Stevens (Eds.), *Mental models* (pp. 15–34). Hillsdale, NJ: Lawrence Erlbaum Associates.

diSessa, A. (1993). Toward an epistemology of physics. *Cognition and Instruction, 10,* 101–104.

diSessa, A. A., & Minstrell, J. (1998). Cultivating conceptual change with benchmark lessons. In J. Greeno & S. Goldman (Eds.), *Thinking practices in mathematics and science learning* (pp. 155–189). Mahwah, NJ: Lawrence Erlbaum Associates.

Du Boulay, B. (2000). Can we learn from ITSs? In G. Gauthier, C. Frasson, & K. VanLehn (Eds.) *Intelligent Tutoring Systems 2000* (pp. 9–17). Berlin, Germany: Springer.

Duncan, S. (1974). Some signals and rules for taking speaking turns in conversation. *Journal of Personality and Social Psychology, 23,* 283–292.

Edelson, D. C. (1996). Learning from cases and questions: The Socratic case-based teaching architecture. *Journal of the Learning Sciences, 5,* 357–410.

Elhadad, M. (1992). *Using argumentation to control lexical choice: A functional unification implementation.* Unpublished doctoral dissertation, Columbia University, New York.

Elhadad, M., & McKeown, K. R. (1990). Generating connectives. In *Proceedings of COLING '90* (Vol. 3, pp. 97–101). Stroudsburg, PA: Association for Computational Linguistics.

Elmi, M. A. (1994). *A natural language parser with interleaved spelling correction supporting lexical functional grammar and ill-formed input.* Unpublished doctoral dissertation, Illinois Institute of Technology, Chicago.

Elmi, M. A., & Evens, M. W. (1998). Spelling correction using context. *Proceedings of COLING 98* (pp. 360–364). East Stroudsburg, PA: Association for Computational Linguistics.

Elsom-Cook, M. (1988). Using multiple teaching strategies in an ITS. In B. Goettl, H. Halff, C. Redfield, & V. J. Shute (Eds.), *Proceedings of Intelligent Tutoring Systems: ITS 88* (pp. 286–290). Berlin, Germany: Springer-Verlag.

Ericsson, K. A., & Simon, H. A. (1993). *Protocol analysis: Verbal reports as data.* Cambridge, MA: MIT Press.

Evens, M., Spitkovsky, J., Boyle, P., Michael, J. A., & Rovick, A. A. (1993). Synthesizing tutorial dialogues. In M. Polson (Ed.), *Proceedings of CogSci '93* (pp. 137–142). Mahwah, NJ: Lawrence Erlbaum Associates.

Evens, M. W. (Ed.). (1988). *Relational models of the lexicon*. Cambridge, England: Cambridge University Press.

Evens, M. W. (2002). Natural language interface for an expert system. In A. Kent & J. G. Williams (Eds.), *Encyclopedia of microcomputers* (pp. 225–254). New York: Marcel Dekker.

Evens, M. W., Litowitz, B., Markowitz, J., Smith, R. N., & Werner, O. (1980). *Lexical-semantic relations: A comparative survey.* Edmonton, Alberta: Linguistic Research, Inc.

Faletti, J. (1982). PANDORA—A program for doing commonsense reasoning and planning in complex situations. *Proceedings of AAAI–82* (pp. 185–188). Menlo Park, CA: AAAI Press.

Feltovich, P. J., Coulson, R., & Spiro, R. (2001). Learners' (mis)understanding of important and difficult concepts. In K. D. Forbus & P. J. Feltovich (Eds.), *Smart machines in education* (pp. 349–375). Cambridge, MA: MIT Press.

Feltovich, P. J., Spiro, R., & Coulson, R. (1989). The nature of conceptual understanding in biomedicine: The deep structure of complex ideas and the development of misconceptions. In D. Evans & V. Patel (Eds.), *Cognitive science in medicine* (pp. 113–172). Cambridge, MA: MIT Press.

Fikes, R., & Nilsson, N. (1971). STRIPS: A new approach to the application of theorem proving and problem solving. *Artificial Intelligence 2,* 189–208.

Fillmore, C. J. (1968). The case for case. In E. Bach & R. Harms (Eds.), *Universals in linguistic theory* (pp. 1–90). New York: Holt, Rinehart & Winston.

Flesch, R. (1955). *Why Johnny can't read and what you can do about it.* New York: Harper.

Forbes, K., & Webber, B. (2002). A semantic account of adverbials as discourse connectives. *Proceedings of the Third SIGDIAL Workshop* (pp. 27–36). East Stroudsburg, PA: Association for Computational Linguistics.

Forbes-Riley, K., & Litman, D. (2004). Predicting emotion in spoken dialogue from multiple knowledge. *Proceedings of the Language Technology Conference: 4th Meeting of the North American Chapter of the Association for Computational Linguistics (HLT/NAACL)* (pp. 201–208). East Stroudsburg, PA: Association for Computational Linguistics.

Forbus, K. D. (1988). Qualitative physics: Past, present, and future. In H. Shrobe (Ed.), *Exploring artificial intelligence* (pp. 239–292), San Mateo, CA: Kaufmann.

Forbus, K. D. (1997). Using qualitative physics to create articulate educational software. *IEEE Expert, 12*(3), 32–41.

Forbus, K. D. (2001). Articulate software for science and engineering education . In K. D. Forbus & P. J. Feltovich (Eds.), *Smart machines in education* (pp. 349–375). Cambridge, MA: MIT Press.

Forbus, K. D., Gentner, D., & Law, K. (1995). MAC/FAC: A model of similarity-based retrieval. *Cognitive Science, 19,* 141–205.

Fox, B. (1987). *Discourse structure and anaphora: Written and conversational English.* Cambridge, England: Cambridge University Press.

Fox, B. (1988a). *Cognitive and interactional aspects of correction in tutoring* (Tech. Rpt. No. 88-2). Boulder, CO: University of Colorado.

Fox, B. (1988b). *Repair as a factor in interface design* (Tech. Rpt. No. 88-4). Boulder, CO: University of Colorado.

Fox, B. (1989). Cognitive and interactional aspects of correction in tutoring. In P. Goodyear (Ed.), *Teaching knowledge and intelligent tutoring* (pp. 149–172). Norwood, NJ: Ablex.

Fox, B. (1990). *Final report on the human tutoring dialogue project* (Tech. Rpt. No. 90-1). Boulder, CO: University of Colorado.

Fox, B. (1993a). Correction in tutoring. In M. Polson (Ed.), *Proceedings of the Fifteenth Annual Meeting of the Cognitive Science Society* (pp. 121–126). Hillsdale, NJ: Lawrence Erlbaum Associates.

Fox, B. (1993b). *The human tutorial dialogue project.* Hillsdale, NJ: Lawrence Erlbaum Associates.

Fox Tree, J. E. (1999). Listening in on monologues and dialogues. *Discourse Processes, 27,* 35–53.

Fraser, J. M., & Smith, P. J. (1992). A catalog of errors. *International Journal of Man–Machine Studies, 37,* 265–307.

Frawley, W. (1988). Relational models in metascience. In M. W. Evens (Ed.), *Relational models of the lexicon* (pp. 343–372). Cambridge, England: Cambridge University Press.

Freedman, R. (1996a). Using a text planner to model the behavior of human tutors in an ITS. *Proceedings of the 1996 Midwest Artificial Intelligence and Cognitive Science Society Conference.* Retrieved May 1, 1996, from http://www.cs.indiana.edu/event/maics96/Proceedings/Freedman/freedman.html

Freedman, R. (1996b). Using tutoring patterns to generate more cohesive text in an intelligent tutoring system. In D. C. Edelson & E. A. Domeshek (Eds.), *Proceedings of the International Conference on Learning Systems (ICLS-96)* (pp. 75–82). Charlottesville, VA: AACE.

Freedman, R. (1996c). *Interaction of discourse planning, instructional planning, and dialogue management in an interactive tutoring system.* Unpublished doctoral dissertation, Northwestern University, Evanston, IL.

Freedman, R. (1997). Degrees of mixed-initiative interaction in an intelligent tutoring system. In S. Haller & S. McRoy (Eds.), *Computational models for mixed initiative interaction. AAAI Spring Symposium* (pp. 44–49). Menlo Park, CA: AAAI Press.

Freedman, R. (2000a). Plan-based dialogue management in a physics tutor. *Proceedings of the Sixth Applied Natural Language Processing Conference* (pp. 52–59). East Stroudsburg, PA: Association for Computational Linguistics.

Freedman, R. (2000b). Using a reactive planner as the basis for a dialogue agent. In J. Etheredge & B. Manaris (Eds.), *Proceedings of FLAIRS 2000* (pp. 203–208). Menlo Park, CA: AAAI Press.

Freedman, R. (2001). An approach to increasing programming efficiency in plan-based dialogue systems. In J. D. Moore, C. L. Redfield, & W. L. Johnson (Eds.), *Proceedings of Artificial Intelligence in Education* (pp. 200–209). Amsterdam: IO Press.

Freedman, R., & Evens, M. W. (1996). Realistic limitations in natural language processing for an intelligent tutoring system. In G. Cottrell (Ed.), *Proceedings of 18th Annual Cognitive Science Conference* (p. 766). Mahwah, NJ: Lawrence Erlbaum Associates.

Freedman, R., & Evens, M. W. (1997). The use of multiple knowledge types in an intelligent tutoring system. In M. Shafto & P. Langley (Eds.), *Proceedings of the Cognitive Science Conference* (p. 920). Mahwah, NJ: Lawrence Erlbaum Associates.

Freedman, R., Haggin, N., Nacheva, D., Leahy, T., & Stilson, R. (2004). Using a domain-independent reactive planner to implement a medical dialogue system. *Systems for Health Communication* (pp. 24–31). Menlo Park, CA: AAAI Press.

Freedman, R., Rosé, C. P., Ringenberg, M., & VanLehn, K. (2000). ITS tools for natural language dialogue: A domain-independent parser and planner. In

G. Gauthier, C. Frasson, & K. VanLehn (Eds.), *Intelligent Tutoring Systems 2000* (pp. 433–442). Berlin, Germany: Springer.

Freedman, R., Zhou, Y., Glass, M. S., Kim, J. H., & Evens, M. W. (1998). Using rule induction to assist in rule construction for a natural-language based intelligent tutoring system. In M. A. Gernsbacher & S. Derry (Eds.), *Proceedings of 20th Annual Cognitive Science Conference* (pp. 362–367). Mahwah, NJ: Lawrence Erlbaum Associates.

Freedman, R., Zhou, Y., Kim, J. H., Glass, M. S., & Evens, M. W. (1998). SGML-based markup as a step toward improving knowledge acquisition for text generation. In J. Chu-Carroll & N. Green (Eds.), *AAAI Spring Symposium on applying machine learning to discourse processing* (pp. 114–177). Menlo Park, CA: AAAI Press.

Fried, D. M., Wilkins, D. C., Grois, E., Peters, S., Schultz, K., & Clark, B. (2003). The Gerona knowledge ontology and its support for spoken dialogue tutoring of crisis decision making skills. *Proceedings of the 3rd workshop on knowledge and reasoning in practical dialogue systems* (pp. 79–89). Menlo Park, CA: AAAI Press.

G. & C. Merriam Company. P. Gove (comp.). (1963). *Webster's seventh collegiate dictionary.* Springfield, MA: Author.

Galdes, D. K., Smith, P. J., & Smith, J. W. (1991). Factors determining when to interrupt and what to say: An empirical study of the case-method tutoring approach. In L. Birnbaum (Ed.), *International Conference on the Learning Sciences* (pp. 194–202). Charlottesville, VA: AACE.

Gamoran, M. (1991, April). *The tutor behind the curtain: Face-to-face and remote tutoring.* Paper presented at the annual meeting of the American Educational Research Association, Chicago.

Gentner, D. (1983). Structure-mapping: A theoretical framework for analogy. *Cognitive Science 7,* 155–170.

Gentner, D. (1998). Analogy. In W. Bechtel & G. Graham (Eds.), *A companion to cognitive science* (pp. 107–113). Oxford, England: Blackwell.

Gentner, D., Holyoak, K. J., & Kokinov, B. N. (Eds.) (2001). *The analogical mind.* Cambridge, MA: MIT Press.

Gentner, D., & Stevens, A. (Eds.). (1983). *Mental models.* Hillsdale, NJ: Lawrence Erlbaum Associates.

Gertner, A. (1998). Providing feedback to equation entries in an intelligent tutoring system for physics. In B. Goettl, H. M. Halff, C. Redfield, & V. J. Shute (Eds.), *Intelligent Tutoring Systems 98,* (pp. 254–263). Berlin, Germany: Springer.

Gertner, A., Conati, C., & VanLehn, K. (1998). Procedural help in Andes: Generating hints using a Bayesian network student model. *Proceedings of the AAAI* (pp. 106–111). Menlo Park, CA: AAAI Press.

Giarratano, J., & Riley, G. (1998). *Expert systems: Principles and practice* (3rd ed.). Boston: PWS Publishing.

Glass, M. S. (1999). *Broadening input understanding in a language-based intelligent tutoring system.* Unpublished doctoral dissertation, Illinois Institute of Technology, Chicago.

Glass, M. S. (2000). Processing language input in the CIRCSIM-Tutor intelligent tutoring system. In C. P. Rosé & R. Freedman (Eds.), *Proceedings of the*

AAAI Fall Symposium on building dialogue systems for tutorial applications (pp. 74–79). Menlo Park, CA: AAAI Press.

Glass, M. S. (2001). Processing language input for an intelligent tutoring system. In J. D. Moore, C. L. Redfield, & W. L. Johnson (Eds.), *Proceedings of Artificial Intelligence in Education* (pp. 210–221). Amsterdam: IOS Press.

Glass, M. S., & Di Eugenio, B. (2002a). MUP: The UIC markup tool. In S. Gordon (Ed.), *Proceedings of the Thirteenth Midwest Artificial Intelligence and Cognitive Science Conference* (pp. 21–27). Chicago: Computer Science Department, Illinois Institute of Technology.

Glass, M. S., & Di Eugenio, B. (2002b). MUP: The UIC standoff markup tool. *Proceedings of the Third SIGDIAL Workshop* (pp. 37–41). East Stroudsburg, PA: Association for Computational Linguistics.

Glass, M. S., Kim, J. H., Evens, M. W., Michael, J. A., & Rovick, A. A. (1999). Novice vs. expert tutors: A comparison of style. In U. Priss (Ed.), *Proceedings of MAICS '99* (pp. 43–49). Menlo Park, CA: AAAI Press.

Goldblum, N. (2001). *The brain-shaped mind.* Cambridge, England: Cambridge University Press.

Golding, A. R., & Roth, D. (1999). A winnow-based approach to context-sensitive spelling correction. *Machine Learning 34,* 107–130.

Goldman, S. R., & Durán, R. P. (1988). Answering questions from oceanography texts: Learner, task and text characteristics. *Discourse Processes, 11,* 373–412.

Goldstein, I. P. (1979). The genetic epistemology of rule systems. *International Journal of Man–Machine Studies 11,* 51–77.

Goldstein, I. P. (1982). The genetic graph: A representation for the evolution of procedural knowledge. In D. H. Sleeman & J. S. Brown (Eds.), *Intelligent tutoring systems* (pp. 51–77). New York: Academic.

Goldstein, I. P., & Carr, B. (1977). The computer as coach: An athletic paradigm for intellectual education. *Proceedings of the ACM77* (pp. 227–233). New York: ACM Press.

Graesser, A. C. (1988). Introduction to cognitive science: Perspectives on question generation. *Questioning Exchange, 2*(1–2).

Graesser, A. C. (1993a). Dialogue patterns and feedback mechanisms during naturalistic tutoring. In M. Polson (Ed.), *Proceedings of the Fifteenth Annual Meeting of the Cognitive Science Society* (pp. 127–130). Mahwah, NJ: Lawrence Erlbaum Associates.

Graesser, A. C. (1993b). *Questioning mechanisms during tutoring, conversation, and human–computer interaction* (Tech. Rpt. R&T 4422576). Arlington, VA: Office of Naval Research, Cognitive Science Program.

Graesser, A. C., Franklin, S., & Wiemer-Hastings, P. (1998). Simulating smooth tutorial dialogue with pedagogical value. In D. Cook (Ed.), *Florida Artificial Intelligence Research Symposium 98.* (pp. 163–167). Menlo Park, CA: AAAI Press.

Graesser, A. C., Lang, K., & Horgan, D. (1988). A taxonomy for question generation. *Questioning Exchange, 2,* 3–15.

Graesser, A. C., & Person, N. K. (1994). Question asking during tutoring. *American Educational Research Journal, 31,* 104–137.

Graesser, A. C., Person, N. K., & Huber, J. (1993). Question asking during tutoring and in the design of educational software. In M. Rabinowitz (Ed.), *Cognitive science foundations of instruction* (pp. 149–172). Hillsdale, NJ: Lawrence Erlbaum Associates.

Graesser, A. C., Person, N. K., & Magliano, J. P. (1995). Collaborative dialogue patterns in naturalistic one-on-one tutoring. *Applied Cognitive Psychology, 9,* 495–522.

Graesser, A. C., Wiemer-Hastings, P., Wiemer-Hastings, K., Harter, D., Person, N., & The Tutoring Research Group. (2000). Using latent semantic analysis to evaluate the contributions of students in AutoTutor [Special Issue]. *Interactive Learning Environments, 8,* 129–148.

Graesser, A. C., Wiemer-Hastings, K., Wiemer-Hastings, P., Kreuz, R., & The Tutoring Research Group. (1999). AutoTutor: A simulation of a human tutor. *Journal of Cognitive Systems Research, 1,* 35–51.

Granger, R. H. (1983). The NOMAD system: Expectation-based detection and correction of errors during understanding of syntactically and semantically ill-formed text. *American Journal of Computational Linguistics, 3,* 188–196.

Green, N., & Carberry, S. (1999). A computational mechanism for initiative in answer generation. *User Modeling and User-Adapted Interaction, 9,* 93–132.

Grice, H. P. (1975). Logic and conversation. In P. Cole & J. Morgan (Eds.), *Syntax and semantics* (pp. 41–58). New York: Academic.

Grimes, J. E. (1975). *The thread of discourse.* The Hague, Netherlands: Mouton.

Grishman, R., Macleod, C., & Meyers, A. (1994). COMLEX syntax: Building a computational lexicon. *COLING 94* (pp. 268–272). East Stroudsburg, PA: Association for Computational Linguistics.

Griswold, R., & Griswold, M. (1997). *The ICON programming language* (3rd ed.). San Jose, CA: Peer-to-Peer.

Grosz, B. J. (1977). The representation and use of focus in a system for understanding dialogs. *Proceedings of the Fifth IJCAI* (pp. 67–76). Pittsburgh, PA: Carnegie-Mellon University.

Grosz, B. J. (1978). Discourse analysis. In D. Walker (Ed.), *Understanding spoken language* (pp. 138–176). New York: Elsevier-North Holland.

Grosz, B. J., & Sidner, C. L. (1986). Attention, intentions, and the structure of discourse. *Computational Linguistics, 12,* 175–204.

Grosz, B. J., & Sidner, C. L. (1990). Plans for discourse. In P. Cohen, J. Morgan, & M. Pollack (Eds.), *Intentions in communication* (pp. 417–444). Cambridge, MA: MIT Press.

Guindon, R. (1988). A multidisciplinary perspective on dialogue structure in user-advisor dialogues. In R. Guindon (Ed.), *Cognitive science and its applications for human–computer interaction* (pp. 163–200). Hillsdale, NJ: Lawrence Erlbaum Associates.

Hake, R. R. (1998). Interactive-engagement vs traditional methods: A six-thousand-student survey of mechanics test data for introductory physics courses. *American Journal of Physics, 66,* 64–74.

Halff, H. M. (1988). Curriculum and instruction in automated tutors. In M. C. Polson & J. J. Richardson (Eds.), *Foundations of intelligent tutoring systems* (pp. 79–108). Hillsdale, NJ: Lawrence Erlbaum Associates.

Halliday, M. A. K., & Hasan, R. (1976). *Cohesion in English.* London: Longman.

Hamburger, H., & Tecuci, G. (1998). Toward a unification of human–computer learning and tutoring. In B. P. Goettl, H. M. Halff, C. L. Redfield, & V. J. Shute (Eds.), *Intelligent Tutoring Systems 1998* (pp. 444–453). Berlin, Germany: Springer-Verlag.

Hammond, K. (1989). *Case-based planning*. New York: Academic.

Hausmann, R. G. M., & Chi, M. T. H. (2002). Self-explaining with a computer interface. *Cognitive Technology, 7,* 4–14.

Hayes, P. J., & Mouradian, G. (1981). Flexible parsing. *American Journal of Computational Linguistics, 7,* 232–242.

Hayes-Roth, B. (1985). A blackboard architecture for control. *Artificial Intelligence, 26,* 251–321.

Heffernan, N. T. (2001). *Intelligent tutoring systems have forgotten the tutor.* Unpublished doctoral dissertation, Carnegie Mellon University, Pittsburgh, PA.

Heffernan, N. T. (2003). Web-based evaluations showing both cognitive and motivational and cognitive benefits of the Ms. Lindquist Tutor. In F. Verdejo, J. Kay, H. Pain, & V. Aleven, *Proceedings of the 11th Conference on AI in Education* (pp. 115–122). Amsterdam: IOS Press.

Heffernan, N. T., & Croteau, E. A. (2004). Web-based evaluations showing differential learning for tutorial strategies employed by the Ms. Lindquist Tutor. In J. C. Lester, R. M. Vicari, & F. Paraguaçu (Eds.), *ITS 2004* (pp. 491–500). Berlin, Germany: Springer-Verlag.

Heffernan, N. T., & Koedinger, K. (2000a). Building a third generation ITS for symbolization: Adding a tutorial model with multiple tutoring strategies. In J. F. Nicaud (Ed.), *Proceedings of the workshop on learning algebra with a computer, ITS 2000* (pp. 12–22). Berlin, Germany: Springer.

Heffernan, N. T., & Koedinger, K. (2000b). Intelligent tutoring systems are missing the tutor: Building a more strategic dialog-based tutor. In C.P. Rosé & R. Freedman (Eds.), *Proceedings of the AAAI Fall Symposium on Building Dialogue Systems for Tutorial Applications* (pp. 14–19). Menlo Park, CA: AAAI Press.

Heffernan, N. T, & Koedinger, K. (2001) The design and formative analysis of a dialog-based tutor. In J. D. Moore, C. L. Redfield, & W. L. Johnson (Eds.), *Workshop at AI-in-Education.* Amsterdam: IOS Press.

Heffernan, N. T., & Koedinger, K. R. (2002). An intelligent tutoring system incorporating a model of an experienced human tutor. In S. Cerri, G. Gouadères, & F. Paraguaçu (Eds.), *International Conference on Intelligent Tutoring Systems 2002* (pp. 596–608). Berlin, Germany: Springer-Verlag.

Heller, L. J., & Mohrman, D. (1981). *Cardiovascular physiology.* Boston: McGraw-Hill.

Hendler, J., Tate, A., & Drummond, M. (1990). AI planning: Systems and techniques. *AI Magazine, 11*(2), 61–77.

Hestenes, D., & Halloun, I. (1995). Interpreting the force concept inventory. *The Physics Teacher, 33,* 504–506.

Hestenes, D., Wells, M., & Swackhamer, G. (1992). Force concept inventory. *The Physics Teacher, 30,* 141–151.

Hill, H., Curt, C., Hier, D., & Evens, M. (1985). The architecture of the IIT-MRH Stroke Consultant. In J. Ackerman (Ed.), *Symposium on Computer Applications in Medical Care* (pp. 314–319). Los Alamitos, CA: IEEE Computer Society Press.

Hirst, G. (1987). *Semantic interpretation and the resolution of ambiguity.* Cambridge, England: Cambridge University Press.

Hix, D., & Hartson, H. R. (1993). *Developing user interfaces: Ensuring usability through product and process.* New York: Wiley.

Hobbs, J., & Moore, R. (Eds.). (1985). *Formal theories of the commonsense world.* Norwood, NJ: Ablex.

Hody, G. L., & Avner, R. A. (1978). The PLATO system: An evaluative description. In E. C. DeLand (Ed.), *Information technology in health science education* (pp. 143–177). New York: Plenum.

Hofstadter, D. R. (2001). Epilogue: Analogy as the core of cognition. In D. Gentner, K. J. Holyoak, & B. N. Kokinov (Eds.), *The analogical mind* (pp. 499–538). Cambridge, MA: MIT Press.

Holland, M., Kaplan, J. D., & Sams, M. R. (1995). *Intelligent language tutors.* Hillsdale, NJ: Lawrence Erlbaum Associates.

Hollingshead, K. (2003). *How OK is used in dialogue*. Unpublished manuscript, Oregon Graduate Center, Computer Speech and Language Understanding.

Holyoak, K. J., & Thagard, P. R. (1995). *Mental leaps: Analogy in creative thought.* Cambridge, MA: MIT Press.

Horn, M. A., Simonett, G., & Webb, G. F. (1999). *Mathematical models in medical and health science.* Nashville, TN: Vanderbilt University Press.

Horowitz, R. (2004, August). *Repetition and engagement*. Paper presented at the annual meeting of the Society for Text and Discourse, Chicago.

Hovy, E. H. (1988a). Planning coherent multisentential text. *Proceedings of the annual meeting of the ACL* (pp. 163–169). East Stroudsburg, PA: Association for Computational Linguistics.

Hovy, E. H. (1988b). Two types of planning in language generation. *Proceedings of the annual meeting of the ACL* (pp. 179–186). East Stroudsburg, PA: Association for Computational Linguistics.

Hovy, E. H. (1988c). Generating language with a phrasal lexicon. In D. McDonald & L. Bolc (Eds.), *Natural language generation systems* (pp. 353–384). New York: Springer-Verlag.

Hovy, E. H. (1991). Approaches to the planning of coherent text. In C. Paris, W. Swartout, & W. Mann (Eds.), *Natural language generation in artificial intelligence and computational linguistics* (pp. 83–102). Dordrecht, The Netherlands: Kluwer.

Hovy, E. H. (1993). Automated discourse generation using discourse structure relations. *Artificial Intelligence, 39,* 341–386.

Hume, G. (1995). *Using student modeling to determine how and when to hint in an intelligent tutoring system.* Unpublished doctoral dissertation, Illinois Institute of Technology, Chicago.

Hume, G., Evens, M. W., Rovick, A. A., & Michael, J. A. (1993). The use of hints as a tutoring tactic. In M. Polson (Ed.), *Proceedings of CogSci '93* (pp. 563–568). Mahwah, NJ: Lawrence Erlbaum Associates.

Hume, G., Michael, J. A., Rovick, A. A., & Evens, M. W. (1995). Controlling active learning: How tutors decide when to generate hints. In J. H. Sherman (Ed.), *Proceedings of FLAIRS '95* (pp. 157–161). Menlo Park, CA: AAAI Press.

Hume, G., Michael, J. A., Rovick, A. A., & Evens, M. W. (1996a). Hinting as a tactic in one-on-one tutoring. *Journal of the Learning Sciences, 5,* 23–47.

Hume, G., Michael, J. A., Rovick, A. A., & Evens, M. W. (1996b). Responses and follow up tutorial tactics in an ITS. In J. Stewman (Ed.), *Proceedings of the 1996 Florida Artificial Intelligence Research Symposium* (pp. 168–172). Menlo Park, CA: AAAI Press.

Hunt, E., & Minstrell, J. (1994). A collaborative classroom for teaching conceptual physics. In K. McGilly (Ed.), *Classroom lessons: Integrating cognitive theory and classroom practice* (pp. 51–74). Cambridge, MA: MIT Press.

Hurst, R. W. & Milkent, M. M. (1996). Facilitating successful prediction problem solving in biology through application of skill theory. *Journal of Research in Science Teaching, 33,* 541–552.

Jackson, G. T., Person, N. K., & Graesser, A. C. (2004). Adaptive tutorial dialogue in AutoTutor. In N. Heffernan & P. Wiemer-Hastings (Eds.), *Proceedings of the Workshop on Dialog-Based Intelligent Tutoring Systems, ITS 2004* (pp. 9–13). Berlin, Germany: Springer-Verlag.

Jackson, G. T., Ventura, M., Chewle, P., Graesser, A. C., & Tutoring Research Group. (2004). The impact of Why/AutoTutor on learning and retention of conceptual physics. In J. C. Lester, R. M. Vicari, & F. Paraguaçu (Eds.), *Proceedings of Intelligent Tutoring Systems, ITS 2004* (pp. 501–510). Berlin, Germany: Springer-Verlag.

Jacobs, G. (1989). Word usage misconceptions among first-year university physics students. *International Journal of Science Education, 11,* 395–399.

Jacobs, P. S. (1988). PHRED: A generator for natural language interfaces. In D. D. McDonald & L. Bolc (Eds.), *Natural language generation systems* (pp. 312–352). Berlin, Germany: Springer.

Jensen, K., Heidorn, G., Miller, L., & Ravin, Y. (1983). Parse fitting and prose fixing: Getting a hold on ill-formedness. *American Journal of Computational Linguistics, 9,* 147–160.

Jeong, I., Evens, M. W., & Kim, Y. K. (1998). Tools for building concept maps. *Korea Telecom Journal, 3,* 11–21.

Johnson, W. L., Beal, C., Fowles-Winkler, A., Lauper, U., Marsella, S., Narayanan, S., et al. (2004). Tactical language training system: An interim report. In J. C. Lester, R. M. Vicari, & F. Paraguaçu (Eds.), *ITS 2004* (pp. 336–345). Berlin, Germany: Springer-Verlag.

Jordan, P. (2004). Using student explanations as models for adapting tutorial dialogue. In D. Dankel (Ed.), *Proceedings of the 17th International FLAIRS Conference* (pp. 905–910). Menlo Park, CA: AAAI Press.

Jordan, P., Makatchev, M., & VanLehn, K. (2003). Abductive theorem proving for analyzing student explanations. In F. Verdejo, J. Kay, H. Pain, & V. Aleven (Eds.), *Proceedings of Artifiical Intelligence in Education* (pp. 73–80). Amsterdam: IOS.

Jordan, P., Makatchev, M., & VanLehn, K. (2004). Combining competing language understanding approaches in an intelligent tutoring system. In J. C. Lester, R. M. Vicari, & F. Paraguaçu (Eds.), *ITS 2004* (pp. 346–357). Berlin, Germany: Springer-Verlag.

Jordan, P., Rosé, C. P., & VanLehn, K. (2001). Tools for authoring tutorial dialogue knowledge. In J. D. Moore, C. L. Redfield, & W. L. Johnson (Eds.), *Proceedings of Artificial Intelligence in Education* (pp. 222–233). Amsterdam: IOS Press.

Jurafsky, D., & Martin, J. H. (2000). *Speech and language processing.* Upper Saddle River, NJ: Prentice Hall.

Justeson, J. S., & Katz, S. M. (1991). Co-occurrences of antonymous adjectives and their contexts. *Computational Linguistics, 17,* 1–19.

Kaplan, R. M. (1999). *The formal architecture of lexical-functional grammar.* Lecture notes of the 11th European Summer School in Logic, Language and Information (ESSLLI), Utrecht University, the Netherlands.

Kaplan, R. M., & Bresnan, J. (1982). Lexical functional grammar: A formal system for grammatical representation. In J. Bresnan (Ed.), *The mental representations of grammatical relations* (pp. 173–281). Cambridge, MA: MIT Press.

Katz, S. (2003). Distributed tutorial strategies. In R. Ackerman & D. Kirsh (Eds.), *Proceedings of the Cognitive Science Conference* (pp. 640–645). Mahwah, NJ: Lawrence Erlbaum Associates.

Katz, S., & Allbritton, D. (2002). Going beyond the problem given: How human tutors use post-practice discussions to support transfer. *Proceedings of Intelligent Tutoring Systems 2002* (pp. 641–650), San Sebastian, Spain, 2002. Berlin, Germany: Springer-Verlag.

Katz, S., Lesgold, A., Eggan, G., & Greenberg, L. (1996). Toward the design of more effective advisors for learning by doing systems. In C. Frasson, G. Gauthier, & A. Lesgold (Eds.), *ITS 1996* (pp. 641–649). Berlin, Germany: Springer-Verlag.

Katz, S., Lesgold, A., Eggan, G., & Gordin, M. (1993). Modeling the student in SHERLOCK II. *Journal of Artificial Intelligence and Education (Special Issue on Student Modeling), 3,* 495–518.

Katz, S., Lesgold, A., Eggan, G., Gordin, M., & Greenberg, L. (1992). Self-adjusting curriculum planning in Sherlock II. In I. Tomek (Ed.), *Proceedings of the Fourth International Conference on Computers in Learning (ICCAL '92)* (pp. 343–355). Berlin, Germany: Springer-Verlag.

Katz, S., Lesgold, A., Hughes, E., Peters, D., Eggan, G., Gordin, M., et al. (1998). Sherlock 2: An intelligent tutoring system built on the LRDC framework. In C. P. Bloom & R. B. Loftin (Eds.), *Facilitating the development and use of interactive learning environments* (pp. 227–258). Mahwah, NJ: Lawrence Erlbaum Associates.

Katz, S., O'Donnell, G., & Kay, H. (2000). An approach to analyzing the role and structure of reflective dialogue. *International Journal of Artificial Intelligence and Education, 11,* 320–343.

Khuwaja, R. A. (1994). *A model of tutoring: Facilitating knowledge integration using multiple models of the domain.* Unpublished doctoral dissertation, Illinois Institute of Technology, Chicago.

Khuwaja, R. A., Evens, M. W., Rovick, A. A., & Michael, J. A. (1994). Architecture of CIRCSIM-TUTOR (v.3): A smart cardiovascular physiology tutor. *Proceedings of Computer-Based Medical Systems CBMS94* (pp. 158–163). Los Alamitos, CA: IEEE Computer Society Press.

Khuwaja, R. A., & Patel, V. (1996). A model of tutoring based on the behavior of effective human tutors. In C. Frasson, G. Gauthier, & A. Lesgold (Eds.), *Proceedings of the Third International Conference on Intelligent Tutoring Systems (ITS '96)* (pp. 130–138). Berlin, Germany: Springer-Verlag.

Khuwaja, R A., Rovick, A. A., Michael, J. A., & Evens, M. W. (1992). Knowledge representation for an intelligent tutoring system based on a multilevel causal model. In C. Frasson, G. Gauthier, & G. I. McCalla (Eds.), *Proceedings of ITS '92* (pp. 217–224). Berlin, Germany: Springer.

Khuwaja, R. A., Rovick, A. A., Michael, J. A., & Evens, M. W. (1994). A tale of three tutoring protocols: The implications for intelligent tutoring systems. In E. A. Ufantis (Ed.), *Intelligent Systems: Proceedings of Golden West* (pp. 109–118). Los Alamitos, CA: IEEE Computer Society Press.

Kieras, D. E. (1985). Thematic processes in the comprehension of technical prose. In B. K. Britton & J. B. Black (Eds.), *Understanding expository text* (pp. 89–108). Hillsdale, NJ: Lawrence Erlbaum Associates.

Kim, J., & Gil, Y. (2002). Deriving acquisition principles from tutoring principles. In S. A. Cerri, G. Gouardères, & F. Paraguaçu (Eds.), *ITS 2002* (pp. 661–670). Berlin, Germany: Springer-Verlag.

Kim, J. H. (1997). *The development of logic forms for CIRCSIM-Tutor v. 3.* Unpublished doctoral qualifying examination paper, Illinois Institute of Technology, Chicago.

Kim, J. H. (2000). *Natural language analysis and generation for tutorial dialogue.* Unpublished doctoral dissertation, Illinois Institute of Technology, Chicago.

Kim, J. H., Freedman, R., & Evens, M. W. (1998a). Relationship between tutorial goals and sentence structure in a corpus of tutoring transcripts. In M. Evens (Ed.), *Ninth Midwest Artificial Intelligence and Cognitive Science Conference* (pp. 124–131). Dayton, OH: AAAI Press.

Kim, J. H., Freedman, R., & Evens, M. W. (1998b). Responding to unexpected student utterances in CIRCSIM-Tutor v.3: Analysis of transcripts. In D. Cook (Ed.), *FLAIRS-98* (pp. 153–157). Menlo Park, CA: AAAI Press.

Kim, J. H., Freedman, R., Glass, M. S., & Evens, M. W. (in preparation). *Tutoring schemas for an intelligent tutoring system. Discourse Processes.*

Kim, J. H., & Glass, M. S. (2004). Evaluating dialogue schemata with the Wizard of Oz computer-assisted algebra tutor. In J. C. Lester, R. M. Vicari, & F. Paraguaçu (Eds.), *Proceedings of ITS 2004* (pp. 358–367). Berlin, Germany: Springer.

Kim, J. H., Glass, M. S., Freedman, R., & Evens, M. W. (2000). Learning the use of discourse markers in tutorial dialogue for an intelligent tutoring system. In L. R. Gleitman & A. K. Joshi (Eds.), *Proceedings of the Cognitive Science Conference 2000* (pp. 262–267). Mahwah, NJ: Lawrence Erlbaum Associates.

Kim, N. (1989). *An intelligent tutoring system for physiology.* Unpublished doctoral dissertation, Illinois Institute of Technology, Chicago.

Kim, N., Evens, M. W., Michael, J. A., & Rovick, A. A. (1989). An intelligent tutoring system for circulatory physiology. In H. Maurer (Ed.), *Proceedings of the International Conference on Computer Assisted Learning* (pp. 254–266). Berlin, Germany: Springer-Verlag.

Kim, Y. C. (2003). *Generation of concept maps from medical index terms for diagrammatic reasoning in physiology tutorials.* Unpublished doctoral dissertation, Illinois Institute of Technology, Chicago.

Kim, Y. C., Evens, M. W., Michael, J. A., & Trace, D. A. (2002). Physiology tutorials using concept mapping. In S. Conlon (Ed.), *MAICS 2002* (pp. 61–64), Chicago Institute of Technology.

Kintsch, W. (1974). *The representation of meaning in memory.* Hillsdale, NJ: Lawrence Erlbaum Associates.

Kirchhoff, K. (2001). A comparison of classification techniques for the automatic detection of error corrections in human-computer dialogues. *Proceedings of the NAACL Workshop on adaptation in dialogue systems* (pp. 33–40). East Stroudsburg, PA: Association for Computational Linguistics.

Knuth, D. (1972). *The art of computer programming, Vol. 3: Sorting and searching*. Reading, MA: Addison-Wesley.

Koedinger, K. R., Corbett, A. T., Ritter, S., & Shapiro, L. (2000). *Carnegie Learning's cognitive tutor summary research results.* Retrieved March 1, 2001, from http://www.carnegielearning.com

Kuipers, B. J. (1987a). New reasoning methods for artificial intelligence in medicine. *International Journal of Man–Machine Studies, 26,* 707–718.

Kuipers, B. J. (1987b). Qualitative simulation as causal explanation. *IEEE Transactions on Systems, Man, and Cybernetics, 17,* 432–444.

Kuipers, B. J. (1987c). Causal reasoning. In S. Shapiro (Ed.), *Encyclopedia of artificial intelligence* (pp. 817–832). New York: Wiley.

Kuipers, B. J., & Kassirer, J. P. (1984). Causal reasoning in medicine: Analysis of a protocol. *Cognitive Science, 8,* 363–385.

Kukich, K. (1992). Techniques for automatically correcting words in text. *ACM Computing Surveys, 24,* 377–439.

Kulik, J. A., & Kulik, C. C. (1988). Timing of feedback and verbal learning. *Review of Educational Research, 58,* 79–97.

Kwasny, S. (1981). Relaxation techniques for parsing grammatically ill-formed input in natural language understanding systems. *American Journal of Computational Linguistics, 7,* 99–108.

Lajoie, S. P., & Lesgold, A. (1989). Apprenticeship training in the workplace: Computer-coached practice environment as a new form of apprenticeship. *Machine-Mediated Learning 3,* 7–28.

Lakoff, G. (1972). Structural complexity in fairy tales. *The Study of Man, 1,* 128–150.

Lakoff, R. (1975). *Language and woman's place.* New York: Harper & Row.

Lane, H. C., & VanLehn, K. (in press). Teaching the tacit knowledge of programming to novices with natural language tutoring. In S. Fitzgerald & M. Guzdial (Eds.), special issue of *Computer Science Education.*

Lavoie, B., & Rambow, O. (1997). A fast and portable realizer for text generation. *Fifth Applied Natural Language Processing* (pp. 265–268). East Stroudsburg, PA: Association for Computational Linguistics.

Lee, C. H., & Evens, M. W. (2003). Interleaved syntactic and semantic processing for CIRCSIM-Tutor dialogues. In A. Radescu (Ed.), *Proceedings of Midwest Artificial Intelligence and Cognitive Science '03* (pp. 69–73). Madison, WI: Omni Press.

Lee, C. H., & Evens, M. W. (2004). Using selectional restrictions to parse and interpret student answers in a cardiovascular tutoring system. In E. Bertkowitz (Ed.), *Proceedings of Midwest Artificial Intelligence and Cognitive Science '04* (pp. 63–67). Schaumburg, IL: Roosevelt University.

Lee, C. H., Evens, M. W., & Glass, M. S. (2004). Looking at the student input to a natural language-based tutoring system. In N. Heffernan & P. Wiemer-Hastings (Eds.), *ITS 2004 Workshop on dialogue-based tutoring Systems* (pp. 15–22). Berlin, Germany: Springer-Verlag.

Lee, C. H., Seu, J. H., & Evens, M. W. (2002a). Building an ontology for CIRCSIM-Tutor. In S. Conlon (Ed.), *Midwest Artificial Intelligence and Cognitive Science 2002* (pp. 161–168). Chicago: Illinois Institute of Technology.

Lee, C. H., Seu, J. H., & Evens, M. W. (2002b). Automating the construction of case frames for CIRCSIM-Tutor. *International Conference on Advanced Science and Technology 2002* (pp. 59–65). Chicago: CAPAMA.

Lee, Y. H. (1990). *Handling ill-formed natural language input for an intelligent tutoring system.* Unpublished doctoral dissertation, Illinois Institute of Technology, Chicago.

Lee, Y. H., & Evens, M. W. (1998). Natural language interface for an expert system. *Expert Systems (International Journal of Knowledge Engineering), 15,* 233–239.

Lehnert, W. G. (1997), Information extraction: What have we learned? *Discourse Processes, 23,* 441–470.

Leinhardt, G., & Greeno, J. G. (1986). The cognitive skill of teaching. *Journal of Educational Psychology, 78,* 75–95.

Lemke, J. (1990). *Talking science: Language, learning, and values.* Norwood, NJ: Ablex.

Lepper, M. R., & Chabay, R. W. (1985). Intrinsic motivation and instruction: Conflicting views on the role of motivational processes in computer-based education. *Educational Psychologist, 20,* 217–230.

Lepper, M. R., & Chabay, R. W. (1988). Socializing the intelligent tutor: Bringing empathy to computer tutors. In H. Mandl & A. M. Lesgold (Eds.),

Learning issues for intelligent tutoring systems (pp. 242–257). Berlin, Germany: Springer.

Lepper, M. R., Woolverton, M., Mumme, D. L., & Gurtner, J. L. (1993). Motivational techniques of expert human tutors: Lessons for the design of computer-based tutors. In S. Lajoie & S. Derry (Eds.), *Computers as cognitive tools* (pp. 75–105). Hillsdale, NJ: Lawrence Erlbaum Associates.

Lesgold, A. M. (1988). Toward a theory of curriculum for use in designing intelligent instructional systems. In H. Mandl & A. M. Lesgold (Eds.), *Learning issues for intelligent tutoring systems* (pp. 114–123). Berlin, Germany: Springer-Verlag.

Lesgold, A. M. (1992). Assessment of intelligent training systems: Sherlock as an example. In E. Baker & H. O'Neil Jr. (Eds.), *Technology assessment: Estimating the future* (pp. 97–116). Hillsdale, NJ: Lawrence Erlbaum Associates.

Lesgold, A. M., Eggan, G., Katz, S., & Rao, G. (1992). Possibilities for assessment using computer-based apprenticeship environments. In W. Regian & V. J. Shute (Eds.), *Cognitive approaches to automated instruction* (pp. 49–80). Hillsdale, NJ: Lawrence Erlbaum Associates.

Lesgold, A. M., Katz, S., Greenberg, L., Hughes, E., & Eggan, G. (1992). Extensions of intelligent learning paradigms to support collaborative learning. In S. Dijkstra, H. Krammer, & J. J. G. Van Merrienboer (Eds.), *Instructional design models in computer-based learning environments* (pp. 291–311). Hillsdale, NJ: Lawrence Erlbaum Associates.

Lesgold, A. M., Lajoie, S., Bunzo, M., & Eggan, G. (1992). SHERLOCK: A coached practice environment for an electronics troubleshooting job. In J. Larkin, R. Chabay, & C. Scheftic (Eds.), *Computer-aided instruction and intelligent tutoring systems: Establishing communication and collaboration* (pp. 201–238). Hillsdale, NJ: Lawrence Erlbaum Associates.

Lesh, R., & Kelly, A. E. (1997). Teachers' evolving conceptions of one-on-one tutoring: A three-tiered teaching experiment. *Journal for Research in Mathematics Education, 28*(4), 398–430.

Li, J., Rovick, A. A., & Michael, J. A. (1992). ABASE: A hypermedia-based tutoring and authoring system. In I. Tomek (Ed.), *Fourth International Conference on Computer Assisted Learning, ICCAL '92* (pp. 380–390). Berlin, Germany: Springer-Verlag.

Li, J., Seu, J., Evens, M. W., Michael, J. A., & Rovick, A. A. (1992). Computer Dialogue System (CDS): A system for capturing computer-mediated dialogues. *Behavior Research Methods, Instruments, and Computers (Journal of the Psychonomic Society), 24,* 535–540.

Lindgren, A. (1999). *Pippi goes to school.* New York: Viking for Puffin Books.

Litman, D. J. (1996). Cue phrase classification using machine learning. *Journal of Artificial Intelligence Research, 5,* 53–94.

Litman, D. J., & Allen, J. F. (1987). A plan recognition model for subdialogues in conversations. *Cognitive Science, 11,* 163–200.

Litman, D. J., & Forbes-Riley, K. (2004). Annotating student emotional states in spoken tutoring dialogues. *Proceedings of the fifth workshop on discourse and dialogue (SIGDIAL)* (pp. 144–151). East Stroudsburg, PA: Association for Computational Linguistics.

Litman, D. J., Hirschberg, J. B., & Swerts, M. (2000). Predicting automatic speech recognition performance using prosodic cues. *Proceedings of the first Annual Meeting of the North American Chapter of the Association for Computational Linguistics* (pp. 218–225). East Stroudsburg, PA: Association for Computational Linguistics.

Litman, D. J., Rosé, C. P., Forbes-Riley, K., VanLehn, K., Bhembe, D., & Silliman, S. (2004). Spoken versus typed human and computer dialogue tutoring. In J. C. Lester, R. M. Vicari, & F. Paraguaçu (Eds.), *Intelligent Tutoring Systems 2004* (pp. 368–379). Berlin, Germany: Springer-Verlag.

Littman, D., Pinto, J., & Soloway, E. (1991). The knowledge required for tutorial planning: An empirical analysis. *Interactive Learning Environments, 1,* 124–151.

Louwerse, M. M., & Mitchell, H. H. (2003). Toward a taxonomy of a set of discourse markers in dialogue: A theoretical and computational linguistic account. *Discourse Processes, 35,* 199–239.

Luksa, F. (1994). *Pathophysiology tutor: Problem solving environment and content authoring tool.* Unpublished master's thesis, Illinois Institute of Technology, Chicago.

Lulis, E., & Evens, M. (2003). The use of analogies in human tutoring dialogues. In R. K. Freedman & C. Callaway (Eds.), *AAAI Symposium: Natural language generation in spoken and written dialogue* (pp. 178–183). Menlo Park, CA: AAAI Press.

Lulis, E., Evens, M. W., & Michael, J. A. (2003). Representation of analogies found in human tutoring sessions. In W. Chei (Ed.), *Proceedings of the Second IASTED International Conference on Information and Knowledge Sharing* (pp. 88–93). Anaheim, CA: ACTA Press.

Lulis, E., Michael, J. A., & Evens, M. W. (2004a). How human tutors employ analogy to facilitate understanding. In K. Forbus, D. Gentner, & T. Regier (Eds.), *Proceedings of COGSCI 2004* (pp. 861–866). Mahwah, NJ: Lawrence Erlbaum Associates.

Lulis, E., Michael, J. A., & Evens, M. W. (2004b). Using qualitative reasoning in the classroom and in electronic teaching systems. In F. de Kleer & K. Forbus (Eds.), *Workshop on qualitative reasoning* (pp. 121–127). Evanston, IL: Northwestern University. Berlin, Germany: Springer-Verlag.

Lulis, E., Michael, J. A., & Evens, M. W. (2004c). Implementing analogies in an electronic tutoring system. In J. C. Lester, R. M. Vicari, & F. Paraguaçu (Eds.), *ITS 2004* (pp. 751–761). Berlin, Germany: Springer-Verlag.

Ma, H. N., Evens, M. W., Trace, D. A., & Naeymi-Rad, F. (1992). A productive user environment for generating progress notes. *Fifth IEEE Symposium on computer-based medical systems* (pp. 486–493). Los Alamitos, CA: IEEE Computer Society Press.

Maloney, D. P., O'Kuma, T. L., Heiggelke, C. J., & Van Heuvelen, A. (2001). Surveying students' conceptual knowledge of electricity and magnetism. *American Journal of Physics, Physics Education Research Supplement, 69,* S12–S23.

Mann, W., & Thompson, S. A. (1986). Relational propositions in discourse. *Discourse Processes, 9,* 57–90.

Mann, W., & Thompson, S. A. (1987). *Rhetorical structure theory: A theory of text organization* (Tech. Rpt. No. ISI/RS-87-190). Marina del Rey: University of Southern California/Information Sciences Institute.

Mark, M. A., Koedinger, K. R., & Hadley, W. S. (1998). Elaborating models of algebraic expression-writing. In B. Goettl, H. Halff, C. Redfield, & V. J. Shute (Eds.), *Proceedings of Intelligent Tutoring Systems '98* (pp. 524–533). Berlin, Germany: Springer.

Markman, A. B. (1999). *Knowledge representation.* Mahwah, NJ: Lawrence Erlbaum Associates.

Martin, J., & VanLehn, K. (1995). Student assessment using Bayesian nets. *International Journal of Human–Computer Interaction, 42,* 575–591.

Matthiessen, C. M. I. M. (1991). Lexico (grammatical) choice in text generation. In C. Paris, W. Swartout, & W. Mann (Eds.), *Natural language generation in artificial intelligence and computational linguistics* (pp. 249–292), Dordrecht, The Netherlands: Kluwer.

Mayer, G. (1992). *Creating a structured knowlege base by parsing natural language text.* Unpublished doctoral dissertation, Illinois Institute of Technology, Chicago.

Mayer, G., Yamamoto, C., Evens, M., & Michael, J. (1989). Constructing a knowledge Base from a natural language text. *Proceedings of the 2nd Annual IEEE Symposium on Computer based medical systems* (pp. 98–107). Los Alamitos, CA: IEEE Computer Society Press.

Mazur, E. (1997). *Peer instruction*. Upper Saddle River, NJ: Prentice Hall.

McArthur, D., Stasz, C., & Zmuidzinas, M. (1990). Tutoring techniques in algebra. *Cognition and Instruction, 7,* 197–244.

McCarthy, J. (1960). Recursive functions of symbolic expressions and their computation by machine. *Communications of the Association for Computing Machinery, 3*, 184–195.

McCarthy, J. (1962). *Lisp 1.5 programmer's manual.* Cambridge, MA: MIT Press.

McCawley, J. D. (1979). *Adverbs, vowels, and other objects of wonder.* Chicago: University of Chicago Press.

McCawley, J. D. (1988). *The syntactic phenomena of English* (Vol. 2, pp. 754–768). Chicago: University of Chicago Press.

McCloskey, M. (1983). Naïve theories of motion. In D. Gentner & A. Stevens (Eds.), *Mental models* (pp. 103–120). Hillsdale, NJ: Lawrence Erlbaum Associates.

McDonald, D. D. (1980). *Natural language production as a process of decision making under constraint*. Unpublished doctoral dissertation, MIT, Cambridge, MA.

McDonald, D. D. (1983). Natural language generation as a computational problem: An introduction. In M. Brady & R. C. Berwick (Eds.), *Computational models of discourse* (pp. 209–265). Cambridge, MA: MIT Press.

McDonald, D. D. (1991). On the place of words in the generation process. In C. Paris, W. Swartout, & W. Mann (Eds.), *Natural language generation in artificial intelligence and computational linguistics* (pp. 227–247). Dordrecht, The Netherlands: Kluwer.

McElwain, C. K., & Evens, M. W. (1962). The Degarbler—a program for correcting machine-read Morse code. *Information and Control, 5,* 368–384.

McEwan, H., & Bull, B. (1991). The pedagogic nature of subject matter knowledge: The community of teaching and scholarship. *American Educational Research Journal, 28,* 316–334.

McKelvie, D., Brew, C., & Thompson, H. (1997). Using SGML as a basis for data-intensive NLP. *Fifth Annual Natural Language Processing* (pp. 229–236). East Stroudsburg, PA: Association for Computational Linguistics.

McKeown, K. R. (1985). *Text generation: Using discourse strategies and focus constraints to generate natural language text.* Cambridge, England: Cambridge University Press.

McNamara, D. S. (2004). SERT: Self-explanation reading training. *Discourse Processes, 38,* 1–30.

McRoy, S., & Hirst, G. (1995). The repair of speech act misunderstandings by abductive inference. *Computational Linguistics, 21,* 435–478.

Merrill, D. C., & Reiser, B. J. (1994). Scaffolding effective problem-solving strategies in interactive learning environments. In A. Ram and K. Eisell (Eds.), *COGSCI '94* (pp. 629–634). Mahwah, NJ: Lawrence Erlbaum Associates.

Merrill, D. C., Reiser, B. J., Ranney, M., & Trafton, J. G. (1992). Effective tutoring techniques: A comparison of human tutors and intelligent tutoring systesm. *Journal of the Learning Sciences, 2*(5), 277–305.

Meyer, B. J. (1975). *The organization of prose and its effect on memory.* Amsterdam: North-Holland.

Meyer, B. J. (1985). Prose analysis: Purposes, procedures, and problems. In B. K. Britton & J. B. Black (Eds.), *Understanding expository text* (pp. 11–64). Hillsdale, NJ: Lawrence Erlbaum Associates.

Michael, J. A. (1993). Teaching problem solving in small groups. In H. I. Modell & J. A. Michael (Eds.), Promoting active learning in the life science classroom. *Annals of the New York Academy of Sciences. 701,* 37–48.

Michael, J. A. (1998). Students' misconceptions about perceived physiological responses. *American Journal of Physiology, 274 (Advances in Physiology Education, 19),* S90–S98.

Michael, J. A. (2001). In pursuit of meaningful learning. *Advances in Physiology Education, 25,* 145–158.

Michael, J. A. (2002). Misconceptions—what students think they know. *Advances in Physiology Education, 26,* 5–6.

Michael, J. A., Haque, M. M., Rovick, A. A., & Evens, M. W. (1989). The pathophysiology tutor: A first step toward a smart tutor. In H. Maurer (Ed.), *International conference on computer assisted learning* (pp. 390–399). Berlin, Germany: Springer-Verlag.

Michael, J. A., & Modell, H. I. (2003). *Active learning in the college and secondary science classroom: A model for helping the learner to learn.* Mahwah, NJ: Lawrence Erlbaum Associates.

Michael, J. A., & Rovick, A. A. (1999). *Problem-solving in physiology.* Upper Saddle River, NJ: Prentice Hall.

Michael, J. A., Rovick, A. A., Evens, M. W., Shim, L., Woo, C., & Kim, N. (1992). The uses of multiple student inputs in modeling and lesson planning in

CAI and ICAI programs. In I. Tomek (Ed.), *Computer assisted learning, International Conference on Computer-Assisted Learning* (pp. 441–452). Berlin, Germany: Springer-Verlag.

Michael, J. A., Rovick, A. A., Glass, M. S., Zhou, Y., & Evens, M. (2003). Learning from a computer tutor with natural language capabilities. *Interactive Learning Environments, 11,* 233–262.

Michael, J. A., Wenderoth, M. P., Modell, H. I., Cliff, W., Horwirz, B., McHale, P., et al. (2002). Undergraduates' understanding of cardiovascular phenomena. *Advances in Physiology Education 26,* 72–84.

Miller, G. A., Beckwith, R., Fellbaum, C., Gross, D., & Miller, K. J. (1991). WordNet, an online lexical database. *Journal of Lexicography, 4,* 1–75.

Miller, L. A., Heidorn, G. E., & Jensen, K. (1981). Text-critiquing with the EPISTLE System: An author's aid to better syntax. In A. Orden & M. Evens (Eds.), *Proceedings of the National Computer Conference* (pp. 649–655). Reston, VA: AFIPS Press.

Mills, B. (2001). Using the Atlas Planning Engine to drive an intelligent tutoring system. In J. Kolen & I. Russell (Eds.), *Proceedings of the Florida Artificial Intelligence Research Symposium, FLAIRS 2001* (pp. 211–215). Menlo Park, CA: AAAI Press.

Mills, B., Evens, M. W., & Freedman, R. (2004). Implementing directed lines of reasoning in an intelligent tutoring system using the Atlas Planning Environment. In S. Latifi (Ed.), *Proceedings of the International Conference on Information Technology Coding and Computing* (pp. 729–733). Los Alamitos, CA: IEE Computer Society Press.

Minstrell, J., & Kraus, P. (2001). The teaching and learning of physics. In J. Brophy (Ed.), *Subject-specific instructional methods and activities, 8* (pp. 215–238). Greenwich, CT: JAI.

Mittal, V. O. (1999). *Generating natural language descriptions with integrated text and examples.* Mahwah, NJ: Lawrence Erlbaum Associates.

Modell, H. I. (2002). How to help students understand physiology? Emphasize general models. *Advances in Physiology Education, 23,* 101–107.

Modell, H. I., Michael, J. A., Adamson, T., Goldberg, J., Horwitz, B. A., Bruce, D. S., et al. (2000). Helping undergraduates repair faulty mental models in the student laboratory. *Advances in Physiology Education, 23,* 82–90.

Moore, J. D. (1993). What makes human explanations effective? In M. Polson (Ed.), *Proceedings of the fifteenth annual meeting of the Cognitive Science Society* (pp. 131–136). Hillsdale, NJ: Lawrence Erlbaum Associates.

Moore, J. D. (1995). *Participating in explanatory dialogues.* Cambridge, MA: MIT Press.

Moore, J. D., Foster, M. E., Lemon, O., & White, M. (2004). Generating tailored, comparative descriptions in spoken dialogue. In V. Barr & Z. Markov (Eds.), *Proceedings of the Seventeenth International Florida Artificial Intelligence Research Society Conference* (pp. 917–922). Menlo Park, CA: AAAI Press.

Moore, J. D., Lemaire, B., & Rosenblum, J. (1996). Discourse generation for instructional applications: Identifying and using prior relevant explanations. *Journal of the Learning Sciences, 5,* 49–94.

Moore, J. D., & Paris, C. L. (1989). Planning text for advisory dialogues. *Proceedings of the 27th annual meeting of the Association for Computational*

Linguistics (pp. 203–211). East Stroudsburg, PA: Association for Computational Linguistics.

Moore, J. D., & Paris, C. L. (1993). Planning text for advisory dialogues: Capturing intentional and rhetorical structure. *Computational Linguistics, 19,* 651–695.

Moore, J. D., & Pollack, M. (1992). A problem for RST: The need for multi-level discourse analysis. *Computational Linguistics, 18,* 537–544.

Moore, J. D., Porayska-Pomsta, K., Varges, S., & Zinn, C. (2004). Generating tutorial feedback with affect. In T. Barr & Z. Markov (Eds.), *Proceedings of the Seventeenth International Florida Artificial Intelligence Research Society Conference* (pp. 923–928). Menlo Park, CA: AAAI Press.

Moser, M., & Moore, J. D. (1995). Investigating cue selection and placement in tutorial discourse. *Proceedings of the 33rd annual meeting of the Association for Computational Linguistics* (pp. 130–135). East Stroudsburg, PA: Association for Computational Linguistics.

Murray, E. (2002). Challenges in educational research. *Medical Education, 36,* 110–112.

Murray, T., Schultz, K., Brown, D., & Clement, J. (1990). An analogy-based computer tutor for remediating physics misconceptions. *Journal of Interactive Learning Environments, 1,* 79–101.

Murray, W. R. (1989). Control for intelligent tutoring systems: A blackboard-based instructional planner. In D. Bierman, J. Breuker, & J. Sandberg (Eds.), *Proceedings of the Fourth International Conference on Artificial Intelligence in Education, AI-ED 89* (pp. 150–168). Amsterdam: IOS Press.

Nakatani, C., & Traum, D. (1998, May). *Draft: Discourse coding manual.* Paper presented at the meeting of the Discourse Resource Initiative, Chiba, Japan.

Nakatani, C., Grosz, B., Ahn, D., & Hirschberg, J. (1995). *Instructions for annotating discourses* (Tech. Rpt. No. 21-95). Cambridge, MA: Harvard University, Center for Research in Computing Technology.

Nathan, M. J., & Petrosino, A. (2003). Expert blind spot among preservice teachers. *American Educational Research Journal, 40,* 905–928.

Norman, D. A. (1990). *The design of everyday things.* New York: Doubleday.

Norman, D. A. (1992). *Turn signals are the facial expressions of automobiles.* Reading, MA: Addison-Wesley.

Norman, D. A., & Draper, S. W. (1986). *User centered system design: New perspectives on human–computer interaction.* Hillsdale, NJ: Lawrence Erlbaum Associates.

Novak, J. D., & Gowin, D. B. (1984). *Learning how to learn*. Cambridge, England: Cambridge University Press.

Nyberg, E. H., & Tomita, M. (1988). *Generation kit and transformation kit Version 3.2 User's Manual* (Rpt. No. CMU-CMT-88, Memo from the Center for Machine Translation). Carnegie-Mellon University, Pittsburgh, PA.

Ohlsson, S. (1987). Some principles of intelligent tutoring. In R. Lawler & M. Yazdani (Eds.), *Artificial intelligence and education* (Vol. I, pp. 203–297). Norwood, NJ: Ablex.

Ohlsson, S. (1992). Constraint-based student modeling, *Artificial Intelligence in Education, 3,* 429–447.

Ottesen, J. T., & Danielsen, M. (2000). *Mathematical modelling in medicine.* Amsterdam: IOS Press.

Oversteegen, L. (1997). On the pragmatic nature of causal and contrastive connectives. *Discourse Processes, 24,* 51–86.

Palmer, M. (1990). *Semantic processing for finite domains.* Cambridge, England: Cambridge University Press.

Paris, C. (1985). Description strategies for naive and expert users. *Proceedings of the 23rd annual meeting of the Association for Computational Linguistics* (pp. 238–245). East Stroudsburg, PA: Association for Computational Linguistics.

Paris, C. (1988). Tailoring object descriptions to the user's level of expertise. *Computational Linguistics, 14,* 64–78.

Patel, N., Glass, M. S., & Kim, J. H. (2003). Data collection applications for the NCA&T algebra tutoring (Wooz Tutor) project. In A. Ralescu (Ed.), *Proceedings of the Fourteenth Midwest Artificial Intelligence and Cognitive Science Conference* (pp. 120–125). Madison, WI: Omni Press.

Pea, R. (2004). The social and technological dimensions of scaffolding and related theoretical concepts for learning, education, and human activity. *Journal of the Learning Sciences, 13,* 423–452.

Pellegrino, J. W., Chudowsky, N., & Glaser, R. (Eds.). (2001). *Knowing what students know: The science and design of educational assessment.* Washington, DC: National Academy Press.

Penberthy, J. S., & Weld, D. (1992). UCPOP: A sound, complete, partial order planner for ADL. *Proceedings of the Third International Conference on Knowledge Representation and Reasoning* (pp. 103–114). Los Altos, CA: Kaufmann.

Person, N. K., Bautista, L., Graesser, A. C., Mathews, E. C., & The Tutoring Research Group. (2001). Evaluating student learning gains in two versions of Auto-Tutor. In J. D. Moore, C. L. Redfield, & W. L. Johnson (Eds.), *Proceedings of Artificial Intelligence in Education* (pp. 246–255). Amsterdam: IOS Press.

Person, N. K., Graesser, A. C., Harter, D. C., Mathews, E. C., & The Tutoring Research Group. (2000). Dialog move generation and conversation management in Auto-Tutor. In C. P. Rosé & R. K. Freedman (Eds.), *Proceedings of the AAAI Fall Symposium on building dialogue systems for tutorial applications* (pp. 87–94). Menlo Park, CA: AAAI Press.

Person, N. K., Graesser, A. C., Magliano, J. P., & Kreuz, R. J. (1994). Inferring what the student knows in one-to-one tutoring: The role of student questions and answers. *Learning and Individual Differences, 6,* 205–229.

Person, N. K., Kreuz, R. J., Zwaan, R. A., & Graesser, A. C. (1995). Pragmatics and pedagogy: Conversational rules and politeness strategies may inhibit effective tutoring. *Cognition and Instruction, 13,* 161–188.

Peterson, J. (1986). A note on undetected typing errors. *Communications of the ACM, 29*(7), 633–637.

Plato (1937). *The dialogues of Plato.* B. Jowett (Trans.). New York: Random House.

Pon-Barry, H., Clark, B., Schultz, K., Bratt, E. O., & Peters, S. (2004a). Advantages of spoken language in dialogue-based tutoring systems. In J. C. Lester, R. M. Vicari, & F. Paraguaçu (Eds.), *Intelligent Tutoring Systems 2004* (pp. 390–400). Berlin, Germany: Springer-Verlag.

Pon-Barry, H., Clark, B. Z., Schultz, K., Bratt, E. O., & Peters, S. (2004b). Evaluating the effectiveness of SCoT—a spoken conversational tutor. In N. Heffernan & P. Wiemer-Hastings (Eds.), *Proceedings of the workshop on dialog-based intelligent tutoring systems, ITS 2004* (pp. 23–32). Berlin, Germany: Springer-Verlag.

Pon-Barry, H., Clark, B. Z., Schultz, K., Bratt, E. O., & Peters, S. (2004c). Contextualizing learning in a reflective conversational tutor. *Proceedings of the Fourth IEEE International Conference on Advanced Learning Technologies* (pp. 236–240). Los Alamitos, CA: IEEE Computer Society Publishing Services.

Portele, T. (2002). Data-driven classification of linguistic styles in spoken dialogues. In S. C. Tseng (Ed.), *COLING 2002* (pp. 807–813). East Stroudsburg, PA: Association fo Computational Linguistics.

Propp, P. (1968). *The morphology of the folktale* (L. Scott, Trans.). Austin: University of Texas Press.

Quinlan, R. J. (1993). *C4.5 programs for machine learning.* Los Altos, CA: Kaufmann.

Quintana, C., Reiser, B., Davis, E., Krajcik, J., Fretz, E., Duncan, R. J., et al. (2004). A scaffolding design framework for software to support science inquiry. *Journal of the Learning Sciences, 13,* 337–386.

Ramachandran, K. (1994). *Lexical choice in surface generation.* Unpublished masters' thesis, Illinois Institute of Technology, Chicago.

Ramachandran, K., & Evens, M. (1995). Lexical choice for an intelligent tutoring system. In M. Evens (Ed.), *Proceedings of MAICSS '95* (pp. 53–57). Carbondale, IL: Division of Continuing Education, Southern Illinois University.

Ramaswami, S. (1993). *User interface for an intelligent tutoring system.* Unpublished paper, Department of Computer Science, Illinois Institute of Technology, Chicago, IL.

Ravid, R. (2000). *Practical statistics for educators* (2nd ed.). Lanham, MD: University Press of America, Inc.

Reiser, B. J. (2004). Scaffolding complex learning: The mechanisms of structuring and problematizing student work. *Journal of the Learning Sciences, 13,* 274–304.

Reiser, B. J., Tabak, I., Sandoval, W. A., Smith, B. K., Steinmuller, F., & Leone, A. J. (2001). BGuILE: Strategic and conceptual scaffolds for scientific inquiry in biology classrooms. In S. M. Carver & D. Klahr (Eds.), *Cognition and instruction: Twenty-five years of progress* (pp. 263–305). Mahwah, NJ: Lawrence Erlbaum Associates.

Reiter, E. (1991). A new model of lexical choice for nouns. *Computational Intelligence, 7,* 240–251.

Reiter, E. (1994). NLG vs. templates. In G. Adomi & M. Zock (Eds.), *Proceedings of the Fifth European Workshop on NLG* (pp. 95–105). Berlin, Germany: Springer-Verlag.

Reiter, E., Cawsey, A., Osman, L., & Roff, Y. (1997). Knowledge acquisition for content selection. In W. Hoeppner (Ed.), *Proceedings of the 1997 European Workshop on NLG* (pp. 117–126), Duisberg, Germany: Gerhard Mercator Universität.

Reiter, E., & Dale, R. (1999). *Building natural language generation systems.* Cambridge, England: Cambridge University Press.

Rich, C., & Sidner, C. L. (1998). COLLAGEN: A collaboration manager for software interface agents. *An International Journal: User Modeling and User-Adapted Interaction, 8,* 315–350.

Rich, E. (1982) Programs as data for their help systems. In H. L. Morgan (Ed.), *Proceedings of the National Computer Conference* (pp. 481–485). Reston, VA: AFIPS Press.

Rickel, J., Lesh, N., Rich, C., Sidner, C. L., & Gertner, A. (2002). Collaborative discourse theory as a foundation for tutorial dialogue. In S. A. Cerri, G. Gouardères, & F. Paraguaçu (Eds.), *ITS 2002* (pp. 542–551). Berlin, Germany: Springer-Verlag.

Robert, J. J. S. (1991). *Design and software engineering of a hypermedia medical record system.* Unpublished doctoral dissertation, Illinois Institute of Technology, Chicago.

Robert, J. J. S., Prakash, S., Naeymi-Rad, F., Trace, D., Carmony, L., & Evens, M. W. (1991). MEDRIS: The hypermedia approach to medical record input—software engineering techniques for developing a hypermedia system. *Proceedings of the Fourth Annual Symposium on computer based medical systems* (pp. 44–51). Los Alamitos, CA: IEEE Computer Society Press.

Robinson, J. J. (1982). DIAGRAM: A grammar for dialogues. *Communications of the ACM, 25*(1), 27–47.

Roche, E., & Schabes, Y. (1997). *Finite-state language processing.* Cambridge, MA: MIT Press.

Rosé, C. P. (1997a). *Robust interactive dialogue interpretation.* Unpublished doctoral dissertation, Carnegie Mellon University, Pittsburgh, PA.

Rosé, C. P. (1997b). The role of natural language interaction in electronic trouble-shooting. *Proceedings of the Energy Week Conference* (pp. 145–152). New York: American Society of Mechanical Engineers Press.

Rosé, C. P. (2000a). A framework for robust semantic interpretation. *First meeting of the North American Chapter of the ACL* (pp. 311–318). East Stroudsburg, PA: Association for Computational Linguistics.

Rosé, C. P. (2000b). Facilitating the rapid development of language understanding interfaces for tutoring systems. In C. P. Rosé & R. K. Freedman (Eds.), *Proceedings of the AAAI Fall Symposium on building dialogue systems for tutorial applications* (pp. 87–95). Menlo Park, CA: AAAI Press.

Rosé, C. P., Bhembe, D., Roque, A., Siler, S., Shrivastava, R., & VanLehn, K. (2002). A hybrid natural language understanding approach for robust selection of tutoring goals. In S. A. Cerri, G. Gouardères, & F. Paraguaçu (Eds.), *ITS 2002* (pp. 552–561). Berlin, Germany: Springer-Verlag.

Rosé, C. P., Di Eugenio, B., & Moore, J. D. (1999). A dialogue based tutoring system for basic electricity and electronics. In S. P. Lajoie & M. Vivet (Eds.), *Proceedings of the Ninth World Conference on Artificial Intelligence in Education* (pp. 759–761). Amsterdam: IOS Press.

Rosé, C. P., Gaydos, A., Hall, B., Roque, A., & VanLehn, K. (2003). Overcoming the knowledge engineering bottleneck for understanding student language input. *Proceedings of Artificial Intelligence in Education* (pp. 315–322). Amsterdam: IOS Press.

Rosé, C. P., Jordan, P., Ringenberg, M., Siler, S., VanLehn, K., & Weinstein, A. (2001). Interactive conceptual tutoring in Atlas-Andes. In J. D. Moore, C. L. Redfield, & W. L. Johnson (Eds.), *Proceedings of Artificial Intelligence in Education* (pp. 256–266). Amsterdam: IOS Press.

Rosé, C. P., & Lavie, A. (2001). Balancing robustness and efficiency in unification augmented context-free parsers for large practical applications. In J. C. Junqua & G. Van Noord (Eds.), *Robustness in language and speech technologies* (pp. 240–269). Dordrecht, The Netherlands: Kluwer.

Rosé, C. P., Moore, J. D., VanLehn, K., & Allbritton, D. (2001). A comparative evaluation of Socratic versus didactic tutoring. In J. D. Moore (Ed.), *Proceedings of the Cognitive Science Society* (pp. 869–874). Mahwah, NJ: Lawrence Erlbaum Associates.

Rosé, C. P., & Torrey, C. (2004). DReSDeN: Toward a trainable tutorial dialogue manager to support negotiation dialogues for learning and reflection. In J. C. Lester, R. M. Vicari, & F. Paraguaçu (Eds.), *Proceedings of Intelligent Tutoring Systems, ITS 2004* (pp. 412–422). Berlin, Germany: Springer-Verlag.

Rosé, C. P., Torrey, C., & Aleven, V. (2004). Guided exploratory learning vs. directed learning in a simulation environment for thermodynamics: A pilot study. In N. Heffernan & P. Wiemer-Hastings (Eds.), *Proceedings of the workshop on dialog-based intelligent tutoring systems, ITS 2004* (pp. 43–47). Berlin, Germany: Springer-Verlag.

Rosé, C. P., Torrey, C., Aleven, V., Robinson, A., Wu, C., & Forbus, K. (2004). CycleTalk: Toward a dialogue agent that guides design with an articulate simulator. In J. C. Lester, R. M. Vicari, & F. Paraguaçu (Eds.), *ITS 2004* (pp. 401–411). Berlin, Germany: Springer-Verlag.

Roth, W.-M., & Lawless, D. (2002). Science, culture, and the emergence of language. *Science Education, 86,* 368–385.

Rovick, A., & Brenner, L. (1983). HEARTSIM: A cardiovascular simulation with didactic feedback. *The Physiologist, 26,* 236–239.

Rovick, A. A., & Michael, J. A. (1986, July). *CIRCSIM: An IBM PC computer teaching exercise on blood pressure regulation*. Paper presented at the XXX IUPS Congress, Vancouver, Canada.

Rovick, A. A., & Michael, J. A. (1992). The prediction table: A tool for assessing students' knowledge. *American Journal of Physiology, 263,* S33–S36.

Rovick, A. A., & Michael, J. A. (1995). Software demonstration: GASP, a computer program for teaching the chemical control of ventilation. *Advances in Physiology Education, 13,* S98.

Russell, D. M. (1988). IDE: The interpreter. In J. Psotka, L. D. Massey, & S. A. Mutter (Eds.), *Intelligent tutoring systems: Lessons learned* (pp. 223–249). Hillsdale, NJ: Lawrence Erlbaum Associates.

Russell, D. M., Moran, T. P., & Jordan, D. S. (1988). The instructional design environment. In J. Psotka, L. D. Massey, & S. A. Mutter (Eds.), *Intelligent tutoring systems: Lessons learned* (pp. 203–228), Hillsdale, NJ: Lawrence Erlbaum Associates.

Sacerdoti, E. D. (1974). Planning in a hierarchy of abstraction spaces. *Artificial Intelligence, 5,* 115–135.

Sacerdoti, E. D. (1977). *A structure for plans and behavior.* Amsterdam: Elsevier-North Holland.

Sager, N. (1981). *Natural language information processing.* Reading, MA: Addison-Wesley.

Sager, N. (1986). Sublanguage: Linguistic phenomenon, computational tool. In R. Grishman & R. Kittredge (Eds.), *Analyzing language in restrictive domains* (pp. 1–17). Hillside, NJ: Lawrence Erlbaum Associates.

Sanders, G. (1995). *Generation of explanations and multi-turn discourse structures in tutorial dialogue based on transcript analysis.* Unpublished doctoral dissertation, Illinois Institute of Technology, Chicago.

Sanders, T. J. M. (1997). Semantic and pragmatic sources of coherence: On the categorization of coherence relations in context. *Discourse Processes, 24,* 119–148.

Sanders, T. J. M., & Noordman, L. G. M. (2000). The role of coherence relations and their linguistic markers in text processing. *Discourse Processes, 29,* 37–60.

Sanders, T. J. M., Spooren, W. P. M., & Noordman, L. G. M. (1992). Towards a taxonomy of coherence relations. *Discourse Processes, 15,* 1–35.

Schank, R. C., & Riesbeck, C. K. (1981). *Inside computer understanding.* Hillsdale, NJ: Lawrence Erlbaum Associates.

Schegloff, E. A., & Sacks, H. (1973). Opening up closings. *Semiotica, 8,* 289–327.

Schiffrin, D. (1987). *Discourse markers.* Cambridge, England: Cambridge University Press.

Schooler, L. L., & Anderson, J. R. (1990). The disruptive potential of immediate feedback. In M. Piatelli-Polmarini (Ed.), *Cognitive Science Conference* (pp. 702–708). Hillsdale, NJ: Lawrence Erlbaum Associates.

Schulze, K. G., Shelby, R. N., Treacy, D. J., Wintersgill, M. C., VanLehn, K., & Gertner, A. (2000). ANDES: An intelligent tutoring system for classical physics. *Journal of Electronic Publishing, 6,* 7227.

Self, J. A. (1990). Bypassing the intractable problem of student modeling. In C. Frasson & G. Gauthier (Eds.), *Intelligent tutoring systems: At the crossroads of artificial intelligence and education* (pp. 107–123). Norwood, NJ: Ablex.

Seu, J. H. (1992). *The development of an input understander for an intelligent tutoring system based on a sublanguage study.* Unpublished doctoral dissertation, Illinois Institute of Technology, Chicago.

Seu, J. H., Chang, R.-C., Li, J., Evens, M., Michael, J. A., & Rovick, A. A. (1991). Language differences in face-to-face and keyboard-to-keyboard sessions. In K. Hammond & D. Gentner (Eds.), *Proceedings of the Cognitive Science Conference* (pp. 576–580). Mahwah, NJ: Lawrence Erlbaum Associates.

Shah, F., Evens, M. W., Michael, J. A., & Rovick, A. A. (2002). Classifying student initiatives and tutor responses in human keyboard-to-keyboard tutoring sessions. *Discourse Processes, 33,* 23–52.

Shanahan, T. (1998). On the effectiveness and limitations of tutoring in reading. *Review of Research in Education, 23,* 217–234.

Sherin, B., Reiser, B. J., & Edelson, D. (2004). Scaffolding analysis: Extending the scaffolding metaphor to learning artifacts. *Journal of the Learning Sciences, 13,* 387–422.

Sherwood, B. A., & Sherwood, J. N. (1988). *The cT language.* Champaign, IL: Stipes Publishing Company.

Sherwood, L. (2001). *Human physiology: From cells to systems* (4th ed.). Pacific Grove, CA: Brooks/Cole.

Shim, L. (1991). *Student modeling for an intelligent tutoring system based on the analysis of human tutoring sessions.* Unpublished doctoral dissertation, Illinois Institute of Technology, Chicago.

Shim, L., Evens, M., Michael, J. A., & Rovick, A. A. (1991).Effective cognitive modeling in an intelligent tutoring system for cardiovascular physiology. *Proceedings of the fourth annual IEEE Symposium on computer based medical systems* (pp. 338–345). Los Alamitos, CA: IEEE Computer Society Press.

Shim, L., Evens, M. W., Rovick, A. A., & Michael, J. A. (1990). Student modeling issues in intelligent tutoring systems. In E. W. Steeg (Ed.), *Proceedings of the third University of New Brunswick Artificial Intelligence Workshop* (pp. 127–136), Fredericton, NB: University of New Brunswick.

Shneiderman, B. (1984). Response time and display rate in human performance with computers. *ACM Computing Surveys, 16,* 265–285.

Shortliffe, E. H. (1976). *Computer-based medical consultations: MYCIN.* New York: Elsevier-North-Holland.

Shulman, L. S. (1986a). Paradigms and research programs for the study of teaching. In M. Wittrock (Ed.), *Handbook of research on teaching* (pp. 3–38). New York: Macmillan

Shulman, L. S. (1986b) Those who understand: Knowledge growth in teaching. *Educational Researcher 15*(2), 4–14.

Siegel, S., & Castellan, N. J. (1988). *Nonparametric statistics for the behavioral sciences.* Boston: McGraw-Hill.

Simon, H. A. (2001). Learning to research about learning. In S. M. Carver & D. Klahr (Eds.), *Cognition and instruction: Twenty-five years of progress* (pp. 205–226). Mahwah, NJ: Lawrence Erlbaum Associates.

Sinclair, J. M., & Coulthard, R. M. (1975). *Towards an analysis of discourse: The English used by teachers and pupils.* Oxford, England: Oxford University Press.

Smadja, F. (1993). Retrieving collocations from text. *Computational Linguistics, 19,* 143–177.

Smith, J. P., III, diSessa, A. A., & Roschelle, J. (1993). Misconceptions reconceived: A constructivist analysis of knowledge in transition. *Journal of the Learning Sciences, 3,* 115–163.

Sperberg-McQueen, C. M., & Burnard, L. (1994). The design of the TEI encoding scheme. *Computers and the Humanities, 29,* 17–39.

Stefik, M. (1981). Planning and meta-planning (MOLGEN: Part 1 and 2). *Artificial Intelligence, 16*(2), 111–140.

Steinberg, E. R. (1984). *Teaching computers to teach.* Hillsdale, NJ: Lawrence Erlbaum Associates.

Stevens, A., & Collins, A. (1977). The goal structure of a Socratic tutor. *1977 national annual conference of the Association for Computing Machinery* (pp. 256–263). New York: ACM Press.

Stevens, A., & Collins, A. (1980). Multiple conceptual models of a complex system. In R. Snow, P. Frederico, & W. Montague (Eds.), *Aptitude, learning, and instruction* (Vol. 2, pp. 177–197). Hillsdale, NJ: Lawrence Erlbaum Associates.

Stevens, A., Collins, A., & Goldin, S. E. (1982). Misconceptions in students' understanding. In D. Sleeman & J. S. Brown (Eds.), *Intelligent tutoring systems* (pp. 13–24). New York: Academic.

Sussman, G. A. (1975). *A computational model of skill acquisition.* New York: Elsevier-North-Holland.

Tabak, I. (2004). Synergy: A complement to emerging patterns of distributed scaffolding. *Journal of the Learning Sciences, 13,* 305–336.

Tamir, P., & Zohar, A. (1991). Anthropomorphism and teleology in reasoning about biological phenomena. *Science Education, 75,* 57–67.

Tate, A. (1975). *Project planning using a hierarchic non-linear planner* (Res. Rpt. No. 25). Edinburgh, Scotland: University of Edinburgh, Department of Artificial Intelligence.

Tate, A. (1977). Interacting goals and their use. *Proceedings of the Fourth International Joint Conference on Artificial Intelligence* (pp. 215–218). Pittsburgh, PA: Carnegie-Mellon University.

Thompson, B. H. (1980). Linguistic analysis of natural language communication with computers. *COLING '80* (pp. 190-201). Kyoto, Japan: Kyoto University.

Thorndyke, P. W. (1977). Cognitive structures in comprehension and memory of narrative discourse. *Cognitive Psychology, 9,* 77–110.

Trace, D. A., Evens, M., Naeymi-Rad, F., & Carmony, L. (1990). Medical information management: The MEDAS approach. In R. A. Miller (Ed.), *Symposium on Computer Applications in Medical Care* (pp. 635–639). Los Alamitos, CA: IEEE Computer Society Press.

Traum, D., & Allen, J. (1994). Discourse obligations in dialogue processing. *Proceedings of the ACL* (pp. 1–8). East Stroudsburg, PA: Association for Computational Linguistics.

U.S. Government, Department of Education. (2001). *No Child Left Behind Act of 2001.* Retrieved January 5, 2005 from www.ed.gov/policy/elsec/leg/esea02/ beginning.html#sec

Van der Linden, K., & Di Eugenio, B. (1996a). A corpus study of negative imperatives in natural language instructions. In F. Tsujii (Ed.), *COLING '96* (pp. 346–351). East Stroudsburg, PA: Association for Computational Linguistics.

Van der Linden, K., & Di Eugenio, B. (1996b). Learning micro-planning rules for preventative expressions. *International Conference on Natural Language Generation 96* (pp. 11–20). East Stroudsburg, PA: Association for Computational Linguistics.

VanLehn, K. (1982). Bugs are not enough: Empirical studies of bugs, impasses, and repairs in procedural skills. *The Journal of Mathematical Behavior, 3,* 3–71.

VanLehn, K. (1988). Student modeling. In M. C. Polson & J. J. Richardson (Eds.), *Foundations of intelligent tutoring systems* (pp. 55–78). Hillsdale, NJ: Lawrence Erlbaum Associates.

VanLehn, K. (1996). Conceptual and meta learning during coached problem solving. In C. Frasson, G. Gauthier, & G. I. McCalla (Eds.), *ITS 96* (pp. 29–47). Berlin, Germany: Springer.

VanLehn, K., Bhembe, D., Chi, M., Lynch, C., Schulze, K., Shelby, R., et al. (2004). Implicit vs. explicit learning of strategies in a non-procedural cognitive skill. In J. C. Lester, R. M. Vicari, & F. Paraguaçu (Eds.), *ITS 2004* (pp. 521–530). Berlin, Germany: Springer-Verlag.

VanLehn, K., Freedman, R., Jordan, P., Murray, C., Osan, R., Ringenberg, et al. (2000). Fading and deepening: The next steps for Andes and other model-tracing tutors. In G. Gauthier, C. Frasson, & K. VanLehn (Eds.), *Proceedings of ITS 2000* (pp. 474–483). Berlin, Germany: Springer.

VanLehn, K., Jordan, P. W., Rosé, C. P., Bhembe, D., Bottner, M., Gaydos, A., et al. (2002a). The architecture of Why2-Atlas: A coach for qualitative physics essay writing. In S. A. Cerri, G. Gouardères, & F. Paraguaçu (Eds.), *ITS 2002* (pp. 158–167). Berlin, Germany: Springer-Verlag.

VanLehn, K., Siler, S., Murray, C., & Baggett, W. (1998). What makes a tutorial event effective? In M. A. Gernsbacher & S. Derry (Eds.), *OGSCI '98* (pp. 1084–1089). Mahwah, NJ: Lawrence Erlbaum Associates.

VanLehn, K., Lynch, C., Taylor, L., Weinstein, A., Shelby, R., Schulze, K., et al. (2002b). Minimally invasive tutoring of complex physics problem solving. In S. A. Cerri, G. Gouardères, & F. Paraguaçu (Eds.), *ITS 2002* (pp. 367–376). Berlin, Germany: Springer-Verlag.

Vasandani, V., & Govindaraj, T. (1994). Intelligent diagnostic problem solving tutor: An experimental evaluation. *IEEE Transactions on Systems, Man and Cybernetics, 3,* 1739–1744.

Vasandani, V., & Govindaraj, T. (1995). Knowledge organization in intelligent tutoring systems for diagnostic problem solving in complex dynamic domains. *IEEE Transactions on Systems, Man and Cybernetics, 25,* 1076–1096.

Vassileva, J. (1995). Reactive instructional planning to support interacting teaching strategies. In J. Greer (Ed.), *Proceedings of the Seventh World Conference on AI and Education (AI-ED '95)* (pp. 334–342). Charlottesville, VA: AACE.

Vicente, A., & Pain, H. (2002). Informing the detection of the students' motivational state: An empirical study. In S. A. Cerri, G. Gourdères, & F. Paraguaçu (Eds.), *Intelligent Tutoring Systems 2002* (pp. 933–943). Berlin, Germany: Springer-Verlag.

Vockell, E. L., & Rivers, R. H. (1984). *Computerized science simulations: Stimulus to generalized problem solving capabilities*. Paper presented at the annual convention of the American Educational Research Association, New Orleans, LA.

Walker, M., & Whittaker, S. (1990). Mixed initiative in dialogue: An investigation into discourse segmentation. *Proceedings of the 28th annual meeting of the Association for Computational Linguistics* (pp. 77–78). East Stroudsburg, PA: Association for Computational Linguistics.

Walters, J. (1993). *Use of anaphora in human tutoring follows the underlying tutoring plan structure*. Unpublished manuscript, Illinois Institute of Technology, Chicago.

Wandersee, J. H., Mintzes, J. A., & Novak, J. D. (1994). Research on alternative conceptions in science. In D. I. Gabel (Ed.), *Handbook of research on science teaching and learning* (pp. 131–210). New York: Macmillan.

Webber, B. (1982). So what can we talk about now? In M. Brody & R. Berwick (Eds.), *Computational models of discourse* (pp. 331–371). Cambridge, MA: MIT Press.

Webber, C. (2004). From errors to conceptions—An approach to student diagnosis. In J. C. Lester, R. M. Vicari, & F. Paraguaçu (Eds.), *ITS 2004* (pp. 710–719). Berlin, Germany: Springer-Verlag.

Weischedel, R., & Sondheimer, N. (1983). Meta-rules as a basis for processing ill-formed input. *American Journal of Computational Linguistics, 9,* 161–178.

Weld, D. S. (1994). An introduction to least commitment planning, *AI Magazine, 15,* 27–61.

Weld, D. S., & de Kleer, J. (1990). *Readings in qualitative reasoning about physical systems*. San Mateo, CA: Kaufmann.

Wells, G. (1999). *Dialogic inquiry.* Cambridge England: Cambridge University Press.

Wenger, E. (1987). *Artificial intelligence and tutoring systems*. Los Altos, CA: Kaufmann.

Werner, O. (1974). The synthetic informant model: On the simulation of large lexical/semantic fields. In M. Loflin & J. Silverberg (Eds.), *Discourse and difference in cognitive anthropology* (pp. 45–83). The Hague, Netherlands: Mouton.

Wescoat, M. T. (1987). Practical instructions for working with the formalism of LFG. In J. Bresnan, (Ed.), *Lexical functional grammar* (pp. 1–39). Stanford CA: Stanford University, Linguistics Summer Institute.

Wiebe, J., Bruce, R., & O'Hara, T. (1999). Development and use of a gold-standard data set for subjectivity classifications. *Proceedings of the annual meeting of the Association for Computational Linguistics '99* (pp. 246–253). East Stroudsburg, PA: Association for Computational Linguistics.

Wielinga, B. J., & Breuker, J. A. (1990). Models of expertise. *International Journal of Intelligent Systems, 5,* 497–509.

Wiemer-Hastings, P. (2000). Adding syntactic information to LSA. In L. Gleitman & A. Joshi (Eds.), *Proceedings of the 22nd annual conference of the Cognitive Science Society* (pp. 989–993). Mahwah, NJ: Lawrence Erlbaum Associates.

Wiemer-Hastings, P. (2004). The design and architecture of the Research Methods Tutor, a second-generation dialog-based tutor. In N. Heffernan & P. Wiemer-Hastings (Eds.), *Proceedings of the workshop on dialog-based intelligent tutoring systems, ITS 2004* (pp. 55–63). Berlin, Germany: Springer-Verlag.

Wiemer-Hastings, P., & Graesser, A. C. (2000). Supporting composition feedback with LSA in Select-a-Kibitzer. *Interactive Learning Environments, 8,* 149–169.

Wiemer-Hastings, P., & Zipitria, I. (2001). Rules for syntax, vectors for semantics. In J. D. Moore (Ed.), *Proceedings of CogSci 2001* (pp. 1112–1117). Mahwah, NJ: Lawrence Erlbaum Associates.

Wildt, A. R., & Ahtola, O. T. (1978). *Analysis of covariance* (quantitative applications in the social sciences series No. 12). Thousand Oaks, CA: Sage.

Wilensky, R. (1983). *Planning and understanding: A computational approach to human reasoning*. Reading, MA: Addison-Wesley.

Wilensky, R., Arens, Y., & Chin, D. (1984). Talking to Unix in English. *CACM, 27,* 574–593.

Wilensky, R., Chin D., Luria, M., Martin, J., Mayfield, J., & Wu, D. (1988). The Berkeley Unix Consultant project. *Computational Linguistics, 14,* 35–84.

Wilkins, D. E. (1984), Domain-independent planning: Representations and plan generation, *Artificial Intelligence, 22,* 574–584.

Wilkins, D. E. (1988). *Practical planning: Extending the classical AI planning paradigm.* San Mateo, CA: Kaufmann.

Wilkins, D. E., Myers, K., Lowrance, J., & Wesley, L. (1995). Planning and reacting in uncertain and dynamic environments. *Journal of Experimental and Theoretical Artificial Intelligence, 7,* 121–252.

Winkels, R., & Breuker, J. (1990). Discourse planning in intelligent help systems. In C. Frasson & G. Gauthier (Eds.), *Intelligent tutoring systems: At the crossroads of artificial intelligence and education* (pp. 124–139). Norwood, NJ: Ablex.

Winograd, T. (1972). *Understanding natural language.* New York: Academic.

Winograd, T. (1983). *Language as a cognitive process: Syntax.* Reading, MA: Addison-Wesley.

Wolf, A. K., Chomsky, C. S., & Green, B. F. (1963). *The Baseball Program: An automatic question answerer.* Bedford, MA: MIT Lincoln Lab.

Woo, C. W. (1991). *Instructional planning in an intelligent tutoring system: Combining global lesson plans with local discourse control.* Unpublished doctoral dissertation, Illinois Institute of Technology, Chicago.

Woo, C. W., Evens, M. W., Michael, J. A., & Rovick, A. A. (1991a). Instructional planning for an intelligent medical tutoring system. In R. Gamble & W. Ball (Eds.), *Proceedings of the Third Midwest Artificial Intelligence and Cognitive Science Conference* (pp. 31–35). Carbondale, IL: Southern Illinois University at Carbondale.

Woo, C. W., Evens, M. W., Michael, J. A., & Rovick, A. A. (1991b). Dynamic planning in an intelligent cardiovascular tutoring system. *Proceedings of the fourth annual IEEE Symposium on computer based medical systems* (pp. 226–233). Los Alamitos, CA: IEEE Computer Society Press.

Woods, W. A. (1970). Transition network grammars for natural language analysis. *CACM 13,* 5915606.

Woolf, B. P. (1984). *Context-dependent planning in a machine tutor.* Unpublished doctoral dissertation, University of Massachusetts at Amherst.

Woolf, B. P., & McDonald, D. (1985). Building a computer tutor: Design issues. *AEDS Monitor, 23,* 10–18.

Woolf, B. P. (1988). 20 years in the trenches: What have we learned? In B. Goettl, H. Halff, C. Redfield, & J. Shute (Eds.), *Proceedings of ITS 88* (pp. 33–39). Berlin, Germany: Springer-Verlag.

Yang, F. J. (2001). *Turn planning and lexical choice in a natural language dialogue-based intelligent tutoring system.* Unpublished doctoral dissertation, Illinois Institute of Technology, Chicago.

Yang, F. J., Kim, J. H., Glass, M. S., & Evens, M. W. (2000a). Lexical issues in the tutoring schemata of CIRCSIM-Tutor: Analysis of variable references and discourse markers. In M. Benedict (Ed.), *Human Interfaces to Complex Systems* (pp. 26–31). Urbana, IL: Beckman Institute.

Yang, F .J., Kim, J. H., Glass, M. S., & Evens, M. W. (2000b). Turn planning in CIRCSIM-Tutor. In J. Etheredge & B. Manaris (Eds.), *Proceedings of the Florida Artificial Intelligence Symposium* (pp. 60–64). Menlo Park, CA: AAAI Press.

Yanofsky, N. M. (1978). NP utterances. In D. Farkas, W. Jacobsen, & K. Todrys (Eds.), *Papers from the fourteenth regional meeting of the Chicago Linguistics Society* (pp. 491–502). Chicago: University of Chicago Linguistics Department.

Young, R. M. (1994). *A developer's guide to the Longbow discourse planning system* (Tech. Rpt. No. 94-4). Pittsburgh: University of Pittsburgh Intelligent Systems Program.

Young, R. M., & Moore, J. D. (1994a). Does discourse planning require a special-purpose planner? *Proceedings of the AAAI workshop on planning for inter-agent communication* (pp. 83–90). AAAI Press.

Young, R. M., & Moore, J. D. (1994b). DPOCL: A principled approach to discourse planning, *Proceedings of the Seventh International Workshop on Natural Language Generation* (pp. 13–20). East Stroudsburg, PA: Association for Computational Linguistics.

Young, R. M., Moore, J. D., & Pollack, M. (1994). Towards a principled representation of discourse plans. In A. Ram & K. Eiselt (Eds.), *Proceedings of CogSci '94* (pp. 946–951). Atlanta, GA:

Yusko, J. A. (1994, August). *The reality of change* (Internal tech. rep.). Lombard, IL: Unlimited Solutions, Inc.

Yusko, J. A., & Evens, M. W. (2002). The knowledge collective: Using microdroids to turn metadata into metaknowledge. In S. Conlon (Ed.), *Proceedings of Midwest Artificial Intelligence and Cognitive Science Conference 2002* (pp. 56–60). Chicago: Illinois Institute of Technology.

Yusko, J. A., & Evens, M. W. (2004). Dynamic ontological support for qualitative reasoning in The Knowledge Collective (TKC). In J. De Kleer & K. Forbus (Eds.), *Workshop on qualitative reasoning* (pp. 187–193). Berlin, Germany: Springer-Verlag.

Zhang, Y. (1991). *Knowledge-based discourse generation for an intelligent tutoring system.* Unpublished doctoral dissertation, Illinois Institute of Technology, Chicago.

Zhang, Y., Evens, M. W., Michael, J. A., & Rovick, A. A. (1987). Knowledge compiler for an expert physiology tutor. *Proceedings of the Electrostatic Dis-*

charge/Semiconductor Manufacturing International Conference on Expert Systems (pp. 153–169). Dearborn, MI: ESD/SMI.

Zhang, Y., Evens, M. W., Michael, J. A., & Rovick, A. A. (1990). Extending a knowledge base to support explanations. *Proceedings of the third IEEE Conference on computer-based medical systems* (pp. 259–266). Los Alamitos, CA: IEEE Computer Society Press.

Zhao, J., Kim, J. H., & Evens, M. W. (2003). Comparison of student initiatives in keyboard-to-keyboard and face-to-face tutoring sessions. In A. Relescu (Ed.), *Proceedings of the Midwest Artificial Intelligence and Cognitive Science Conference, MAICS '03* (pp. 178–183). Madison, WI: Omni Press.

Zhou, Y. (2000). *Building a new student model to support adaptive tutoring in a natural language dialogue system.* Unpublished doctoral dissertation, Illinois Institute of Technology, Chicago.

Zhou, Y., & Evens, M. W. (1999). A practical student model in an intelligent tutoring system. *Proceedings of the 11th IEEE International Conference on tools with artificial intelligence* (pp. 13–18). Los Alamitos, CA: IEEE Computer Society Press.

Zhou, Y., Freedman, R. K., Glass, M. S., Michael, J. A., Rovick, A. A., & Evens, M. W. (1999a). What should the tutor do when the student cannot answer a question? In A. Kumar & I. Russell (Eds.), *Proceedings of the 12th Florida Artificial Intelligence Symposium (FLAIRS-99)* (pp. 187–191). Menlo Park, CA: AAAI Press.

Zhou, Y., Freedman, R., Glass, M., Michael, J. A., Rovick, A. A., & Evens, M. W. (1999b). Delivering hints in a dialogue-based intelligent tutoring system. *Proceedings of AAAI* (pp. 128–134). Menlo Park, CA: AAAI Press.

Zinn, C., Moore, J. D., & Core, M. G. (2002). A 3-tier planning architecture for managing tutorial dialogue. In S. A. Cerri, G. Gouardères, & F. Paraguaçu (Eds.), *ITS 2002* (pp. 574–584). Berlin, Germany: Springer.

This page intentionally left blank

Author Index

C

D

E

F

M

N

O

P

Q

R

S

Y

Z

Subject Index

A

B

J, K

L

M

N

T

U

V

W